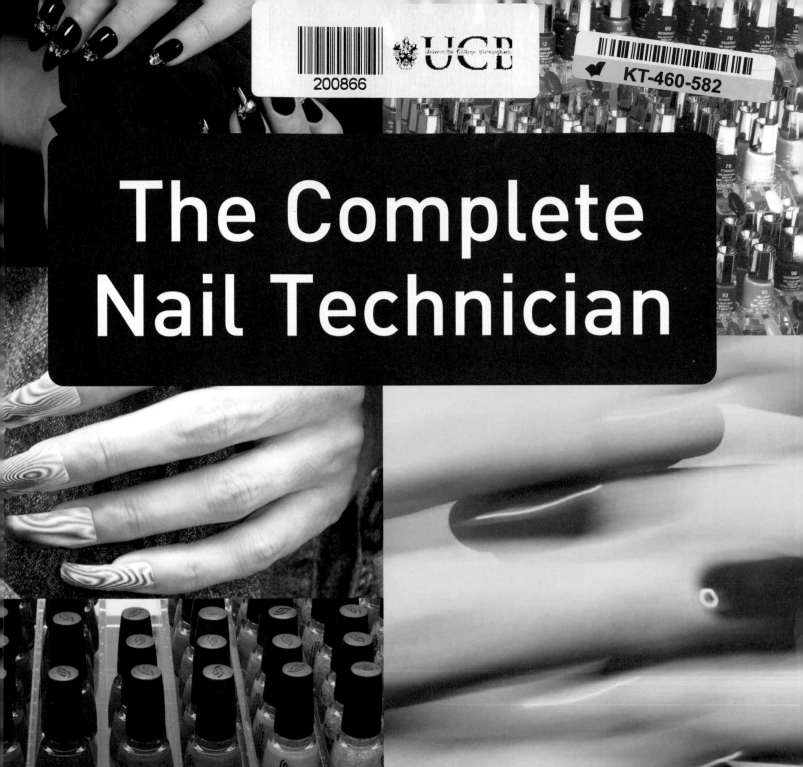

The Complete Nail Technician

HAIRDRESSING AND BEAUTY INDUSTRY AUTHORITY SERIES

Hairdressing

Student textbooks

Begin Hairdressing: The Official Guide to Level 1 2e *Martin Green*

Hairdressing – The Foundations: The Official Guide to Level 2 6e *Leo Palladino and Martin Green*

Professional Hairdressing: The Official Guide to Level 3 6e *Martin Green and Leo Palladino*

The Official Guide to the City & Guilds Certificate in Salon Service 1e *John Armstrong with Anita Crosland, Martin Green and Lorraine Nordmann*

The Colour Book: The Official Guide to Colour for NVQ Levels 2 and 3 1e *Tracey Lloyd with Christine McMillan-Bodell*

eXtensions: The Official Guide to Hair Extensions 1e *Theresa Bullock*

Salon Management *Martin Green*

Men's Hairdressing: Traditional and Modern Barbering 2e *Maurice Lister*

African-Caribbean Hairdressing 2e *Sandra Gittens*

The World of Hair Colour 1e *John Gray*

The Cutting Book: The Official Guide to Cutting at S/NVQ Levels 2 and 3 *Jane Goldsbro and Elaine White*

Professional Hairdressing titles

Trevor Sorbie: The Bridal Hair Book 1e *Trevor Sorbie and Jacki Wadeson*

The Art of Dressing Long Hair 1 e *Guy Kremer and Jacki Wadeson*

Patrick Cameron: Dressing Long Hair 1e *Patrick Cameron and Jacki Wadeson*

Patrick Cameron: Dressing Long Hair 2 1e *Patrick Cameron and Jacki Wadeson*

Bridal Hair 1e *Pat Dixon and Jacki Wadeson*

Professional Men's Hairdressing: The art of cutting and styling 1e *Guy Kremer and Jacki Wadeson*

Essensuals, The Next Generation Toni and Guy: Step by Step 1e *Sacha Mascolo, Christian Mascolo and Stuart Wesson*

Mahogany Hairdressing: Step to Cutting, Colouring and Finishing Hair 1e *Martin Gannon and Richard Thompson*

Mahogany Hairdressing: Advanced Looks 1e *Martin Gannon and Richard Thompson*

The Total Look: The Style Guide for Hair and Make-up Professional 1e *Ian Mistlin*

Trevor Sorbie: Visions in Hair 1e *Trevor Sorbie, Kris Sorbie and Jacki Wadeson*

The Art of Hair Colouring 1e *David Adams and Jacki Wadeson*

Beauty therapy

Beauty Basics; The Official Guide to Level 1 3e *Lorraine Nordmann*

Beauty Therapy – The Foundations: The Official Guide to Level 2 5e *Lorraine Nordmann*

Professional Beauty Therapy – The Official Guide to Level 3 4e *Lorraine Nordmann*

The Official Guide to the City & Guilds Certificate in Salon Services 1e *John Armstrong with Anita Crosland, Martin Green and Lorraine Nordmann*

The Complete Guide to Make-Up 1e *Suzanne Le Quesne*

The Encyclopedia of Nails 1e *Jacqui Jefford and Anne Swain*

The Art of Nails: A Comprehensive Style Guide to Nail Treatments and Nail Art 1e *Jacqui Jefford*

Nail Artistry 1e *Jacqui Jefford*

The Complete Nail Technician 3e *Marian Newman*

Manicure, Pedicure and Advanced Nail Techniques 1e *Elaine Almond*

The Official Guide to Body Massage 2e *Adele O'Keefe*

An Holistic Guide to Massage 1e *Tina Parsons*

Indian Head Massage 2e *Muriel Burnham-Airey and Adele O'Keefe*

Aromatherapy for the Beauty Therapist 1e *Valerie Worwood*

An Holistic Guide to Reflexology 1e *Tina Parsons*

An Holistic Guide to Anatomy and Physiology 1e *Tina Parsons*

The Essential Guide to Holistic and Complementary Therapy 1e *Helen Beckmann and Suzanne Le Quesne*

The Spa Book 1e *Jane Crebbin-Bailey, Dr John Harcup, and John Harrington*

SPA: The Official Guide to Spa Therapy at Levels 2 and 3, *Joan Scott and Andrea Harrison*

Nutrition: A Practical Approach 1e *Suzanne Le Quesne* Hands on Sports Therapty 1e *Keith Ward*

Encyclopedia of Hair Removal: A Complete Reference to Methods, Techniques and Career Opportunities, *Gill Morris and Janice Brown*

The Anatomy and Physiology Workbook: For Beauty and Holistic Therapies Levels 1–3. *Tina Parsons*

The Anatomy and Physiology CD-Rom

Beautiful Selling: The Complete Guide to Sales Success in the Salon *Ruth Langley*

The Official Guide to the Diploma in Hair and Beauty Studies at Foundation Level 1e *Jane Goldsbro and Elaine White*

The Official Guide to the Diploma in Hair and Beauty Studies at Higher level 1e *Jane Goldsbro and Elaine White*

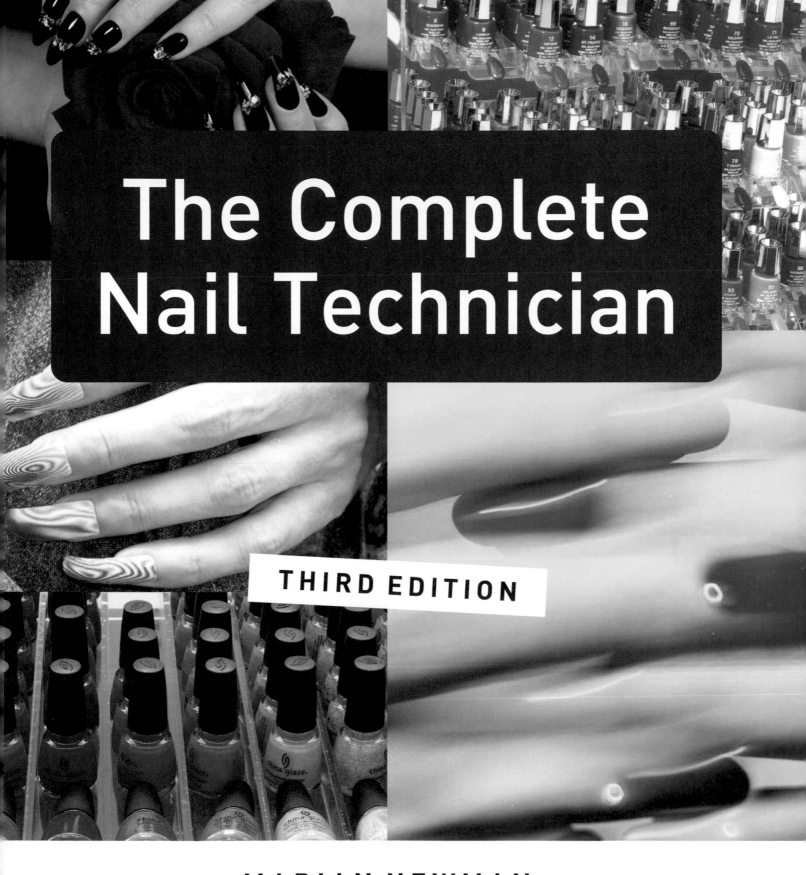

The Complete
Nail Technician

THIRD EDITION

MARIAN NEWMAN

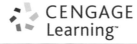

CENGAGE
Learning™

Australia • Brazil • Japan • Korea • Mexico • Singapore • Spain • United Kingdom • United States

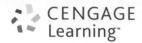

The Complete Nail Technician, Third Edition
Marian Newman

Publishing Director: Linden Harris

Commissioning Editor: Lucy Mills

Development Editor: Juliet Smith

Editorial Assistant: Claire Napoli

Content Project Editor: Alison Cooke

Production Controller: Eyvett Davis

Marketing Manager: Lauren Redwood

Typesetter: MPS Limited, a Macmillan Company

Cover design: HCT Creative

Text design: Design Deluxe

For product information and technology assistance,
contact **emea.info@cengage.com.**.

For permission to use material from this text or product,
and for permission queries,
email **clsuk.permissions@cengage.com.**

The Author has asserted the right under the Copyright, Designs and Patents Act 1988 to be identified as Author of this Work.

This work is adapted from *The Complete Nail Technician*, 2nd Edition, published by Cengage Learning, Inc. © 2005.

British Library Cataloguing-in-Publication Data
A catalogue record for this book is available from the British Library.

ISBN 10: 1-4080-3244-9

ISBN 13: 978-1-4080-3244-2

Cengage Learning EMEA
Cheriton House, North Way, Andover, Hampshire, SP10 5BE.
United Kingdom

Cengage Learning products are represented in Canada by Nelson Education Ltd.

For your lifelong learning solutions, visit
www.cengage.co.uk

Purchase your next print book, e-book or e-chapter at
www.cengagebrain.co.uk

Printed in China
1 2 3 4 5 6 7 8 9 10–13 12 11

Contents

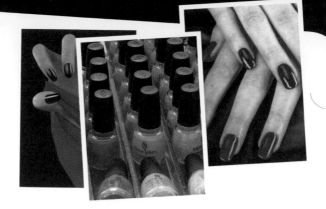

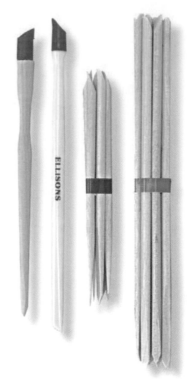

12 Business matters 238

13 Nail art, basic and advanced 259

14 Media work and special occassions 289

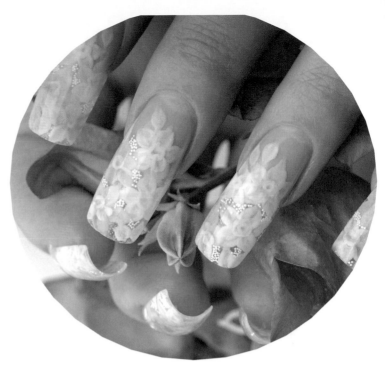

15 Using electric files 310

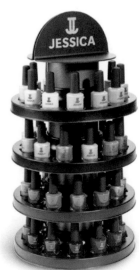

Acknowledgements

The author and publishers would like to thank the following people and organizations for their assistance in producing this book:

Cover Image courtesy of **Nick Knight / Vogue** © The Condé Nast Publications Ltd.

Sweet Squared and CND

Kelly Winterburn

Georgie Smedley

Aet Kase

Aircare Europe

Mundo

Scratch Magazine

Alex Fox

Tom Wandrag

Nail Delights

Beauty Concepts Int

Nick Knight

Vogue

Odyssey

Nail Creations

Nail Art

Nail Systems

Ralph Lopez

Val Garland and Jade Parfitt

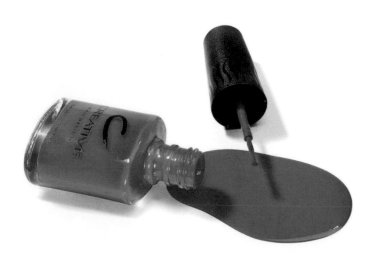

Foreword from Habia

Marian Newman is one of the most inspirational people I have ever met. When I first met Marian in 1995 she was the leading force and passion driving the nail industry forward. Her direct approach, never afraid to question or challenge pre-conceived ideas, has given her an immense knowledge of the industry. She is recognised today by her peers and the media as the most influential person in UK nails.

Marian creates many of the beautiful nails that are used on the covers of fashion magazines; one look at her work and you will soon see why she is so much in demand from film stars and celebrities all over the world. Marian is clearly an inspiration who never stops promoting the industry over and above her own work.

The third edition of *The Complete Nail Technician* is an absolute must for anyone in the industry. From basics to master techniques – it's here for all budding nail technicians and industry professionals who want to see what happens when learning never stops.

Alan Goldsboro
Chief Executive Officer
HABIA

Note from the author

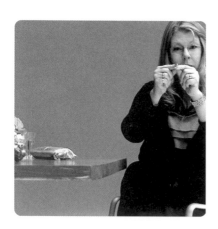

I was delighted to be invited to write a third edition of my textbook, The Complete Nail Technician. I feel very strongly about the standards of education and skills of nail technicians working in the professional industry. The National Occupational Standards have provided the basis for this education but they are only a start. There is a lot more learning needed after the completion of 'job ready' qualifications.

This book covers all the requirements of the NOS but what I have tried to achieve is to take the learning process a little further. I hope it provides the nail technician not only with a good learning tool but also a useful reference book during their personal development. A lifetime of learning is essential for a technical subject that also requires a large 'dose' of creativity. Hopefully, this book provides many answers but I also hope it encourages further research. The internet is a wonderful thing and so much information is just a 'click' away for those that want to take their career seriously.

In previous editions I have thanked all the people that make it possible for me to work as I do. I receive enormous support, loyalty and commitment. Once again, I thank you all most sincerely. You know who you are!

Marian Newman

About the book

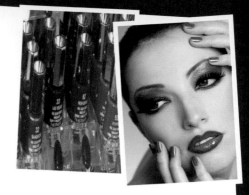

PLUS POINTS

- can be carried out part-time and provide additional income and interest
- a very good way of maintaining high standards
- job satisfaction (and often frustration) in teaching new skills to students
- if connected to a product company, there is involvement with the industry as a whole.

Plus Points boxes draw your attention to the positive aspects of specific industry scenarios.

MINUS POINTS

- full-time jobs are rare so will have several applicants
- part-time jobs may be casual (that is, only when required).

Minus Points boxes draw your attention to the negative aspects of specific industry scenarios.

HEALTH & SAFETY

Always sit square to the desk without crossing your legs or leaning on one arm.

Health and Safety boxes draw your attention to related health and safety information essential for each technical skill.

ALWAYS REMEMBER

DO NOT cut the proximal nail fold! It is living and will protect itself by thickening!

Always Remember boxes draw your attention to key information or helpful hints that will help you prepare for assessment.

TOP TIP

For further information visit these websites:

www.businesslink.gov.uk

www.direct.gov.uk.

Top Tips share the author's experience and provide positive suggestions to improve knowledge and skills for each unit.

BEST PRACTICE

At the end of the consultation and discussion on treatments, the information should be recorded in writing on the client's record card. This should include all the information about the client and the condition of their nails and skin, their expectations of the treatment, the recommendations of the technician and the treatment that has been agreed. The client should then sign this and a note made of which technician carried out the treatment.

Best Practice boxes suggest good working practice and help you develop your skills and awareness during your training.

ACTIVITY

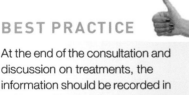

Make a chart listing all the products you are using. Create a column for:

- safe storage
- safe and correct usage (e.g. methods of decanting, personal protective equipment (PPE) if required, etc.)
- spillage removal from hard surfaces
- any specific health hazard
- comments.

Activity boxes feature within all chapters and provide additional tasks for you to further your understanding

> ❝ ANECDOTE
> A client of mine always kept a small bottle of nail adhesive in her bag in case of accidents. One night she was on her way to dinner with her husband; they were in the car, it was dark and she was in the passenger seat. She felt a bit tired and her eyes were 'gritty'. She knew she had some eye drops with her, so rummaged in her bag to find the bottle. She opened it and tipped her head back to use the eye drops. Out came a drop but … she had mistaken the eye drop bottle for the nail adhesive bottle. She didn't go to dinner, but spent the night in casualty! Luckily although her eye was sore for a few days, there was no permanent damage done.

Industry Anecdote are included throughout a number of core chapters. Each anecdote provides valuable insight into the world of work, providing helpful and practical advice about working in such a varied and innovative industry.

EQUIPMENT LIST

hand sanitizer	hoof stick
varnish remover	hand cream
nail wipes	towels
file	orange sticks
cuticle softener	three-way buffer
bowl of warm water with softener	base and top coats
cuticle knife	coloured varnish
cuticle nippers	

Equipment lists help you prepare for each practical treatment and show you the tools, materials and products required.

Step-by-step: Manicure 1

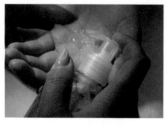

1 After washing the hands with soap and water, sanitize both the client's and your own hands.

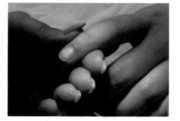

2 Examine the hands and nails in order to diagnose their condition and to look for any contra-indications.

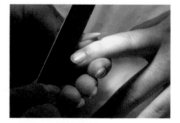

3 Shape the nails on one hand with a 240 grit (or higher) file after discussing with the client as to what shape they prefer. Keep the file angled slightly under the free edge.

Step-by-step sequences demonstrate the featured practical skills using colour photographs to enhance your understanding.

ASSESSMENT OF KNOWLEDGE AND UNDERSTANDING

1 What are the correct methods of filing natural nails?

2 Describe the nail plate with regard to the layers.

3 Why should the nail plate layers be kept sealed and how can this be achieved?

4 What is the cuticle and why should it be removed?

5 Name three ways of softening the cuticle.

6 What are the benefits and effects of massage?

7 What is a paraffin wax treatment and what are the benefits?

8 What would be your recommendations to a nail biter?

9 How would you treat:
 • weak nails?
 • brittle nails?
 • peeling nails?

10 Why is aftercare advice important to the client?

Assessment of knowledge and understanding questions are provided at the end of all core chapters. You can use the questions to prepare for oral and written assessments and help test your knowledge throughout. Seek guidance from your supervisor/assessor if there are any areas you are unsure of.

1

Starting out: you and your industry

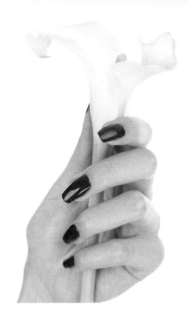

Learning objectives

In this chapter you will learn about:

- a brief history of the nail industry

- the education and qualifications available today

- the career routes open to a technician

- the benefits and pitfalls of each career route

- how to start your career

- how to promote your services.

Introduction

This chapter introduces the world of 'nails'. It is an amazingly fast-growing section of the service industry that includes beauty and hair. What used to be an 'add-on' service for some therapists and hairdressers is now a booming business that has its own identity, with many dedicated salons all over the country. There are even many nail salons that offer beauty or hair treatments as an 'add-on' service to their main business of 'nails'. This chapter provides a brief history of the industry, describes the training available and the possible career routes for the nail technician.

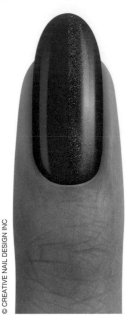

Painted fingernails

Artificial nails: a brief history

The art of lengthening nails has been around for centuries, and in many cultures long nails are a symbol of wealth. The ancient Egyptians had shapes made from gold, bone or ivory that could be attached to the end of the finger to indicate wealth and class. Far Eastern cultures have, over the centuries, displayed their social standing by growing their own nails to extreme lengths. The ability to grow nails or wear extended decorations on fingers is meant to show that the person does not do any manual work and has servants or slaves to attend to all their needs.

There are lots of people who have been doing 'nails' for 40 years who claim to have been the first to offer artificial nail services in the UK and Europe. They are probably all correct if their concept of the UK and Europe is scaled down to mean their own particular area. Artificial nails as a practice appeared almost simultaneously in many places, but it was in the US before any other country where it became big business. The idea of creating artificial nails came from the dental and hearing aid industries as inventive people started experimenting with the **polymers** and **adhesives** that dental technicians used to create crowns, moulds and other dental appliances. These materials, when mixed, could be formed into a strong solid structure that could go into the mouth, but could also be moulded onto a nail to lengthen or protect it. Small quantities could be applied with a brush and shaped to look like a natural nail. Pigments were already being added to match the colours of teeth or skin, and a method of etching tooth enamel to allow the material to bond could be modified to work with nails.

The earliest experiments and resultant artificial nails used a **monomer** and polymer mix applied to the nail and extended over a supporting form. This structure hardened and, when the support was removed, was then shaped to look like a natural extension of the nail plate. These dental materials were chemicals that came under the 'family' name of **acrylics**: thus the acrylic artificial nail was created. All materials subsequently used also belong to the acrylic family, but the term 'acrylic nails' has stuck to the method of using a **liquid** monomer and **powder** polymer.

Plastic nail shapes that could be stuck onto natural nails with an adhesive had been available for some time so it was not long before the shape of these was adapted to create the support for the acrylic structure. Lots of other tools and equipment were used or created to assist this skill. Even dental drills found their way into the equation, as the early acrylics could be so hard that help was needed to shape the nails. An industry grew up to provide nail technicians with a whole range of accessories.

The modern nail technician
Education and skills training

In the US, technicians utilized these new materials very well and the public loved the resulting long, painted nails. Eventually colleges included teaching the skill in their cosmetology courses and each of the States included it in their licensing legislation, as it became essential to regulate the practice. This is the situation that remains in the US today; students in cosmetology learn manicure, pedicure and the art of artificial nails and, if they want to be a commercial practitioner, they have to achieve their State licence. Each State has different requirements but, essentially, training is usually carried out in a college environment and a set number of hours learning and practising must be completed, followed by a practical exam. Once they have passed this, individuals receive their licence and this allows them to work and purchase products.

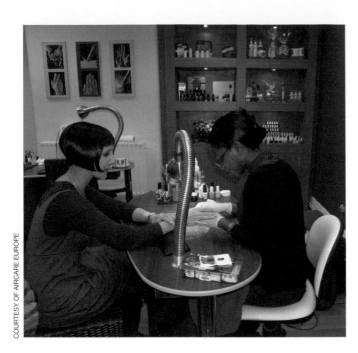

COURTESY OF AIRCARE EUROPE

The nail companies obviously want to sell their products and many of them provide a 'postgraduate' training service to provide qualified technicians with advanced skills and an understanding of their particular product range. Of course this does not apply to all companies, as many find selling to the wholesale outlets and mail order via trade magazines sufficient.

The education programme offered by some nail product companies can be likened to the skincare companies that provide application techniques and product knowledge to the qualified beauty therapists who will be using their ranges. It can be an important aspect of the product range as correct usage is essential for optimum results and there are usually some techniques that have been developed to make a specific product range different from that of a competitor.

It was this type of postgraduate training, typically of 1 or 2 days' duration, that was imported from the US to the UK along with the products. It was training that was designed for qualified technicians who had already learned the basic skills. These short courses were offered in the UK to anyone who was interested in buying products and hundreds of 'technicians' were created who had no theoretical knowledge of the nail and skin, hygiene requirements, legislation or any of the basic information provided in a full qualifying course.

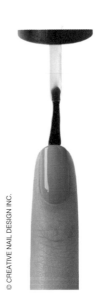

© CREATIVE NAIL DESIGN INC.

For many years this has been the accepted practice; it has always been assumed that 'nails' is an additional service that can be learned in under a week and has a good profit margin. Fortunately for the future of the industry, it has been becoming apparent that there is more to it than that. A therapist or hairdresser can learn how to apply nails but not in the same way as learning a new massage technique or a new hair colour range. It is more like adding aromatherapy to a therapist's services or a stylist learning how to perm. Many clients will only ever go to a specialist and many are happy to have one person provide all treatments. There will always be plenty of room for both types of technicians.

As the industry grows, so does the number of nail salons. It is becoming an industry in its own right, recognized by employers, insurers and local authorities. 'Nails' has its own magazines and trade shows, and it now has its own qualifications.

The industry is an exciting place to work in, as it is still so new. It is developing and growing, and opportunities for those working within it are becoming wider. 'Nails' is a creative and practical skill and, as such, needs education, practice and dedication. It cannot be learned in a day or two. There are some 'natural' technicians who have good coordination and an 'eye' for form, shape, balance and symmetry. Others need to learn how to use the tools and materials and develop their 'eye'. Good training and education is the first step; a dedication to practise is the second; the acceptance that no one ever stops learning and improving is the final step to a whole new career and skill.

Qualifications

The qualification structure evolved over time and now the professional nail industry has full qualifications dedicated to the required skills.

The **National Occupational Standards (NOS)** are a set of requirements drawn up by **Habia** (the Hairdressing and Beauty Industry Authority) with the help of professionals in the sector, following an analysis of the sector's needs, and approved by a wide range of relevant establishments and individuals. They are a set of skills, knowledge and understanding that those experienced in the sector believe are the *minimum* requirements for an individual working in the sector and providing services for paying clients.

They also make sure that individuals have a knowledge and understanding in areas such as health and safety, legislation and customer service issues. The formal qualifications in the UK that are based on the NOS fall into two categories:

- *Job ready*. These are qualifications that have taught the learner an understanding of the subject, theoretical knowledge and a wide variety of relevant skills that they have proved to be competent in. The qualified person is then ready to be employed in a junior capacity (NOT an unqualified Junior) with the potential to build their own clientele. More training and experience is needed but this should be easily achievable while working as a valuable member of a salon or as a freelance technician. An example of this type of qualification is the National Vocational Qualification (NVQ).

- *Prepared for work*. It has been demonstrated over the past few years that some employers prefer to educate their employees in their own methods of working themselves. This will be in the practical skills side of the profession. There is still a vast amount of knowledge and understanding to be learnt plus a limited amount of practical skills. This can be achieved in a variety of ways including distance learning. The individuals achieving these qualifications are then 'prepared for work'. This is very different from 'job ready' but suitable for assistants or, perhaps, receptionists who want to become a technician. It is NOT suitable for a freelance technician. These are known as Vocationally Recognized Qualifications (VRQs).

The NOS are used in a variety of ways to measure skills but, most importantly for the purposes of this book, they are used to create recognized qualifications that students and experienced individuals who do not already possess a suitable qualification can achieve for the purposes of employment, further education, insurance purposes and local authority licensing. They can also be used in most European Union (EU) countries as proof of competence. Habia own the NOS and have many overseas partners who use Standards to structure their own version of education in this sector.

The **NVQ** is understood by most people as a recognized and widely available qualification (they are known as SVQs in Scotland). The NOS are used to create these NVQs. In Beauty Therapy, of which Nail Services is a specialist route, there are currently 2 levels. (There is no Level 1 as this does not relate to a position that is recognized in the sector.)

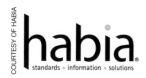

standards • information • solutions

NVQ Level 2 in Nail Services is a qualification for nail technicians and will allow them to work unsupervised for services such as manicure and pedicure, the application of one method of nail enhancements and basic nail art. There are also certain general subjects to be achieved, such as health and safety issues, reception duties and good working practices.

Level 3 in Nail Services is the advanced qualification for technicians. This also has general areas of knowledge covering aspects of the salon that demonstrate more responsibility. The nails sections, for both artificial nails and nail art, are more advanced.

This Level now has a structure that allows learners to choose a 'business' route (perfect for freelance technicians) or the more 'creative' route with nail art.

A new method of training and one that is very suited to the industry is the apprenticeship route. There are many ways this will be offered around the country but, basically, it is like the old apprentice system where a person is employed straight from school and learns while working. The apprentice technician will work in a salon for a small wage and go to college or other type of training provider for, perhaps, 1 day a week or a few days a month. All the theoretical learning will be done in college together with the basic skills. All the practice and experience will be gained in the real salon environment. Details about this excellent option is on the Habia website (www.habia.org).

How qualifications are created

Habia create the NOS in a process that is mostly funded by Government sponsorship (as the industry authority, Habia is the only organization recognized for this role. For every industry sector there is only one set of NOS). An organization can only be recognized as an industry authority following exhaustive proof of their suitability and Habia achieved this many years ago.

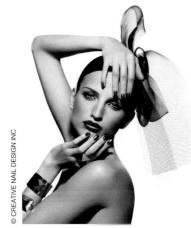

The creation of a NOS takes a very long time and a process that ensures it truly suits the sector it is representing. It starts with a group of experienced industry professionals from a variety of areas, e.g. technicians, employers, teachers, product suppliers, etc. led by an expert in the creation of NOS (in any sector) to make sure it fits with the relevant criteria laid down by the relevant governmental department. When a first draft is ready it is sent out to a very wide 'audience' for a consultation process. Anyone working in the industry can take part in this consultation and it is 'advertised' in trade magazines and the Habia website together with 100's of questionnaires sent to professionals.

This process is repeated until a final draft is put forward to the relevant Habia committee for approval. Then this is submitted to the governmental department and, eventually, the NOS are officially changed and the new version is put into place.

Awarding bodies (these are accredited to award qualifications by the regulating body of the industry, in this instance, Habia) then use the NOS to structure the qualifications that they provide. These may be an NVQ that follow the NOS exactly. They may be a VRQ or they may create a qualification specific to them. This could be an award or certificate or diploma.

Some of the are awarding bodies are City & Guilds, ITEC, VTCT, CIBTAC, Edexcel. An NVQ or VRQ achieved through any of the accredited awarding bodies is an identical qualification as it will follow the NOS and be verified by an approved method with strict guidelines. Other qualifications from the individual awarding bodies will differ but only perhaps in the combination of subjects. The content will still follow the NOS.

Awards, certificates and diplomas are now being based on the number of credits they achieve. Credits are based on the number of hours a specific unit of part of the qualification requires for competency with awards being the smallest achievement and a diploma the highest. It is also possible to collect a certain number of awards or certificates that will make a diploma.

Private training providers in the professional nail industry create their own courses and qualifications. These are sometimes based on the NOS but are more than likely associated with a specific brand, like the training courses in the subject were years ago. This type of training for beginners is not accredited by the regulating body and there is no real check on the quality of training or accuracy of the information being taught. Some courses are accredited by trade associations for insurance purposes. Some are also accredited by Habia for continuing personal development (CPD) purposes which as the title implies, is not for beginners.

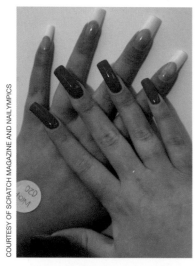

Any person preferring to take the route of private training from an unaccredited provider should make sure the company has a good reputation and teaches all the aspects of the specific subject as described in the NOS. Important areas such as health and safety and anatomy and physiology should not just be a hand-out! There should be some discussion on the subjects and, in particular, relating the subjects to the practical skills being taught.

The **NOS** are available as a download on the Habia website: www.habia.org. The required notional learning hours for each of the units are also on the site which can act as a guideline to the length a course should be.

As an approximate guideline the hours for manicure are 60 hours of any type of learning (theory, skill training, practicing, etc.) and for advanced enhancements of one system is 100 hours.

This book covers all the necessary knowledge for the specialist nail qualifications, regardless of level, the title of the qualification or the awarding body. It is based on the NOS and they are based on all the essential skills, knowledge, information and understanding required by a beginner in the field of nails, or an experienced technician needing a reference or to revise areas of their work. The book also includes the skills and knowledge necessary for earning a living in the sector. It also deals with real situations and scenarios in the commercial world and gives some specific guidelines in starting a business.

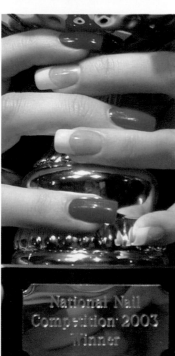

Winning nails

Career routes

Doing 'nails' is not just about sitting behind a desk and buffing for 8 hours a day. A qualified and experienced technician has a wide range of choices available. The best starting point to choosing one of these routes, however, is to put in the time at that nail desk. Nails is a public service and experience of working with the public is invaluable. Eight career routes are common today: mobile technician; working from home; being self-employed or employed in a salon; running a salon of your own; teaching or demonstration work; or being a media technician. We shall briefly look at all of these.

For information and help on all the career routes, an excellent website is www.habia.org. The sales department has numerous publications for all personnel and businesses. There are many other useful sections and it is a generally interesting site to explore.

All technicians should get public and products liability insurance, whether they are employed or not. If a client decides to take legal action they could sue the salon and the individual technician separately. This type of insurance is inexpensive and will protect the technician from most situations involving products, whether as a result of an accident or an allergic reaction, for example. It often covers for accidental damage to property and loss of products and tools. This form of insurance is readily available from trade associations and some trade publications.

Mobile technicians

Like hairdressing and most beauty treatments, 'nails' can be a service that can be carried out in a client's home, as the equipment can be carried. It is a popular career route for newly-trained technicians as start-up costs are low. There are many technicians who have made a successful career with a good income this way.

Requirements   A qualification that is suitable for insurance purposes and local authority licensing if needed, for example the NVQ Level 2 in Nail Services. Experience is not essential as this may be the way a newly-qualified technician can gain practice. NVQ Level 3 is ideal as it covers all subjects for a technician including a commercial route for being self-employed.

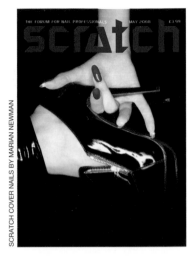

SCRATCH COVER NAILS BY MARIAN NEWMAN

Scratch cover May 2008

PLUS POINTS

- low start-up costs (no property deposits/mortgages, legal costs, decoration, salon equipment)
- low overheads (no rent, council taxes, utility bills)
- flexible working time (no set opening times).

MINUS POINTS

- lots of travelling time that is not paid for
- client expectation of lower charges
- lots of kit carrying
- less than ideal working situation (working on a dining room or kitchen table).

Things to consider

- the cost of a car, petrol and car insurance when used for business and carrying your kit (make sure you are insured to do this as not all insurance policies cover business use and you may find you are not insured if you are travelling to a client)

- maintaining good working standards without the stimulus of salon colleagues

- working in unfavourable conditions that could cause back strain

- problems of promotion of services, advertising

- working in a salon is invaluable experience and advisable for a beginner

- perception: however good the service, a mobile service is frequently perceived as having a lower professional status. There are many mobile technicians who do not bother with basic requirements like insurance, and over time this has led to a public view that 'mobile' can mean 'amateur'.

Where to start   Anyone thinking of starting to work in this way should approach it as a business and seek advice from those who understand financial matters. A bank manager can often recommend or be aware of schemes to help a business start up. Some extremely useful websites: www.businesslink.gov.uk, www.direct.gov.uk.

When you have decided what services you plan to offer you will need to create a price list (see Chapter 3 p. 84) and you must decide how you are going to promote your services. This need not be expensive (see Chapter 12 Business Matters). Leaflets handed out to all your friends and family with a request to pass them onto their friends and colleagues can sometimes start the ball rolling. You could put them through letterboxes in your local area. In addition, you can have some small posters printed and ask to put them up in local shops, waiting rooms of doctors and dentists, village halls (especially if they hold women's interest group meetings), on supermarket notice boards, etc. For a little extra money, you can place a small advert in the classified section of your local paper or, if you have some money to invest in your new business, you could have a larger boxed advert.

Monitor the effectiveness of each method you try, as there is no point in continuing with a method that does not bring you clients.

When designing cards, posters and price lists the best piece of advice is to look at examples everywhere you go, including adverts in magazines. Notice the ones that grab your attention, their colour and layout. Notice the words that make you think you must try that product or service or rush out and buy it. Look at notice boards and shop windows and see if one thing stands out more than others.

Think very carefully about how you will organize yourself and your kit for travelling around. You will need to carry enough equipment for all the services you offer but not so much that you need several boxes and bags. Remember your client may be on the fourth floor with no lift! You need to remember all the rules of hygiene and you and your kit must look immaculate at all times. You may find that your kit evolves over time as you discover better ways to arrange it, but start off with well-thought out planning and carry spares of everything in your car.

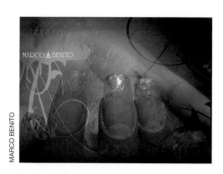

MARCO BENITO

Display your work to promote, the salon

Working from home

A salon can be set up in a private home instead of commercial premises.

Decorate your salon and promote retail

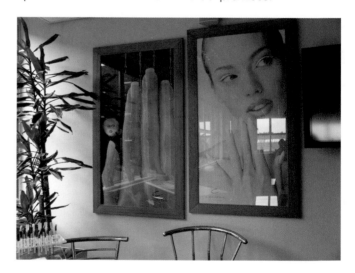

Requirements   A qualification that is suitable for insurance purposes and local authority licensing if needed, such as the NVQ mentioned above. Experience is not essential as this may be the way a newly qualified technician can gain practice.

PLUS POINTS

- low overheads
- no travelling
- can be good for a working parent
- flexible hours
- salon atmosphere can be achieved.

MINUS POINTS

- strangers brought into home
- lack of stimulus from salon colleagues
- can disrupt family life.

Things to consider

- Local authority permission needs to be gained to run a business from a residential property.
- Good working practices and hygiene need to be adhered to, as vapours from products and dust can affect the whole house.
- Is access to the salon going to affect the family or the security of the home?
- As with a mobile technician, this should be set up as a proper business.

Where to start
Careful thought must be given to the salon set-up. Make sure there is sufficient space for what you plan to do and make sure all the necessary health and safety rules are followed. Thoroughly research the best furniture and equipment for the space you have and plan every detail. Consult the Habia website for health and safety help.

Promotion of your services is essential. See the suggestions above for the mobile technician.

Self-employed in a salon

Clients of most salons, whether hair or beauty, will often ask if the salon does 'nails'. Working as a technician in a salon on a self-employed basis can prove to be a good relationship for the technician and the salon. A nail desk takes up so little space that it can usually be squeezed into most salons.

Requirements
These will be the same as for a mobile technician, but a salon may require experience. It is important to get personal public and product liability insurance. The salon may have appropriate insurance, but it may not cover a person who is not employed by them and it is not always easy to get a look at the policy to make sure it is relevant for you.

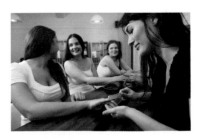

PLUS POINTS

- existing potential clients in a commercial environment
- potential for good promotion, with salon staff having their nails done by you
- professional atmosphere (hopefully!)
- less lonely than working alone
- possibility of sharing promotion and advertising costs and benefits.

MINUS POINTS

- salon owner may be too demanding
- staff may not like 'nails' and be unhelpful in making recommendations.

Things to consider

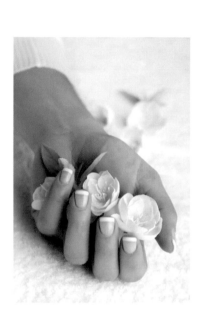

- Care must be taken in making a financial arrangement with the salon owner. Being self-employed is a common arrangement, but it has implications for VAT (if appropriate) and your position with the Inland Revenue. It is often difficult to get definite answers to questions on tax, but the problem usually lies with the salon owner rather than the technician. The technician must ensure that all legal rules for a self-employed person are followed – that is to say, payment of income tax and National Insurance and the keeping of accurate accounts.

- There are several financial arrangements that salon owners can use for this 'rent a space' idea. A weekly or monthly fixed rent is one way; the rent can often be high for a technician just starting out but, when the technician becomes busy, it may appear low to the salon owner who can see how much business the technician is doing. Under this arrangement, it is best to keep payments from clients separate so that both parties have an accurate record of client payments.

- Another possibility is to share clients' payments as a form of rent, for example 40 per cent to the salon and 60 per cent to the technician. This can help the technician in the early days as there is no rent to pay if there are no clients, but a lot of 'rent' will be paid when the technician becomes busy. It can, however, cause tax problems for the owner. There is sometimes an added complication if a salon owner provides the nail products. In this instance, the percentage of payments as 'rent' are usually reversed.

- As with a mobile or home-based technician, this is a business, and should be set up properly.

Where to start Research the salons in your area. Find out what services they offer and see how busy they are. Before you approach a proprietor, make sure there is enough room for a nail desk and have a plan of what you would like to offer in that salon. Think of how you can impress the proprietor so that they cannot afford to miss out on what you can offer them. Have some projected figures ready of how many clients you could accommodate in a day and an estimated turnover. Decide how much you can invest in your new venture, for example, have pictures of the equipment you would like to work with and will provide, how much you are willing to pay for promotional materials, etc. Convince the proprietor that you are serious about making your proposal work for you and the salon and it is worth their while giving you a chance.

Employed in a salon

Many employers now require qualified technicians who can provide specialist services for their clients. Many therapists and hairdressers can do 'nails', but they are often too busy or do not like doing it. Also, as nail work is a practical skill, it needs to be done frequently and with enjoyment to result in good work. It can often make sense for a busy salon to employ a specialist technician.

Requirements Qualifications are required and, depending on the salon, experience may be necessary. A potential employer may ask you to carry out a trade test where you can demonstrate your skills. This can be nerve-wracking, but just imagine you are dealing with a new client. Again, it is worth having personal insurance, as a client can sue both technician and salon and having the correct cover will give you peace of mind.

PLUS POINTS

- guaranteed income
- the salon handles all promotion
- no worries about products, stock and equipment
- colleagues to work with.

MINUS POINTS

- no independence.

Things to consider

- Many salons in the service industries pay a basic salary and then commission on treatments and sales on top. In this way, therapists and technicians are encouraged to work well and keep their clients.

- If the 'nails' service is new to the salon, the onus would be on the technician to make it work. As long as the salon is prepared to promote the treatments, the technician should produce good work and keep their clients happy and rebooking.

Where to start Write yourself a CV if you do not already have one. There are many ways of writing a good CV and, if you do not have experience of this, there is a lot of help on the following website: www.direct.gov.uk.

Look in the local papers and trade magazines for vacancies or contact specialist employment agencies that often advertise in trade magazines.

When going for an interview, try to have examples of your work such as before and after pictures or examples of nail art you have done on tips. Make sure your appearance is clean and tidy and that your own nails are immaculate. If possible, do some research on the salon to find out what they offer already and be knowledgeable about their services and products. If nails are new to the salon, have plenty of ideas about how to promote a nail service.

Opening a salon

There are nail salons opening all over the country now and many of them are very successful. Clients often prefer to go to a specialist for a specific service and 'nails' is no exception.

Requirements Some salon owners have no experience of the services offered and rely on their staff. For working owners it is advisable to have experience of working in a commercial environment together with practical experience. A salon owner will have to deal with difficult clients and no amount of training in a school or college can be a substitute for experience. It is also advisable to have some knowledge of the legal requirements for salons – PAYE, National Insurance, the responsibilities of employers, book-keeping, retailing and promotion, health and safety of staff and premises.

PLUS POINTS

- total control
- satisfaction of owning your own business.

MINUS POINTS

- large financial investment required
- potential problems with staffing
- permanent commitment
- the need to work long hours or stand in for staff to cover sickness and holidays.

Things to consider

- As with any new business, there is a great deal of work to do before the doors of the salon open. This work, such as researching the area, creating a viable business plan, making any necessary applications to the local authority, decorating the salon, printing promotional material, recruiting staff and so on, must be done thoroughly and time must be taken to get it right. So many businesses fail because the groundwork has not been properly done. (See Chapter 12 Business Matters.)

- Your own business is an exciting prospect and will have a better chance of succeeding if you have spent some time working in a good salon. This experience is invaluable and ensures that a lot of mistakes can be avoided.

Where to start Never underestimate the value of professional advice. If you are starting a business for the first time, get as much professional help and advice as you can. This does not have to cost much money. Speak to your bank, as they may recommend schemes to help new businesses. Also, you will probably have a business link in your area and they have many different types of help for new businesses, including help with creating your business plan, marketing and promotion. Do not rush into it and take time to plan every detail.

Consult the Habia website (www.habia.org). The Business Advice and Guidance section has a very useful free download: Habia Guide to Business Success for Beauty Therapy Salons. Plus the Official Health & Safety Implementation Pack available in the online store is an invaluable tool for salons.

Teaching

The way in which the nail industry has grown has produced a lot of 'nail' trainers, both good and bad. It has been traditional for product companies to have trainers in various parts of the country usually on a self-employed basis and often connected with sales of the products. Many training schools have opened (and many have closed) on the strength of income received from short courses and product sales. Private schools and colleges of further education who offer qualifications in beauty therapy often have the facility to teach 'nail' qualifications and many bring in technicians to teach the subject rather than relying on their beauty therapy lecturers. Usually a minimum of 3 years' industry experience is required to provide training on behalf of a product company. When teaching candidates for formal qualifications, most teachers need to have achieved, at least, the qualification of **assessor** (your local Further Education college will have details on how to achieve this). This requires a minimum of 5 years' industry experience, that is working in a commercially active salon for 5 years before becoming an assessor and holding the relevant qualifications in the sector. All assessors must also undertake CPD throughout their career. (Guidelines for assessors and verifiers are on the following website, www.habia.org.)

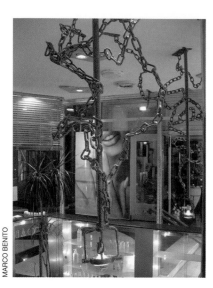

MARCO BENITO

Salons do not have to be traditional

TOP TIP

For further information visit these websites:

www.businesslink.gov.uk

www.direct.gov.uk.

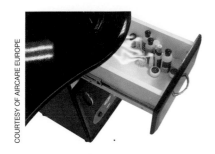

COURTESY OF AIRCARE EUROPE

Keep your desk and products clean and tidy

PLUS POINTS

- can be carried out part-time and provide additional income and <u>interest</u>
- a very good way of maintaining high standards
- job satisfaction (and often frustration) in teaching new skills to students
- if connected to a product company, there is involvement with the industry as a whole.

MINUS POINTS

- full-time teaching of 'nails' is hard to find
- if self-employed and connected to a company, there is no guaranteed income.

Things to consider

- A good technician does not necessarily make a good teacher, and vice versa.

- To become a good teacher, it is worth learning teaching skills in addition to 'nail' skills. If working in a college, it is usually necessary to be a qualified vocational assessor and a teaching qualification is required.

- Part-time teaching can often fit very well with working in a salon. You will be bringing real experience to your students, supplementing your income and gaining variety in your working life.

Where to start Product companies usually expect a minimum number of years' experience, and teaching for formal qualifications requires 5 years' experience before the relevant assessor qualification can be achieved.

If company training is an option, send an up-to-date CV to the company with a covering letter explaining that you are interested in becoming a trainer. If formal teaching is preferred, it is important to understand that, in order to achieve the assessors qualification, actual teaching needs to be done. Therefore a teaching job must be found first. Also Further Education colleges that run courses in Beauty Therapy often have vacancies for specialist teachers, especially those with extensive experience in a nail salon. Both product companies and colleges will be able to advise you on how to achieve an assessors qualification.

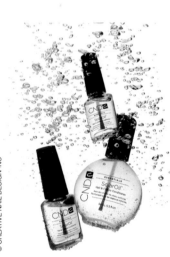

Sales/demonstrator

Product companies often have a salesperson who visits salons to sell and demonstrate products and technicians who demonstrate on stands at trade shows.

Requirements A skilled technician with a good understanding of how products work would be suited to this job. Experience in sales would also be a bonus.

Personality is very important; this job needs an outgoing person who communicates well with people. Qualifications are always desirable and personal insurance is recommended. It is unlikely that a set period of experience would be required, but it is obviously preferable.

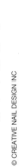

PLUS POINTS

- variety of work
- involvement in the wider industry
- usually part-time, so could fit around clients.

MINUS POINTS

- full-time jobs are rare so will have several applicants
- part-time jobs may be casual (that is, only when required).

Things to consider

- There are not many companies that are large enough to employ full-time sales reps. Many have part-time technicians who are either employed or self-employed and work on a commission basis. Demonstrators are often technicians connected with the company who are prepared to work at trade shows.

Where to start
Research the companies to see what they sell and who to. Look in trade magazines for vacancies. Have a good CV prepared.

Media technicians

The nail industry is beginning to achieve a higher profile in the market and people are becoming more aware of 'nails' as part of grooming and fashion. A separate person to do 'nails' on photographic shoots and catwalk shows is now the norm (if the budget allows).

Requirements
A high level of skill, creativity and imagination is needed and insurance is essential. Patience, adaptability and discretion are essential commodities. The level of skill is more important than time spent working, but this technician will often be called upon to solve many different problems and nothing takes the place of experience.

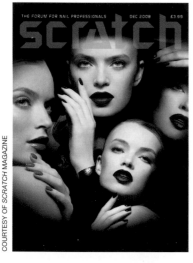

Nails by Marian Newman for Nails Inc.
Photographer Joachim Norvik.

PLUS POINTS

- wide variety of work
- chance of meeting and working with famous people
- high fees for some types of work
- high profile for technician.

MINUS POINTS

- work not regular
- long hours of waiting around following frantic working sessions
- dealing with sometimes difficult people
- carrying a very heavy kit
- working very long hours on some jobs
- lots of free or low-paid work in order to achieve the recognition needed to get paid work.

Things to consider
At the present time, there are very few technicians who get 'published' in the media. Lots appear in trade magazines. Media work is a very different world and technicians need to be like make-up artists and hairdressers who can help create images for advertising, editorial work and fashion shows. A portfolio of work needs to be compiled to show prospective clients. As a general 'rule of thumb', work that receives credits (that is, the person's name with the pictures) is usually low-paid or even free; work

that does not receive credit is usually paid for by way of a fee. It is advisable to use the services of an agent as most magazines, advertising agencies, designers and photographers are used to using an agent to arrange the creative team. Agents obviously charge a fee, but the potential earnings of this kind of work are very high.

Where to start There are many 'special occasion' opportunities for technicians. These may be weddings, fancy dress parties, local fashion shows held by shops or colleges. Keep a lookout for local activities and approach relevant outlets (e.g. fancy dress hire shops, fashion shops, colleges) to offer your services. Keep pictures of work you have done.

A way of gaining experience for this type of work is to contact hair and make-up agencies, usually based in London but there are some provincial ones, to find out if they represent any technicians. If they do, offer to assist the technician. There is not usually any payment for this type of work but the experience will be invaluable.

This list of career routes is not exhaustive; there are many variants and combinations. The nail industry is an exciting place to be and there is a place for everyone. Artificial nails is not the only skill and treatment involved; there are many who specialize in natural nail care, and it seems that the majority of European women prefer natural nails to artificial ones, even if they have used the artificial variety to help them on their way.

The most important message is that recognized qualifications, practice, dedication and a lifetime of learning are essential for real success.

Summary

This chapter has sketched the education and skills training required by a modern nail technician and outlined the eight most common career paths the technician can follow, highlighting the advantages and disadvantages of each.

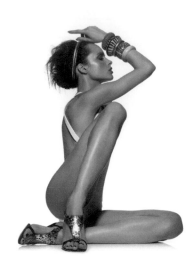

2

Anatomy and physiology as related to nail treatments

Learning objectives

In this chapter you will learn about:

- why anatomy and physiology is important knowledge for technicians

- the structures and functions of the skin

- an understanding of the skin as an organ and its relevance in all nail treatments

- the basic structure and functions of the cardiovascular system

- the basic structure and functions of the lymphatic system

- the basic structure and functions of the skeletal system

- the basic structure and functions of the muscular system

- the basic structure and functions of the nervous system

- some common conditions relating to each of the body systems

- the nail unit in depth.

Introduction

This chapter provides all the essential theoretical information about the skin and nails, the parts of the body that may be affected by any nail services. It covers all the requirements of the NOS and puts nail services into the context of the potential problems of an individual client.

Essential knowledge

Hairdressers learn about the structure of hair, how it grows and where it comes from; beauty therapists learn about the structure of skin, the underlying muscles and bones and the basic workings of the human body. They do this in order to understand the area that is being treated, how to vary treatments for individuals, how to recognize potential problems and how to put right something that has gone wrong. Nail technicians must do the same. They must learn about the area of the human body they deal with. This will ensure that they work safely, understand when and how to adapt treatments, give the best possible advice to their clients and know how to deal with problems.

Areas of the body are not isolated. The body functions because several systems within the human body work together. When one of these systems does not work properly, many areas of the body and other systems are affected. The main 'systems' in the human body are: nervous system; cardiovascular system (heart, lungs and circulation); digestive system; skeletal system; endocrine system (glands); urinary system; and reproductive system. Many organs are concerned with and form part of these systems and, when they all function correctly and efficiently, we have a healthy body.

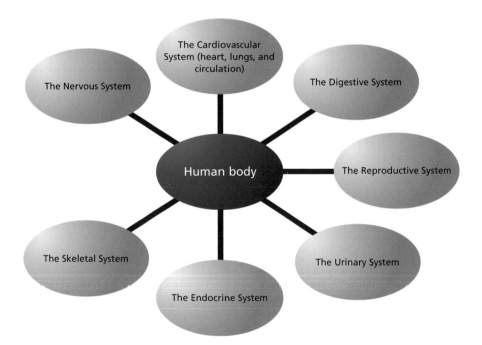

Although it is not necessary to have an in-depth understanding of all the workings of the human body, it is useful to have a basic understanding of how all areas affect the parts relevant to a nail technician. It can help to explain such things as how a poor diet can affect nail growth, why a **systemic disorder** (a disorder of the body as a whole but arising from one of the systems) can be noticed in the condition of the nails.

A **natural nail** is an adaptation of skin **cells** and is surrounded by skin. Like hair and sweat glands they are considered to be appendages of the skin. By understanding how the skin is formed and why, helps us to understand how a nail is created and what may be happening if the nail is growing less than perfectly. The hands and feet are a collection of bones, connected by muscles, nourished by a blood supply and surrounded by skin. A thorough knowledge of this part of the body is a good basis for a nail technician because it will:

- help you to *recognize any disorders* and understand what may have caused them

- assist your understanding of how these specific parts of the body function

- demonstrate a knowledge and understanding of the area being worked on during treatments by answering any question the client may ask; this will *promote professionalism and generate confidence*

- help you to choose the *most suitable products* for the client and *understand their effects* on the skin and nails.

The skin

The skin is the largest organ of the human body and plays many essential roles. It weighs 6–10 lb (3–4 kg) and measures approximately 20 sq feet in an adult. It is protective, helps with temperature control and is involved in one of the senses: touch–it is a giant, washable, stretchable, tough, waterproof sensory apparatus covering your whole body.

A body's skin has basically the same structure all over, but with some local variations, e.g. thickness, blood and nerve supply, colour, etc. Hair and nails are made of modified skin cells.

Cross-section through the skin

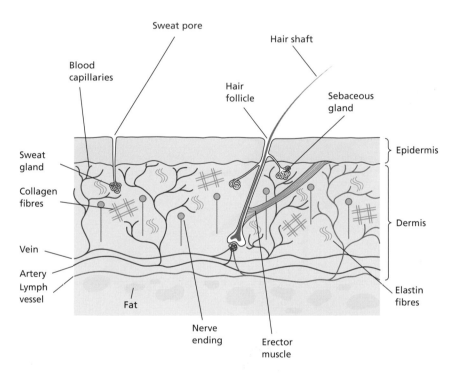

Functions

The skin performs eight main functions for the body.

1. Protection Skin provides a waterproof coat that acts as a barrier to protect the body from dirt, minor injuries, bacterial infection and chemical attack. It does this in a number of ways.

- The first barrier is a mixture of oil (**sebum**) and **sweat** which forms a slightly acidic film over the skin's surface. This discourages the growth of unwanted **bacteria** and **fungus**. (There is plenty of bacteria that lives very happily on the skin but this is of the 'wanted' variety.) The sebum, the natural oil produced by sebaceous glands in the

TOP TIP

The best moisture for the skin is its own natural level of water. Helping to prevent the loss of natural moisture is the best treatment to avoid dry skin.

hair follicles of the skin, creates a waterproof coating which helps prevent the skin lose essential water and, to a certain extent, also prevents the skin from absorbing too much water. This effect is minimal, as the skin can be quite absorbent, especially when it suffers from dryness, i.e. a lack of natural oil and moisture due to a skin condition or due to a lifestyle that destroys or removes too much oil and moisture.

- The second barrier is the uppermost layer of the skin (**stratum corneum**) that can act as a filter against invading bacteria. The healthy construction of this barrier provides good protection but it is very easily damaged. It relies on a good level of natural moisture to hold the **keratinized** skin cells together. On the hands, especially, this moisture is very often lost through environmental damage (detergents, water and so on).

- The third barrier is the production of a pigment called **melanin** in the skin; this protects lower-level tissues against **ultraviolet (UV) light** damage. Darker skins have more melanin which is a genetic modification. Darker skins have evolved from hot countries where the skin needs a lot of UV protection. Paler skins evolved from cooler countries. Whatever the melanin content, the skin needs extra protection in the sun. Even an overcast day has plenty of UV rays around so a minimum of sun protection factor (SPF) 15 should be used. Hands are especially susceptible to UV damage and are often forgotten in a sun protection regimen.

- In addition to these barriers, the skin has an early warning system against invasion by a chemical that the body will not tolerate or is sensitive or allergic to. **Irritation** on any part of the skin is usually a sign that an **allergic reaction** is starting. If an **allergen** (substance that is causing the reaction) is promptly removed, the reaction should subside. This reaction is more common when a substance is applied to the skin as part of a treatment, as it can be absorbed by the skin, but can also be the result of a substance getting inside the body either by **ingestion** (via the mouth) or **inhalation** (by breathing it in).

2. Sensation   There are several different nerve endings carried in the skin that respond to heat, cold, touch, pressure and pain. These are the sensory nerve fibres that end in the skin and send messages to the brain detecting the various sensations. Motor nerve fibres are connected to the arrector pili muscles of the hair follicles. These cause the muscle to contract and lift the hair when the person is cold or frightened causing 'goose bumps'.

3. Heat regulation   The skin helps to keep the body at a constant temperature of 37°C. It is able to do this in several ways: by **dilation** or **constriction** (vasodilation or vasoconstriction) of the blood vessels (**capillaries**) near the surface of the skin thus retaining heat or allowing it to escape; through sweat, produced by the sweat glands, which evaporates and cools the body; and by having fat in the **subcutaneous layer** that insulates the body. Sensory nerve fibres control this process as well as the skin's reaction to the 'fright, fight or flight' mechanism that results in sweaty palms.

4. Excretion   Perspiration and some waste products, such as water and salt, are lost through the skin.

5. Secretion   Sebum, which moisturizes and protects, is produced in the **sebaceous glands**.

6. Vitamin D formation   The skin is able to produce **vitamin D** through the action of UV light. This vitamin is essential to the absorption of calcium in the digestive system.

7. Storage The skin stores fat and water that can be used by any part of the body as necessary.

8. Absorption Some substances can be absorbed through the skin and will stay in that area or enter the bloodstream and be carried throughout the body. (The effect of over-absorption can be seen after a good soak in the bath!) This absorbency can be useful when applying nourishing products to the skin but it can also be quite the reverse: the skin can sometimes allow penetration of harmful substances. **Absorption** through the skin is one of the routes of entry to the human body for chemicals, together with inhalation and ingestion. The skin should be protected when using potentially harmful substances so that the chances of absorption are minimized.

Classes of skin

There are two main classes of skin; both of which can be found on the hands and feet. (The other types are the **mucous membrane** that lines the inside of the body's orifices and **mucocutaneous** skin, which is found at the junction of the mucous membrane, e.g. lips and nostrils.) We are mainly concerned here with the two major types.

Thick, hairless skin **Hairless skin** is found on the palms of the hands and the soles of the feet. As the name suggests, this type does not have any hair follicles and therefore has no oil-producing glands, which makes it prone to dryness. It has many sweat glands, which assist in gripping objects, and heightens **sensitivity**. Certain layers of the skin in this type are thicker and ridged to allow for wear and tear and to give a 'non-slip' surface. It has an **epidermis** of about 1.5 mm in thickness and a **dermis** of about 3 mm.

Thin, hairy skin **Hairy skin** covers much of the body and, along with the many structures found in all skin, has hair follicles. Its epidermal layer is about 0.07 mm in thickness (half the thickness of hairless skin) and a dermis of about 1–2 mm.

Layers of skin

It can be seen from the earlier diagram that there are three main layers of skin: the epidermis, the dermis and the subcutaneous layer. In carrying out hand, feet and nail treatments, we are more concerned with the structure of the epidermis although the dermis does play some part.

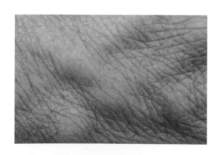

Surface of the Skin (epidermis)

The epidermis The epidermis is of special interest as nails are evolutionary adaptations of this cell-producing area, as are hair, hooves, horns, scales and feathers. It is this layer that is treated in manicures and pedicures and an improvement to the condition of this layer is what is most sought by clients who request a manicure.

The epidermis consists of layers of skin cells in various stages of development, growth, adaptation and death. The adaptation will depend on where in the body the skin is situated:

● in a hair follicle the cells will form a hair

● in the **matrix** of the nail, they will form a **nail plate**

● in areas exposed to UV light, they will produce more melanin

● on the palms of the hands and soles of the feet, the clear layer (**stratum lucidum**) will be much thicker.

This progression of cells takes place from the lower level of the epidermis up through to the surface of the skin. The cells go through many changes during this journey. The progression of a skin cell in an area of skin that does not require any adaptations and is normal and healthy takes around 4–6 weeks. Skin disorders or other general health problems can influence this process. The little skin cell ends up keratinized, flat and non-living and part of the protective stratum corneum. It is eventually shed from the skin and often found in house dust (or the inside of a pair of tights!).

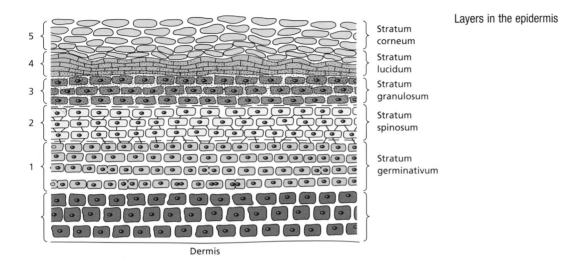

Layers in the epidermis

5 — Stratum corneum
4 — Stratum lucidum
3 — Stratum granulosum
2 — Stratum spinosum
1 — Stratum germinativum

Dermis

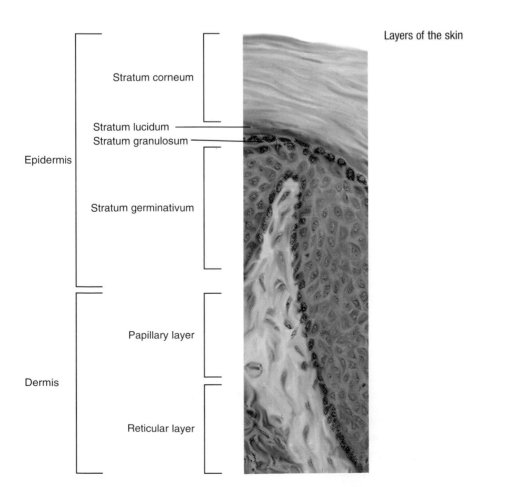

Layers of the skin

Epidermis
- Stratum corneum
- Stratum lucidum
- Stratum granulosum
- Stratum germinativum

Dermis
- Papillary layer
- Reticular layer

Layers in the epidermis

1 The base layer or **stratum germinativum** is where the skin cells are formed and is responsible for the growth of the epidermis. These cells contain the early stages of **keratin**, which is a protein, and will eventually form either a protective layer on the top of the skin or be adapted to form nails or hair. Some of the cells are melanocytes forming melanin. The cells here are continually dividing and reproducing themselves. This is a process called **mitosis**. The cells are plump, surrounded by the porous cell membrane, full of cellular fluid called **cytoplasm** and with an active nucleus that is responsible for cell reproduction and function and carries the genes inherited from our parents.

As these cells divide and reproduce themselves, they are pushed up and into the next layer of the epidermis.

2 The **stratum spinosum**, or prickle-cell layer, is where most of the cells have developed spines that connect them to surrounding cells. The nucleus is becoming less active as reproduction has slowed down or stopped.

Some of the cells, **melanocytes** that produce the pigment melanin, are extending through the spines to other cells. These are the cells that help protect the lower layers of the skin from UV damage from the sun. The amount of melanocytes depends on our skin colour. Black skins that have evolved from very hot countries, for example, have significantly more melanin for maximum protection. Fairer-skinned people who tend to come from the colder countries have much less pigment. Fair-skinned people who have been sunbathing or using a sunbed have developed extra melanocytes for their protection and this is what appears as a suntan. All skin colours will develop some degree of colour with unprotected exposure to UV radiation. Sunburn is where too much radiation from the sun has been on the skin before melanocytes have been formed to protect it. This radiation has been able to penetrate to lower levels and could cause problems in later life. There is a great deal of advice becoming available now as the effects of overexposure to the sun's radiation are further understood.

The amount of melanin can vary in the same area of skin. Patches of darker skin can be evident, sometimes on the back of the hands, the face or chest. This can be due to an over-production of melanin and is stimulated by UV radiation, or caused by a hormone imbalance, for example during pregnancy or when taking a contraceptive pill. In older people, 'liver spots' on the back of the hand are caused by minor sun damage throughout their life. Freckles are triggered by exposure to sunlight and the amount of them can be genetic. They can also be the result of **sun damage** and are often found on lighter skin as this type is more prone to suffer from overexposure.

There is an opposite effect to the over-production of melanin that results in lighter patches on the skin. This is called **vitiligo** or **leucoderma**, and it is where the skin has lost its ability to produce melanin. There is also a condition where the whole of the skin is unable to produce melanin, called **albinism**. People with this condition have very light skin and their hair and eyes lack colour.

None of these conditions is infectious, but the skin often needs extra protection and the hands are the areas that tend to suffer the most.

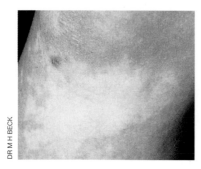

DR M H BECK

Vitiligo

3 The **stratum granulosum**, or granular layer, is where the cells are beginning to die. They appear much less plump and the nucleus begins to break up. The cytoplasm (or cellular fluid) is thickening and becoming granular where keratin is beginning to form.

4 The stratum lucidum, or clear layer, is an adapted layer that is found only on the palms of the hand and soles of the feet—that is, the thick hairless class of skin. This extra layer gives specific characteristics to these areas. The hands and feet need to grip: the hands to hold things and the feet to grip the ground. This clear layer helps to form the dips and ridges in our hands and feet that are known as our 'finger or hand prints' (our feet also have the same 'prints'). The skin in these areas does not produce sebum (natural oil) as it does not have any hair follicles: oil would make our hands and feet slippery. This area of skin only produces sweat from millions of sweat glands. A small amount of sweat, together with the ridges and dips, helps our grip. Too much sweat makes our skin slippery and is usually a hormonal effect arising from an emotional moment such as fright or nervousness. Some people produce an excess amount of sweat on the palms of their hands. If 'slippery' hands are noticed, then the technician should take extra care in preparing the nail (see Chapter 5).

5 The stratum corneum, or cornified layer, is the uppermost layer of skin. The cells have flattened, lost their nucleus and all the cytoplasm and have become keratinized. The flat cells are held together in a type of 'brick-wall' arrangement by intercellular cement, which is mostly composed of lipids, a natural fat produced by the skin together with sebum and sweat and keratin bonds. This forms a wonderful barrier and protection for the skin but it is easily damaged, especially on the hands. As newly keratinized cells are pushed up, the older flakes of dead skin are shed in a process called **desquamation** in which the bonds are broken down. This will happen naturally but can be speeded up by environmental excesses such as pollution or hard water that break down the intercellular cement.

There are many conditions that affect this whole cycle and there are skin disorders that can speed up the process, such as **psoriasis**, or slow it down.

It is very important for a nail technician to understand this process just described, for two reasons. First it shows us why the skin surrounding the nail and that on the hand must be cared for and, second, it is the basis of how nails are formed.

Below the epidermis is another part of the skin that is very different and much thicker; this is called the dermis.

The dermis

This layer carries the many structures that exist within the skin, such as nerves, blood capillaries, nerve endings, sweat ducts that open onto the surface of the skin as pores and sebaceous glands that open into hair follicles. It helps to serve the epidermis by carrying a vast network of capillaries and it gives the epidermis structural support.

Fibres in the dermis One of the main features of the dermis is the network of strong fibres, of which there are two types: **collagen** and **elastin**. They are both made of protein.

Collagen acts as a support to the skin, keeps it firm and gives it a plump, youthful appearance. Elastin gives the skin its elastic properties, allowing it to move and stretch but then return to its original position. In young skin, both types of fibres are plentiful, but as the skin ages, the fibres start to break down and are not replaced so readily. A lack of collagen allows the skin to form into wrinkles between muscles and a lack of elastin allows the skin to become softer and less firm.

The skin on the back of the hands does not always demonstrate a person's exact biological age as it is prone to misuse and damage and can look older than necessary. The skin

TOP TIP

Women, in particular, sometimes find patches of darker skin at the sides of their neck. This is often due to a reaction of the sun on the area of skin that has perfume sprayed on to it regularly. Also hormonal disturbances, such as taking the contraceptive pill, pregnancy and the menopause, can cause discoloration of the cheeks or the face.

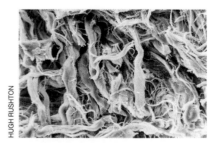

HUGH RUSHTON

Collagen and elastin fibres in the dermis

of the face is usually given more care and can often appear younger than the person's actual age. The skin on the backs of the hands has very little support in the way of muscles and stored fat. It does, however, have some very strong tendons that move the fingers and large blood vessels that supply the hand. As the elastin and collagen become less effective, owing to age and damage from UV light and weather, the tendons and blood vessels become more apparent and thus add to the ageing appearance.

Other structures in the dermis

- Nerves. The dermis carries a vast network of nerve endings that send a whole host of messages back to the brain where the messages are 'decoded' and any work that the body needs to do is undertaken. Nerves give us our sense of touch and our fingertips are some of the most sensitive areas of our body because they have a large number of sensory nerves. In addition to the ability to feel, the nerves also provide a form of protection. If extreme heat is touched, sensory nerves send an emergency message to the brain; the brain recognizes the emergency and sends another message, via the nervous system and motor nerves, to the muscles that will then move the relevant area of the body away from danger. The type of nerve that sends a message to a muscle is a motor nerve. This procedure can take place in a fraction of a second.

- Blood vessels. These make up a network of fine arteries, veins and capillaries that carry blood around the body to maintain the health of all the organs, including the skin. Blood carries nutrients (food) and oxygen to every cell in the body and removes waste products. The blood plays several essential roles in the working of the whole body. With regard to the skin, its main role is connected with heat regulation. If the body is becoming too hot, the blood vessels dilate (become bigger) in the skin. This assists heat loss. The reverse happens if the body is becoming cold: the vessels constrict, keeping the blood deeper within the body to conserve heat.

  If the skin is damaged by a superficial cut, the tiny capillaries are severed and the skin bleeds. Some of the cells that make up the blood are capable of forming together and creating a clot that blocks the ruptured vessels and prevent further blood loss. The redness seen around a cut or other damage is an increase in the blood supply that helps the cells to repair themselves.

  Increased blood supply in the skin causing redness without any obvious damage could be the body's defence mechanism in action. A harmful item (such as a splinter) or chemical could have entered the skin and be causing an irritation. Cells within the dermis called mast cells release a chemical called **histamine** that increases the blood supply to the area and attempts to destroy the invader. This defence mechanism can progress from a slight redness, to itching and even to blisters and swelling. If the allergen (the substance that is causing the allergic reaction) or irritant is removed at the first hint of trouble, the reactions will often subside. If not, the condition can continue and result in a painful and distressing type of **dermatitis**.

- Lymph vessels. Like the network of blood vessels, another system carries a fluid called lymph around the body. **Lymph** is similar in many ways to blood, in that it circulates to all the cells and carries a certain amount of nutrients, but its main role is as our body's defence mechanism. The lymph fights and removes bacteria and other invasive substances and carries excess fluid away from cells and surrounding tissue. The lymphatic fluid is 'filtered' by lymph glands situated all over the body. When the body is fighting an infection glands, often in the neck, can feel swollen and tender.

TOP TIP

A gentle pinch to the skin on the backs of the hands demonstrates age and skin condition. A young and hydrated skin recovers immediately. Older and/or dehydrated skin takes longer to recover. Experiment on different ages of skin to discover the difference.

The lymphatic system does not have a pump to move it around in the way that the blood has the heart. It relies, instead, on muscular movement to push it along. The flow of lymph can sometimes be sluggish and excess fluid and waste can build up in certain areas.

There are no lymph glands sited near the feet and gravity will often cause excess fluid to collect in this area. The nearest glands are at the top of the leg in the groin and behind the knee. The nearest glands to the hands are on the inside of the elbows. Massage in these areas, with movements towards the glands, can help to increase circulation and reduce excess fluid in the hands and feet.

● **Sweat glands**. Sweat glands, with their own blood supply, are sited in the dermis and a tube, or duct, leads directly from the gland through the dermis and epidermis to open onto the surface and is seen as a pore in the skin. There are more sweat glands on the palms of the hands and soles of the feet than anywhere else on the body.

The most common type of gland, **eccrine glands**, are found all over the body and help to regulate the body's heat by secreting small amounts of sweat all the time. This function also helps to regulate the body's salt levels and eliminates some waste products. It helps to keep the skin hydrated and is part of the acid mantle that helps protect the skin. The level of sweat produced can be affected by the nervous system, for example emotions can raise the level, you may have noticed how anxiety often makes your palms very sweaty.

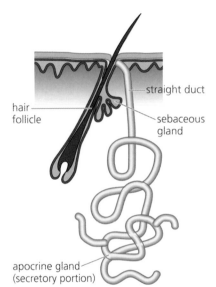

hair follicle — straight duct — sebaceous gland

apocrine gland (secretory portion)

Apocrine gland

Another, less common type, are **apocrine glands**, which are situated under the arm and groin. The sweat secreted from these has a different chemical composition and **hormones** control its production.

● Hair follicles. Another structure found in the dermis of the skin are **hair follicles** (with the exception of the palms of the hands, the soles of the feet and the lips). A follicle is a long sack-like shape where epidermal tissue extends from the surface of the skin down through the epidermis and dermis to its own blood supply. At the base of the follicle is an area called the germinal matrix where certain epidermal cells are 'instructed' by their nucleus to adapt their growth and form together to create a hair. As in the epidermis, the new cells push the older ones upward and the hair grows up the follicle and out through the surface of the skin. Different types of hair grow on different areas of the skin. Although the same structure, the hairs have different characteristics, for example hair on the head has a longer life span than the hair of an eyelash. This is why eyelashes only grow to a certain length before falling out.

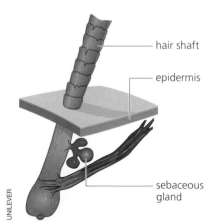

hair shaft — epidermis — sebaceous gland

Sebaceous gland

● Sebaceous glands. Connected to the follicle is another structure: the sebaceous gland. This secretes a natural oil, sebum, onto the hair shaft and the skin's surface. The oil helps to lubricate the hair shaft and plays an important role in the skin's protective functions. It helps create a waterproof barrier and therefore keep moisture in the cells of the skin and it also, together with sweat, creates a slightly acidic covering on the skin that acts as a bactericide and discourages the growth of unwanted microorganisms. This covering is known as the **acid mantle**.

● pH values. For the skin to remain healthy it needs to maintain the degree of acidity created by the sebum and sweat. If this changes too much the skin can become dry and if it changes drastically the skin is damaged. A scale called the **pH value** measures acidity and alkalinity. Low numbers (1–6) are acidic, 7 is neutral and high numbers (8–14) are **alkaline**. A value of 7 is neutral. Examples of acids can be

UNILEVER

found in citrus fruits, such as lemons. This level of acidity would not damage the skin unless it were left on it for a period of time. Fruit acids are usually the base of a popular ingredient in skin care: alpha hydroxy acids (**AHA**). These can be useful in skin-care as they help to remove dead skin cells and debris from the surface of the skin and generate cell renewal in areas that need assistance, such as the face and backs of the hands. **Acids** with low pH values would 'burn' the skin, causing extreme irritation and blisters.

At the other end of the scale are the alkalines that can have a similar effect on the skin. The milder alkalines are often used in skin treatments. Sodium hydroxide is sometimes used to soften and remove unwanted skin cells, for example in a cuticle remover. Soap is alkaline and is very drying to the skin. Extreme alkalines, such as houschold bleach, will damage skin in the same way that acids will.

The pH value of the skin is naturally 5.5–5.6–that is, slightly acidic, and skin pre-parations that are called 'pH balanced' will have a similar pH value.

Another structure attached to the hair follicle is a tiny muscle, the arrector pili mus-cle. When this contracts it causes the hair to stand upright in the skin. It does this to help trap heat and also as a response to some emotional reactions. The effect is usually known as 'goose bumps'.

Below the level of the dermis is a layer of stored fat. This fat is a supply of energy for the body and also helps contain heat within the body.

Common conditions of the skin

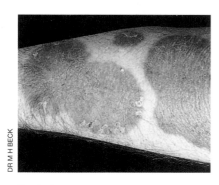

DR M H BECK

Psoriasis

- One of the most common skin conditions a nail technician is likely to come across is dermatitis. This literally means an inflammation of the skin and is non-specific (meaning the cause of the inflammation is not necessarily known). It is caused by an irritant to the skin or other part of the body activating the body's immune system so that white blood cells fight the invasion. Removing the cause can cure it.

- Eczema, on the other hand, has symptoms very similar to dermatitis, in that it is an inflammation of the skin, but it is usually a genetic condition.

- Psoriasis is a condition where there is an over-production of skin cells and scaly patches of dry, dead skin can be seen.

- There is a more detailed discussion of skin conditions in Chapter 4.

Blood circulation

Blood needs to be carried to every cell of the body. It is the internal transport system that keeps the body functioning. It links every part of the body with every other part.

- The blood carries food in the form of nutrients extracted from the digestive system and oxygen from the lungs to every cell, where they are converted into the fuel necessary to the functioning of the cell.

- Waste products produced by every cell are carried away: **carbon dioxide** to the lungs, and the other waste products to the liver and kidneys where they are extracted from the blood.

- Many different glands around the body secrete hormones. These are controlled by the brain and are the chemical messengers that instruct the organs and tissues how and when to function. Hormones are transported by the blood system.

- The body's defence mechanism to fight the invasion of foreign bodies, such as bacteria, **viruses**, harmful chemicals, etc. is also a major function of the blood. Cells in the blood are able to recognize any invasion and decide whether it needs fighting or whether it is harmless. If it needs to be fought, other cells in the blood attack and, if necessary, bring other systems of the body into the fight to help defend against **disease** or damage.

- Blood circulation also helps with the control of heat. It distributes heat evenly around the body and, when necessary, helps it to cool down by dilating (opening) vessels near the skin surface to lose some heat, or contracting those vessels to keep the heat nearer the centre of the body.

- If the skin is damaged by a superficial cut, the tiny capillaries are severed and the skin bleeds. Some of the cells that form blood are capable of forming together and creating a clot that blocks the ruptured vessels and prevents further blood loss. The redness seen around a cut or other damage is an increase in the blood supply as it helps the cells to repair themselves.

The heart

The circulation of the blood needs a pump: the **heart**, a four-chambered, muscular organ. The muscles of the heart are of a special type; instead of being individual fibres bundled together, they are connected so that a contraction in one area stimulates a wave of contractions throughout. Its muscle function is controlled by the autonomic nervous system, that is it happens without any conscious effort on our part.

The upper right chamber (right **atrium**) of the heart receives **deoxygenated blood** that has travelled all around the body providing oxygen to the cells via two major veins: the superior and inferior **vena cava**. This travels into the lower right chamber (right **ventricle**) where strong muscles pump it directly to the lungs, close by, via the **pulmonary** arteries. The blood, low in oxygen but high in carbon dioxide that has been collected from the cells, collects oxygen from the tiny air sacks in the lungs that are filled when we breathe in and releases the carbon dioxide into the air sacks that is then dispersed when we breathe out.

When the blood has passed through the lungs, it is delivered back to the upper left chamber of the heart (left atrium) via the pulmonary veins. This blood, high in oxygen and low in carbon dioxide, passes into the lower left chamber (left ventricle) where very powerful muscles send it on its journey around the body again via a huge blood vessel, the **aorta**.

The heart beats on average 70–80 times a minute in a healthy body. This pump starts when we are an embryo in the womb and continues until we die. Quite literally, our lives depend on it!

The blood travels along three main types of vessels: **arteries**, **veins** and **capillaries**.

1   Arteries are the vessels that carry the blood away from the heart (remember: A = artery and away). The blood is oxygenated and bright red. The structure of the artery has a thick muscular wall that helps maintain the pressure of blood in order for it to travel to all areas of the body. If an artery is cut, this pressure causes the blood to pump out with each heartbeat. Arteries are usually situated deeper within the body to protect them from this kind of damage.

2   Veins carry blood that is returning from all parts of the body to the heart. These vessels do not have the muscular walls of arteries but they do have 'non-return' valves to keep the blood flowing in one direction, that is to the heart. The movement of the blood is mainly affected by the movement of the muscles in the areas around

TOP TIP

Some general terms when relating to the positioning within the body:

Distal: furthest away from the body

Proximal: closest to the body

Lateral: at the side

Medial: middle

Anterior: front

Posterior: back

the veins and by the flow generated by the heart. This is one important reason why exercise and movement is essential for a healthy body. There are more veins than arteries and many are situated closer to the surface of the skin. If a vein is cut, the blood is seen to well out rather than the way it pumps out of an artery.

3   Capillaries are the link between the arteries and veins and allow the blood to reach every cell in the body. They are tiny, thread-like vessels with very thin walls and they branch out to every extremity. Their walls are so thin that the nutrients and oxygen carried in the blood are able to pass through the wall and into the tissue fluid that bathes the spaces between cells. Red blood cells are too large to pass through the capillary walls, just the clear blood **plasma** carrying the nutrients is transferred. These substances, which are essential for life, flow naturally through the wall from an area of high level (the blood) into an area with a lower level (the tissues). Waste materials from the cells, in the same way, flow from the tissues into the blood to be carried away for elimination.

For the purposes of manicure and pedicure, an understanding of how the blood circulation works is required. However, you will only need to remember the main arteries and veins in the hand, arm, leg and foot.

The heart

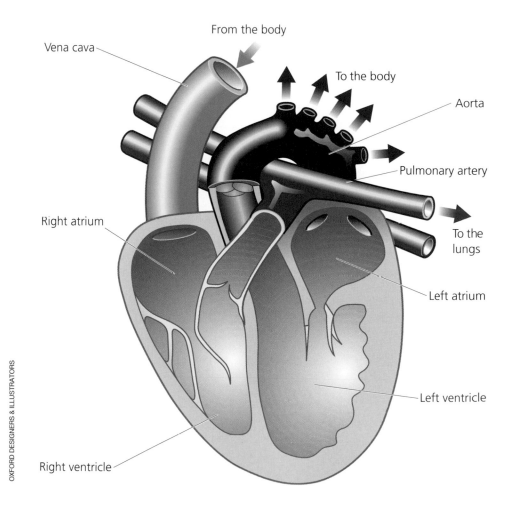

OXFORD DESIGNERS & ILLUSTRATORS

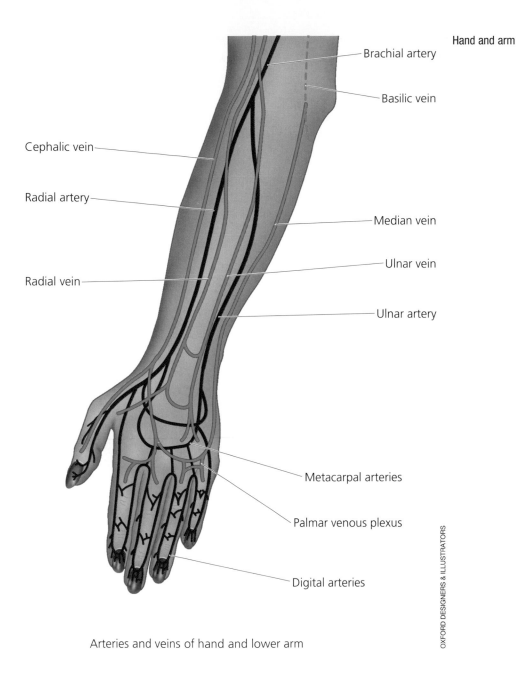

Hand and arm

Brachial artery

Basilic vein

Cephalic vein

Radial artery

Median vein

Ulnar vein

Radial vein

Ulnar artery

Metacarpal arteries

Palmar venous plexus

Digital arteries

Arteries and veins of hand and lower arm

OXFORD DESIGNERS & ILLUSTRATORS

Hand and arm

The artery that serves the arms branches indirectly from the aorta and is known as the **brachial artery**. It runs down the middle of the inside of the upper arm, quite deep, to just below the elbow where it branches into:

- The **radial artery** running down the thumb side of the lower arm where it supplies oxygenated blood to that side of the hand and the back of the hand. It is commonly used as a pulse point as it is quite close to the surface in the wrist and the beat of the heart can be felt.

- The **ulnar artery** that runs down the other side of the lower arm, crosses the wrist and supplies that side of the hand and the palm.

There are interconnections between the radial and ulnar arteries that form the **palmar arches**: known as the deep and superficial arches. Branches from these serve the main areas of the hand (**metacarpal arteries**) and more branches run down the fingers (**digital arteries**) to end under each nail to supply the nail unit with blood.

The hand and arm are served by more veins than arteries to carry away the **deoxygenated blood** from the area. The deeper veins have the same names as the relevant arteries, that is the **radial vein** serving the thumb side of the hand and lower arm and the **ulnar vein** serving the outside of the hand and lower arm, plus the digital, **metacarpal and palmar veins**.

In addition to the major vessels, there are veins closer to the skin, known as superficial veins. Many of these can be seen through the skin on the back of the hand (**dorsal** venous network) and the palm (palmar venous plexus) and lead into the main superficial veins:

- basilic vein, seen on the back of the hand on the little finger side and up the centre of the forearm

- cephalic vein seen on the back of the hand around the thumb and up the forearm to the elbow

- median vein from the palm of the hand up the forearm where it joins the basilic vein.

Foot and lower leg

A large and important artery branches into each leg around the groin area: the **femoral artery**. It goes to behind the knee where it becomes the **popliteal artery** and branches into the main lower leg arteries:

Foot and lower leg

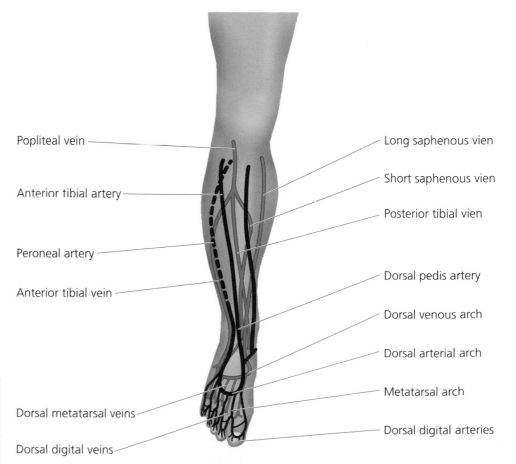

Popliteal vein

Anterior tibial artery

Peroneal artery

Anterior tibial vein

Dorsal metatarsal veins

Dorsal digital veins

Long saphenous vien

Short saphenous vien

Posterior tibial vien

Dorsal pedis artery

Dorsal venous arch

Dorsal arterial arch

Metatarsal arch

Dorsal digital arteries

Arteries and veins of the foot and lower leg

- The anterior tibial artery passes between the bones of the lower leg towards the front of the leg to the ankle and from there to the top of the foot at the dorsal pedis artery. This branches to form the dorsal arterial arch and dorsal digital arteries. It then passes through the foot to form part of the **plantar arch** on the sole of the foot.

- The posterior tibial artery passes down the centre of the back of the leg, past the ankle to the inside of the sole. Here it branches to form the **lateral and medial plantar arteries**, which in turn supply the arteries to the toes. It also branches near the knee to form the peroneal artery running down the outside of the leg towards the heel.

Like the hand and arm, there are deep and superficial veins serving this area. The deep veins follow and have the same names as the main arteries. The two main superficial veins are the long **saphenous vein** which begins at the dorsal venous arch on the top of the foot and runs up the inside of the lower leg and thigh to join the femoral vein, and the short saphenous vein from the ankle up the back of the calf to the popliteal vein at the knee.

Obviously, there are many branches and smaller veins in the area that remove the deoxygenated blood and take it on its journey back to the heart and from there to the lungs.

Some common conditions involving the blood system

- Heart disease, even if it is minor, can cause a problem with circulation, leading to poor circulation at the extremities of the body. Weak nails and dry skin can result and nails can appear bluish in colour due to poor delivery of red, oxygenated blood.

- A lack of essential vitamins and minerals in the blood can affect the condition of skin and nails.

- **Anaemia**: this is a condition that results in a shortage of red blood cells, that is the cells that carry oxygen. This shortage affects the whole body. The most common symptoms are extreme tiredness and pale skin (and nail beds). In some instances, the body just needs extra iron. This condition is especially common in young girls who don't have a proper diet and women whose periods are heavy (for example during early stages of the menopause).

- **Varicose veins**: this is an impaired functioning of the valves in the veins. The veins can become swollen and tender and can result in ulcers in extreme cases. They should be avoided during a leg massage.

As with all conditions, a nail technician must never diagnose for their client. Understanding how the systems of the body work helps technicians to decide the best type of treatment for their client together with informed aftercare advice.

The lymphatic system

The **lymphatic system** is a second system of circulation, closely associated with the blood circulation. It is just as complex and just as essential to the survival of the human body.

The system carries a fluid known as lymph. Lymph is a clear fluid that bathes every cell in the body and is the carrier of all the cellular requirements and waste products. Lymph carries white blood cells that are transported in and out of the bloodstream as necessary. It is the main 'ingredient' of the human body's immune system. Like veins in the blood system, the vessels carrying the lymph do not have muscular walls and the pressure of a heart to act as a pump. The movement of the lymph relies on movement in nearby muscles and close arteries.

The main functions of the lymphatic system are to:

- drain the **intercellular fluid**; approximately 15 per cent of this fluid is not reabsorbed by the capillaries

- be responsible for the transportation and absorption of dietary fats

- initiates and regulates the immune responses.

The network of lymphatic vessels contains approximately 100 **lymph nodes** around the body and lymph fluid passes through at least one of these before eventually draining into venous blood. The nodes are small, kidney-shaped structures and have two main functions:

1 They are filters of the fluid and will remove any unwanted microorganisms and other foreign materials. The unwanted organisms are stored here and specialist cells (called **macrophages**) engulf and destroy the invaders.

2 They store several types of white blood cells needed for the fight and destruction of infections and release them as required.

When a harmful microorganism enters the body, the lymph nodes usually become swollen with large amounts of the white blood cells (**lymphocytes**) that are ready to be released to destroy the invader.

If lymph nodes or vessels become blocked or the movement of lymph becomes sluggish for any reason (for example, lack of exercise, low metabolism, etc.) then local swelling may be noticed: known as **oedema**. Excess fluid is not being efficiently removed from the tissues and is very often experienced around the ankles. **Massage** techniques provided during a manicure and pedicure can encourage an efficient circulation of lymph and help to remove excess waste productions from the area.

All of the organs and systems of the human body are connected with and are influenced by each other. Some of the organs that are specifically associated with the lymphatic system are:

- The **spleen**, which is located in the abdomen. It filters the blood by breaking down old red blood cells and also manufactures the lymphocytes essential to the immune system.

- The **tonsils** are patches of lymphatic tissue at the back of the throat. Their function is to help trap harmful materials trying to enter the body via breathing, eating and drinking.

- **Peyer's patches** – similar in function and structure to the tonsils – are located in the small intestine to destroy the bacteria that could thrive in that environment.

Some common conditions concerning the lymphatic system

- The condition that a technician is most likely to come across is dermatitis, where the immune system rushes to protect the body at one of its 'routes of entry' (see Chapter 4), that is absorption through the skin.

- Blisters are usually filled with a clear fluid; this is lymph where is collects to protect the skin.

- Oedema is a condition where fluid collects in certain areas. This is often seen in the feet and ankles as they are so far away from the heart. Exercise and stimulation by lymph drainage massage will help.

- **Lymphoedema** is similar to oedema but is due to an obstruction of the lymph vessels draining the area.

The bones of the hands and feet

The skeleton of the human body is a living structure and the framework that supports and protects the whole body. It functions in the following ways.

- Support: the skeleton creates the shape of the body allowing it to function, that is stand erect and move via the attachment of muscles. There are also other types of connections that provide support for the organs of the body.

- Protection: sections of the skeleton create cavities that encase and protect some essential structures of the body. The skull provides an exceptionally strong cavity for the brain; the spine provides a canal for the spinal cord that connects the brain to all other parts of the body; the rib cage provides a cavity and protective structure for some of the most important and delicate organs, e.g. the heart, lungs, spleen.

- Manufactures red blood cells. The central part of many bones is filled with a substance called bone marrow and is where red blood cells are manufactured.

- The skeleton also stores minerals.

The bones of a very young person are relatively soft and slightly bendy. As the body ages, the bones calcify and become harder and more brittle. Babies are born with 270 soft bones (64 more than an adult). Many of these will fuse together by their early twenties into the 206 hard, permanent bones.

All the bones articulate (move) against each other in order that the body can move. The areas where two or more bones come together are called joints. There are three types of joint:

1   Immoveable joints or **fibrous joints**. These are the skull and the pelvis. Each of these skeletal structures is created from several separate bones that are joined together with strong fibrous tissue. There are certain times when these need to have some movement. The skull needs to change shape during birth and a woman's pelvis can sometimes slightly enlarge during pregnancy and birth.

2   Slightly moveable joints or **cartilaginous joints**. These joints are found between the many bones in the spine where some movement is needed but is restricted.

3   Moveable joints or **synovial joints**. There are many more of these and they also fall into different categories depending on their range of movement:

    -   ball and socket joints allows circular movement, for example the shoulder and hip joints

    -   hinge joints allow a movement of approximately 90°, these are found in the elbows, knees and fingers

    -   gliding joints allow surfaces to glide over each other, for example the wrist and ankle joints

    -   pivot joints allow rotation around an axis, for example the movement allowed by the bones in the lower arm (radius and ulna) that gives the hand its circular movement when the palm is turned up and down.

For the purposes of hand and foot treatments, it is only the moveable (synovial) joints that are relevant.

The ends of the bones need protection from articulating against each other and there is a system in each joint that allows this movement and offers protection. The joint is surrounded by the synovial membrane that secretes synovial fluid and lubricates the joint to allow free movement. The bones are protected by **cartilage**, a gel-like substance, that also provides some cushioning.

There are several disorders and diseases that affect joints and therefore have implications during a hand or foot treatment. One of the most common is **arthritis** that can be caused by an illness or by wear and tear. Arthritis can cause the joints to become inflamed, painful and, in later stages, deformed.

For the purposes of massage, it is necessary to understand the positioning of the bones in the hands, lower arms, feet and lower legs and how they move against each other.

The forearm

The elbow joint is where the large upper arm bone, the **humerus**, articulates mainly with one of the two forearm bones, the **ulna**, creating a hinge joint. The other forearm bone is the **radius**, attached to the ulna at the elbow.

The presence and positioning of two bones in the forearm allows the hand to rotate, that is, the palm can be turned uppermost or it can rotate at the wrist so the back of the hand is uppermost. This is achieved by the articulation of the bone on the thumb side of the arm, the radius, rotation over the bone on the little finger side of the arm, the ulna (the radius rotates). This is a pivot joint.

The end of the radius articulates with the bones in the wrist, which, together, provide a wide range of movement for the hand.

The hand

At the wrist there are several small bones, **carpals**, that glide over each other (gliding joint) allowing a great range of movement for the hand. There are eight carpals arranged in two rows of four. These bones fit closely together and are held in place by **ligaments**.

The palm of the hand has five bones, the **metacarpals**, which can be felt along the back of the hand and these articulate with the finger bones, the **phalanges**.

The hand has four fingers, each with three phalanges, and a thumb with two phalanges. Each bone of the fingers and thumb comes together in a hinge joint, which allows for the vast amount of dexterity a human hand can demonstrate. There is a certain amount of rotation at the joint between the metacarpals and the phalanges that allows further movement for the fingers and thumb. The hand has in total 27 bones.

Our nearest relations in the animal kingdom, the apes, are very close to us in terms of anatomy and physiology. One of the main differences, which some evolutionists believe is the main reason humans evolved much further than the apes, is the movement we have in our thumb. A human thumb has a wide range of movement allowing us to become much more dextrous. An ape, as indeed a young baby learning to control their hands, can only move their thumb towards the hand and away in a pincer movement. The full movement of the human thumb allows for minute control and dexterity.

Bones of the hand

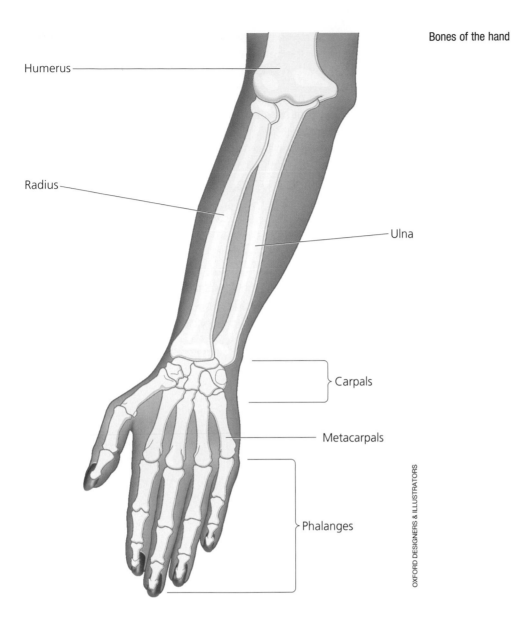

Humerus

Radius

Ulna

Carpals

Metacarpals

Phalanges

OXFORD DESIGNERS & ILLUSTRATORS

The lower leg

The arrangement of bones in the lower leg is, in many ways, similar to the lower arm. The longest bone in the human body, the **femur**, or thigh bone, extends from the hip to the knee. The femur articulates with one of the lower leg bones, the **tibia**, at a hinge joint, the knee. The knee has an extra bone that acts as a protective, the **patella**.

The lower leg, like the lower arm, has two bones that allow a certain amount of rotation of the foot. The larger one, the tibia, runs down the centre and the inside of the leg and is the one you can feel with a sharp edge as the shinbone. This articulates with the **talus** (one of the ankle bones) at the ankle. The smaller bone, the **fibula**, articulates with the tibia at the knee then runs down the outside of the leg to articulate, like the tibia, with the talus. It is the knobbly ends of these bones that stick out on either side of the ankle.

In the ankle, there are a collection of seven bones, the **tarsals**, that glide over each other to form the ankle. The largest of them, the **calcaneus**, forms the heel of the foot. On top of this is the second largest, the talus which articulates with both the tibia and fibula. There are then two rows of two and three bones, respectively.

The five bones that can be felt on the upper foot are the **metatarsals**. These articulate with the phalanges and, like those in the hand, there are three bones for the smaller toes and two for the big toe. Unlike the fingers, the movement in the toes is more restricted. Their main functions are concerned with grip and balance.

The foot

The foot is obviously essential to the balance and walking movement of the human body. Consider its shape as being similar to a tripod, with the points of contact being the heel, under the big toe and under the little toe. This structure is able to support the weight of the body when standing, walking, running, etc. and gives it balance when the body weight shifts to the various contact points. The arches in the middle of the foot, while being part of this structure, also allow for the free flow of blood to all parts of the foot without any pressure from contact with the surface.

Bones of the feet and lower legs

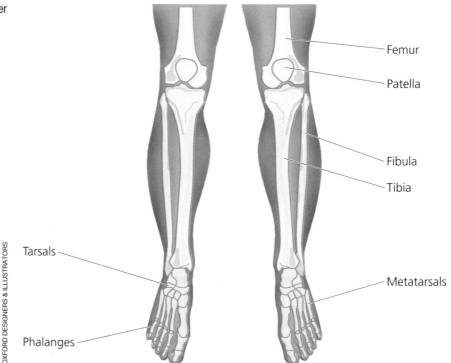

OXFORD DESIGNERS & ILLUSTRATORS

Femur

Patella

Fibula

Tibia

Tarsals

Metatarsals

Phalanges

Some common conditions concerning the bones

- Arthritis is a very common condition affecting the joints.

- Broken bones are relatively common and a technician is likely to come across this condition.

- Bunions are a painful condition affecting the base of the big toe. The big toe leans towards the second toe and there is a deformity of the joint sometimes with a painful, fluid-filled swelling. There are several causes, even heredity, and poorly fitting shoes is just one of them. If severe the only solution is surgery.

- Rheumatoid arthritis is an inflammation of the connective tissue in the joints similar to arthritis but often more aggressive.

Muscles

We have looked at the structure of skin, the blood and lymph circulation systems and the skeleton. Every system in the body relies on every other system to function. Think about how muscles affect the anatomical areas we have looked at so far.

The skin has muscles lying directly beneath it. These muscles in the face provide us with the wide range of facial expressions that is so important to human communication. The loss of muscle tone or substance creates visible signs of ageing and illness. This is especially visible on the face, the backs of the hands and the neck.

Muscles play a very important part in the circulation of blood and lymph. The heart mainly comprises a specialized muscle tissue that keeps it beating and pumping the blood around our body. It is muscle movements in associated areas that encourage the flow of lymph around the body. The skeleton can support and protect but it needs the vast array of muscles to allow it to move.

It would be impossible for a human body to do anything without muscles. Everything you conceive in your brain is expressed in muscular motion: talking, walking, drawing, reading, laughing, etc. Muscles turn energy from nutrition into movement. They are long-lasting, self-healing, and are able to grow stronger with practice.

There are three different types of muscle in the human body:

1. **Skeletal muscle**. This is the type we can see and feel. We are usually aware that they are moving and that we are controlling them. They are attached to the skeleton and work in pairs, that is one muscle moves the joint one way and another moves it back. Muscles can pull but cannot push. The only times we do not control them voluntarily is when our nervous system sends an emergency message of self-protection, such as touching something hot, blinking if something approaches our eye. Skeletal muscles are the body's most abundant tissue and comprise approximately 23 per cent of a woman's body weight and 40 per cent of a man's.

2. **Smooth muscle**. This is the muscle associated with our organs and blood vessels. It is found in the **digestive system** (e.g. stomach and intestines for churning food and pushing it along), blood vessels (for pumping blood along the arteries), bladder, airways and uterus. The body is largely unaware of its control over this type of muscle; it is triggered automatically by signals from the brain.

3. **Cardiac muscle**. This is only found in the heart and is a specialized muscle where the fibres are connected together and are controlled by the brain.

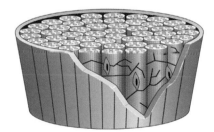

Muscle tissue

For the purposes of treatments, only skeletal muscle is relevant, although an understanding of the basic systems of the body is important.

The basic action of a muscle is contracting. An example of this can be seen in lifting your lower arm. The muscle on the front of your upper arm, the bicep, contracts and lifts the lower arm, and can hold it there. When this action is no longer needed, the bicep relaxes, but the arm needs to be returned to its original position. This is when the tricep, on the back of your upper arm, contracts to bring the lower arm back. This example shows how skeletal muscles work in pairs because their basic action is to contract.

The order to a muscle to contract comes from the brain via the nervous system. The motor nerves situated in all muscle fibres initiate what is actually a chemical reaction that causes the minute fibres to contract and shorten. The chemical reaction needs specific nutrients and oxygen, which are carried to them via the blood system.

There are two types of contraction: isotonic and isometric contraction.

Isotonic contraction is where the length of the muscle shortens, as in the lifting of the forearm. **Isometric contraction** is where the muscle is put under tension but is not necessarily shortened. An example of this would be carrying a heavy bag. The force generated by the muscle allows the arm to do this. The toning of a muscle needs repetitive movements with little associated weight, while the building of muscle needs the tension and force required to move or support heavy weights.

Skeletal muscle is made up of bundles of fibres. It is also called **striated muscle** as stripes can be seen when viewed under a microscope. The fibres can be thought of as long cylinders and can vary in size from 10 per cent up to the full width of a hair. A muscle fibre contains many smaller, long cylinders called **myofibrils** (muscle protein) that surround **filaments**. It is the filaments that actually contract the myofibrils and therefore the fibres that are connected in parallel bundles.

Tired, overworked or slightly damaged muscles have myofibrils that are not fully relaxed and feel like knots in the muscle. Stress often causes a contraction that does not relax. A good massage, using techniques that stroke the fibres and encourage them to relax and return to their resting position, is very helpful and pleasant for the client. This is relatively easy to achieve on the lower arms, hands, lower legs and feet, as the muscles are not large and are close to the surface of the skin. On other parts of the body, such as the back and upper leg, the muscles are large and a much firmer pressure is needed to reach the deep muscles.

Associated with the muscles are two other types of tissue:

1   **Ligament**. This is a short band of fibrous tissue that binds bones together.

2   **Tendon**. This fibrous tissue attaches the muscle to the bone. An example of this is found in the Achilles heel, the tough ridge at the back of the heel that joins the heel to the calf muscle.

Both of the above can be damaged, usually by overstretching.

For massage purposes, it is necessary to know and have a basic understanding of how muscles work and their positions in the arm, hand, leg and foot.

The lower arm and hand

The muscles in the lower arm are concerned with the movements of the hand (the upper arm has the muscles that raise and lower this part of the arm). The muscles work in pairs, as explained above.

● One of the muscles that extends (or straightens) the wrist and helps to turn the hand is the extensor carpi ulnaris. Its name should suggest to you where it is and what it does. It starts at the humerus, runs down the ulna side of the arm to the little finger side of the carpals.

TOP TIP

General terms relating to the action of a muscle:

Extensor: extends or straightens

Flexor: bends

Adductor: bring towards the body

Abductor: move away from the body

Supinator: turns palm of the hand up

Pronator: turns palm of hand down

Muscles of the lower arm and hand

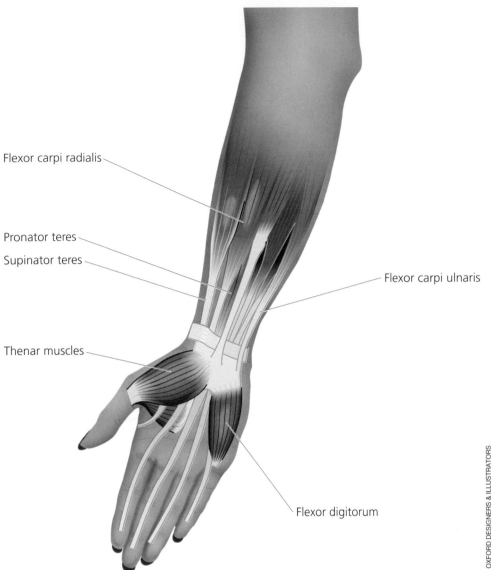

Flexor carpi radialis

Pronator teres

Supinator teres

Thenar muscles

Flexor carpi ulnaris

Flexor digitorum

OXFORD DESIGNERS & ILLUSTRATORS

- The opposing muscle to this, which bends the wrist and turns the hand in the other direction, is the flexor carpi ulnaris.

- There is another muscle that extends the wrist and helps turn the hand that runs down the radius side of the arm: the extensor carpi radialis.

- Its opposing muscle is the flexor carpi radialis.

- The muscle that rotates the hand to bring the palm downwards starts at the humerus and extends down the top of the ulna to the base of the radius and is known as the pronator teres.

- Its opposing muscle, the supinator teres, follows a similar route and connects with the other side of the radius.

Tendons from these muscles run down the hand to each finger:

- Extensor digitorum tendons run down the back of the hand, right along the fingers and allow the fingers to extend. These can be seen and felt as the fingers move and are particularly obvious in older hands as the skin loses its support.

- Flexor digitorum tendons are the opposing tendons that are in the palm of the hand and fingers and allow the fingers to bend.

The hand also has a group of muscles in the palm that gives the thumb and little finger their range of movement.

The wrist has four important ligaments that hold the carpals together, while allowing them to slide over each other during the movements of the wrist.

The lower leg and foot

The muscle groups in the leg and foot have similarities to those in the arm and hand. However, in addition to the range of movements, these muscles are important for walking and balance.

Muscles of the foot and lower leg

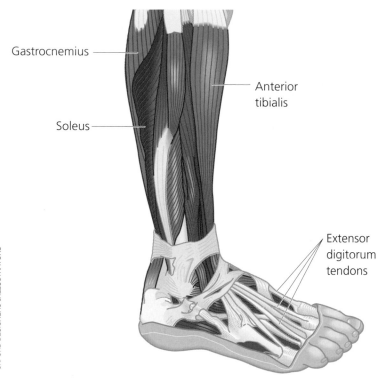

Gastrocnemius

Anterior tibialis

Soleus

Extensor digitorum tendons

OXFORD DESIGNERS & ILLUSTRATORS

- The large calf muscle, which starts at the femur behind the knee, runs down the lower leg to where it joins the heel (calcaneus) via the Achilles tendon and is known as the gastrocnemius. This muscle flexes the ankle to straighten the foot.

- Its opposing muscle, the anterior tibialis, flexes the foot to bring it up towards the leg. It attaches at the upper tibia, runs down the front of the leg to join the metatarsals.

- The muscle that helps to stabilize the body when standing and flexes the foot inwards is the soleus. This starts with the upper tibia and fibula and joins the tendon of the gastrocnemius.

The muscles of the foot that lift the toes are the extensor digitorum brevis and they continue onto tendons for each toe: the extensor digitorum tendons. Under the foot is the flexor digitorum brevis leading to the flexor digitorum tendons.

Some common conditions concerning muscles

- Sprains and strains are a frequent problem with muscles. They mainly involve the ligaments, which can be overstretched and sometimes torn.

- A torn muscle, especially in the leg, is quite common, as are strained muscles that have been overworked.

The nervous system

The organs and tissues that make up the nervous system are the brain, spinal cord, sense organs (eye, ear, skin, nose, tongue) and the nerves. The system can be differentiated into two main structural areas:

1 The **central nervous system (CNS)** comprising the brain and spinal cord.

2 The **peripheral nervous system (PNS)** with all the sensory and motor **neurones**.

The functions of the nervous system can also be differentiated into two categories:

1 The **voluntary nervous system**. These are movements under our conscious control, for example walking, speaking, etc.

2 The **autonomic nervous system**. These movements are out of our conscious control, for example blinking, breathing, and movements in the digestive organs. This system regulates the muscles in the skin (around the hair **follicles** and the smooth muscle of our internal structures), blood vessels, the iris of the eye and the cardiac muscle of the heart.

Messages to and from the brain and spinal cord use the peripheral nervous system and are transmitted along nerve fibres. Along these fibres are neurones. These are cells like tiny batteries that power the electrical circuits in the body (the method by which messages are transmitted). They transmit from cell to cell for communication, control and interpretation of the sensory input.

There are three main types of nerves:

1 **Sensory nerve** fibres that carry impulses from the nerve endings in the sensory organs (for example the skin) back to the brain via the spinal cord. This keeps the brain informed about our external environment.

2 **Motor nerve** fibres that relay messages from the brain and spinal cord to instruct relevant parts of the body to respond, for example bending an arm or jerking away from unexpected heat.

3 The **autonomic nerves** that are working all the time to control the subconscious workings of the body. This includes temperature control that affects the skin.

The skin is the largest sensory organ and responds to touch, pressure and heat. **Receptors** in the epidermis and dermis can detect pressure, vibration, mechanical stimulation, thermal and noxious (harmful) stimulation.

The hands have a plentiful supply of nerves, especially on the fingertips. Although all the skin is involved in the sense of touch, the fingers are especially sensitive.

There are some fairly common disorders, either permanent or temporary, that can affect the nervous system in the hands and feet. They can cause phenomena such as a loss of sensation in the skin and an inability to feel or quickly respond to extreme temperatures. This is why care must be taken when using heated products or equipment. Their temperature must be tested before the client uses them.

Nerves of the hand and lower arm

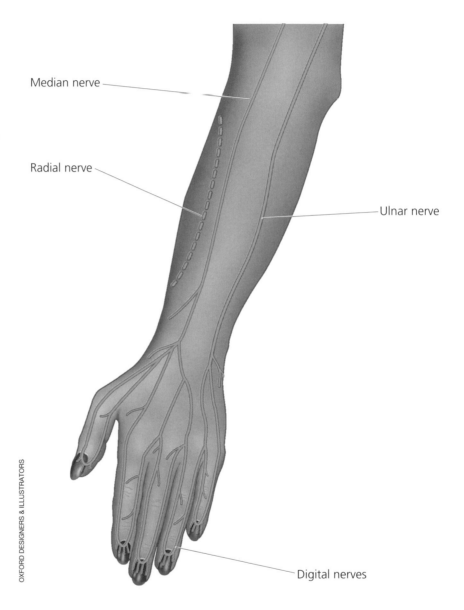

Median nerve

Radial nerve

Ulnar nerve

Digital nerves

OXFORD DESIGNERS & ILLUSTRATORS

Some disorders involving the nervous system

- **Parkinson's disease** affects more than 1 person in 1000 and 1 in 100 of those over 60. It results in shaking and tremors and muscular rigidity. It is a progressive disease.

- **Multiple sclerosis** affects the nerve fibres resulting in a progressive impairment of muscular control.

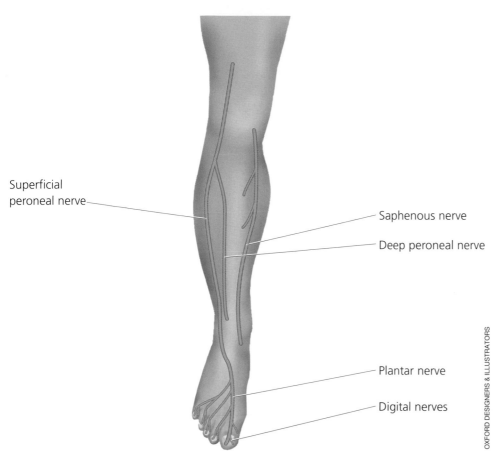

Nerves of the foot and lower leg

Superficial peroneal nerve

Saphenous nerve

Deep peroneal nerve

Plantar nerve

Digital nerves

OXFORD DESIGNERS & ILLUSTRATORS

The nail unit

A thorough understanding of the **nail unit** is absolutely *essential* for the professional nail technician. Information about the structure and physiology of this area of the body has been sketchy in the past. Now there has been so much research that we are able to understand it so much better. Essential reading to get an even better understanding is *Nail Structure and Product Chemistry* by Douglas D Schoon.

A basic understanding of how the skin is structured and how it grows should help with understanding how finger and toenails are formed as a nail unit. Like the hair follicle, the area where the nail starts life is a fold of the epidermal layer where skin cells are instructed by their nucleus to make certain adaptations. In the skin, they become keratinized to form the flattened cells of the stratum corneum. In a hair, they are keratinized and adapted to create a hair shaft. In a nail, they are also keratinized and form flat layers that make up a hard nail plate. Like the upper layer of the epidermis (stratum corneum) and hair, the nail is non-living. Like hair it can be cut without any sensation.

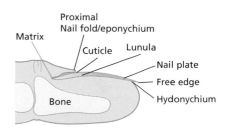

Cross-section of the nail unit

The function of the nail

All species of primate have nails. They are linked to the evolution of using hands (and feet) to manipulate objects. Humans, however, are the only animals able to use the thumb and forefinger in a pincer movement. The higher primates, such as gorillas and chimpanzees,

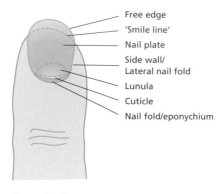

The nail unit

Free edge
'Smile line'
Nail plate
Side wall/
Lateral nail fold
Lunula
Cuticle
Nail fold/eponychium

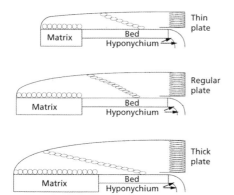

Thin plate

Regular plate

Thick plate

Matrix · Bed · Hyponychium

The longer the matrix, the thicker the nail plate

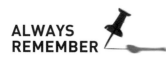

TOP TIP

A way to remember the difference between 'proximal' and 'distal' is to think of proximal as being 'in the proximity of', that is, close to. Distal is at a distance.

ALWAYS REMEMBER

DO NOT cut the proximal nail fold! It is living and will protect itself by thickening!

have hands that are very similar to ours with fingerprints and perfect nails, but they cannot manipulate their thumbs as we can. There is a theory that this arrangement of our thumbs gave our species the opportunity to evolve faster, as we were able to use a wider variety of tools.

Nails are on the ends of our fingers for several reasons and are not just there to paint or chew! They provide a rigid support for the end of the finger, allowing us to pick things up more easily, and they protect the end of the finger and the last bone from countless knocks. The last bone in each finger and toe is actually quite delicate and needs this protection.

Nails start to form in an unborn baby very early in the gestation period and by 17–20 weeks are fully formed. Nails will even appear to 'grow' for a short period after death, as the cycle of adaptation of the skin cells and keratinization will continue, once it has started, without any nourishment from the blood supply plus the surrounding skin shrinks back.

The structure of the nail

Matrix This is the most important area of the nail unit. It is directly under the **proximal nail fold** or **mantle** and it is where the cells are incubated to form the nail plate. New cells push the older cells forward and this is the growth of the nail plate. Keratin is a protein formed of amino acids that is within each cell. As the cells become keratinized, they bond together and lose the other cell contents. Unlike in the epidermis, where the bonds break down and the cells are shed, the bonds in a newly forming nail plate are much stronger and the **lipid** content is retained. The keratinized cells form layers, or lamellar, and several of these bond together to form the nail plate. As the cells move forward they become more compact and the nail plate becomes harder as it moves towards the free edge.

The shape and size of the matrix will determine the thickness and width of the nail. The matrix extends from the base of the nail down towards the first joint. The longer the matrix, the thicker the nail. Thin nails will tend to have a short matrix. The width of the nail will be determined by the width of the matrix. Naturally thin (or thick) nails are hereditary; however, a lot can happen to them once they are grown to change this characteristic. There is no scientific evidence that anything you eat will make a nail plate thicker and stronger but there is evidence that malnutrition can make a nail weaker.

The developing nail in the matrix is very soft until full keratinization has taken place and damage to this area can result in a permanently deformed nail. Examples can be seen in a person who has shut their finger in a door, even as a child. If the area of the matrix is damaged, the base of the nail and the nail plate may have a permanent ridge. Another example would be if someone has had a serious infection in the area. If damage to the area is temporary and heals properly in the matrix, any deformity to the nail should grow out in approximately 6 months after the damage has healed.

Proximal nail fold or eponychium The epidermis of the skin on the finger, above the matrix, folds back on itself and underneath. As in the hair follicle, the deeper area of the fold forms part of the germinal matrix and helps protect the area.

This fold is living skin! The edge of the fold does not look like living skin because it is the epidermis folding back on itself and this does not have any nerve or blood vessels in it. However, it is still living and, if cut, will react like any other area of cut skin and form a scar that will eventually thicken if cutting continues.

This area of skin can often be quite large and unsightly, for example, when it is stuck to the cuticle, the nail grows and pulls the skin with it. When the skin is overstretched it splits, usually at the sides, and appears ragged. These splits can be quite sore and, if pulled, can become infected and inflamed. The split piece of skin can be very carefully removed with cuticle nippers. Proper care of the nails ensures that the nail fold does not stick to the nail plate as it is regularly lifted away. This area should not be pushed as this can cause damage to the underlying soft nail and matrix. The area also forms a seal around the proximal edge of the nail that prevents bacteria from entering. When the nails are soaked in water or softened with oils, the nail fold can be lifted with ease. It is not recommended that the lifted skin is cut on a regular basis. The body is expert at protecting itself and, if an area is removed, the body will often compensate and grow thicker skin. The area should be treated with regular applications of oil or cream to keep the skin soft and prevent it from sticking to the cuticle. Applying nail oil every day will cause this skin to shrink and the problem will disappear.

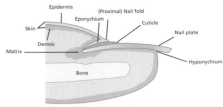

Cross-section of the nail unit

Lateral nail fold or side wall The skin of the finger folds down along the side of the nail and provides the nail plate with protection and a groove to guide the growth of the nail. A seal is formed here to prevent the invasion of unwanted substances or micro-organisms.

TOP TIP To help you remember 'lateral', think of 'lateral thinking', which can be described as sideways thinking.

Eponychium The **eponychium** is an area at the base of the nail plate where the proximal nail fold meets the nail plate. It acts as a seal for that area of the nail and guards against invasive bacteria. During a manicure, this area should be treated gently because, if the seal is broken, not only is it painful, but infection can occur.

The cuticle The nail fold is often called the **cuticle**, but this is inaccurate. The underside of the proximal nail fold constantly sheds a layer of dead skin cells that sits on the nail plate and grows with it. These cells are some of the stickiest in the whole body which is why they stick to the nail and the eponychium stick to them. This is the real cuticle and is not always visible until softened. This is the skin that should be removed during a manicure and always before the application of artificial nails to avoid any lifting problems, as products do not bond with skin, only with the nail plate. When using a cuticle knife, it is usually possible to feel the difference between skin and hard nail even if the skin is not visible. As the epidermis of the nail fold produces this layer continuously, there is always some to be found on the nail plate, however little.

The nail plate As previously explained, keratinized skin cells form the nail plate. These flattened cells stick together and form layers. There are approximately 100 layers of keratinized skin cells (more in thicker toenails). There is less concentration of lipids (fats) in the nail plate compared to the stratum corneum (1 per cent versus 20 per cent) and there are many air spaces; this allows ten times as much water to be absorbed by the nail than by the skin. This can be seen when the nails are soaked in water, e.g. in the bath they become very transparent and flexible.

Oil and moisture can travel through the nail plate in both directions. Secretions from the nail bed travel up from under the nail plate and help keep it flexible. Water and many other chemicals can travel down from the top of the nail plate as long as their chemical structure is small enough to work their way through the gaps created between the cells. Harsh chemicals such as detergents, bleach, etc. can strip away the oils and moisture from the upper layers of seep between the layers at the free edge where the bonds between the layers have broken. Nail oil on the other hand, when applied daily to the nail plate, can penetrate through the layers and fill up the spaces with a useful lubricant that will help keep the nail flexible and prevent unwanted chemicals from invading the nail plate.

The bonds holding the cells together are tougher in the nail plate than in the stratum corneum, as the skin cells are designed to be shed, whereas the nail plate needs to be kept together.

TECH-NOLOGY

MARIAN NEWMAN
Speaks out...
Cuticle care & knowledge

MARIAN NEWMAN reveals all about the definitive cuticle and replaces fiction with fact

The cuticle is an area of anatomy that still gives rise to much confusion. I was taught incorrectly many years ago and so were many others. The reasons for this are the cuticle area was not microscopically investigated for manicure purposes until recent years and the detail wasn't considered important enough to differentiate the structures.

But now, and for several years, its importance has been recognised leading to the structures being identified and quite clearly defined. The general public can be forgiven for not having this knowledge, but there is certainly no excuse for nail professionals who must know the structures, their purpose and suitable treatment.

This article is another attempt to clear up any confusion and persuade a larger section of nail professionals to understand the area, call the structures by the correct name and provide suitable treatment. This is not opinion, mine or any others. It's anatomical and physiological fact.

The definition (from *Merrium-Webster Online Dictionary*) of cuticle is:
1 - an outer covering layer: as **a:** an external envelope (as of an insect) secreted usually by epidermal cells **b:** the outermost layer of animal integument composed of epidermis **c:** a thin continuous fatty or waxy film on the external surface of many higher plants that consists chiefly of cutin **d:** the outermost membranous layer of a hair consisting of overlapping scales of epithelial cells
2 - dead or horny epidermis

The relevant description here is the dead or horny epidermis. So, we know the cuticle is dead or non-living. Also, that it's the dead cells shed from living epidermis.

Dead skin cells cover the skin of the body. The cells of the epidermis evolve through the various layers until they reach the *stratum corneum* where they become non-living (as all the cell contents have become keratinised).

> "The cuticle is dead skin cells and should be gently removed. The skin fold is living skin and should not be removed, gently or otherwise!"

They are shed continuously. This is basic anatomy that every nail professional should know inside out.

Skin on the fingers and toes doesn't just come to an end where it touches the nail. What it does is fold back on itself to form a seal at the sides and base of the nail. This area at the base of the nail is called the eponychium and the seal is there to protect the structures beneath and behind it from pathogens and physical damage. The part of the folded epidermis is called the proximal nail fold at the base and the lateral nail fold at the sides.

The underside of the folded skin still sheds dead cells but, unlike other areas of skin, these cells are very sticky. They stick together and to the nail plate. The nail plate grows forward and takes the sticky cells with it.

THIS IS THE CUTICLE. It is NOT the bit of epidermis that is folded over.

The cuticle is dead skin cells and should be gently removed. The skin fold is living skin and should not be removed, gently or otherwise!

Look at the diagram. The skin is formed of dermis and epidermis. The dermis is where all the blood and lymph vessels and nerve fibres are. The epidermis is supplied by these structures in the dermis, but doesn't have any itself.

The dermis does not fold back, but the epidermis does and this bit is colourless. It's not pink with blood supply and has no feeling as it has no nerves, but it is still living tissue. (Think of a blister. You can peel off that skin without any pain or blood. If the blister goes the skin doesn't fall off; it goes back to normal looking skin because it's still living. This is the epidermis).

If living skin is cut it protects itself by forming a scar. If it's continually cut it grows thicker. It's this folded skin that so many people call the cuticle and cut off. This doesn't necessarily cause

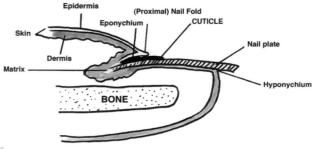

Cross section of the nail unit

damage to underlying structures, but it can. What it does do is make the skin grow thicker.

Those that have been taught to do this during a manicure have been taught incorrectly. There are circumstances where this may be appropriate – I will highlight later.

The cuticle is sticky. The nail fold also sticks to the top of the cuticle and the growth of the nail plate pulls the cuticle out with it along with the 'rider' on top. People have different rates of skin growth, different thickness' of skin, different nail and finger shapes etc so some have the problem of overgrown cuticles and nail fold much more than others.

Cuticle treatment

I'm not going to mention brands or specific products, instead I'll talk about the general 'families'.

Before any treatment can be carried out the skin needs to be softened so it's more pliable and can be moved easily. Three types of 'products' will do this:

1 - **Warm water alone or with a softener:** Water will be absorbed by the skin and make it soft and pliable. It will also take away the 'stickiness' of the cuticle. Do remember that water is one of the most common harmful chemicals for nails.

Nails are 10 times more absorbent than skin and soak up the water, which eventually evaporates taking some of the natural moisture with it. If the free edge has any sign of peeling, however small, water seeps between the layers and breaks hundreds more bonds. The choice of soaking is yours, but an informed choice is better than doing it just because it's in the manicure steps.

"Skin on the fingers and toes doesn't just come to an end where it touches the nail. What it does is fold back on itself to form a seal at the sides and base of the nail."

2 - **Water-based alkaline liquids:** These have sodium or potassium hydroxide that are both very efficient at softening skin quickly and breaking down bonds between the dead skin cells. These need to be thoroughly removed when the job is done as they continue to soften both skin and the nail and can cause irritation.

3 - **Creams/oils:** These have skin softening properties and may also house fruit acids (AHAs) that soften skin and break down bonds as above. They also encourage cellular renewal. It may not be so important to remove these, but manufacturer's instructions should always be followed carefully.

Treating the eponychium and nail fold

Before the cuticle can be dealt with the nail fold must be gently lifted from it. This is easy when softened and it's perfectly acceptable to use a disinfected metal tool. However, it must be a very gentle process that does not push the skin back into the sealed area of the eponychium. The tool must not be angled into the nail plate as the nail is very soft and not fully keratinised in this area and incorrect use results in a horseshoe shaped dent in the nail that will grow up the nail bed. It's also possible to cause permanent damage to the matrix resulting in a damaged nail plate. If the seal is broken the matrix is open to infection and this is not only painful, but could cause permanent damage.

This is the part of the nail unit that's subject to much debate - *to cut or not to cut.*

In the past it was cut routinely and there are still many manicurists that continue to do this. Research has moved the nail industry on and, when you understand the area, it becomes obvious that

routine cutting is not the best way to treat this area. Once it's lifted off the cuticle and kept off, it cannot be dragged along with the nail growth. It can be prevented from sticking back onto the cuticle by regular applications and gentle massage with nail oil and when it's not being dragged it shrinks.

Clients with severely overgrown nail folds could fall into the category of needing cutting. However, you need to be aware that technically, this is an invasive treatment that nail professionals are not qualified or insured to carry out. It's invasive as it involves cutting living skin with a blade and could easily result in infection.

I would be naïve and less than truthful if I said it should never happen. Here I will differentiate between fact and opinion and say that it could be suitable under very specific circumstances:

1 - When the overgrowth is extreme.
2 - Leaving the excess skin could result in hard skin that catches on everything.
3 - You know exactly what you're doing.
4 - Your nippers are very sharp and disinfected.
5 - It's a one-off treatment that will not be repeated.
6 - You're confident your client knows, understands and agrees and will follow your advice with aftercare (i.e. oil applied every day).

Treating the cuticle

The cuticle needs to be removed from the nail plate. Day to day, a lot will be rubbed or exfoliated away naturally, but close to the base of the nail there's usually a layer. During a manicure or nail prep for application of overlays, this needs to be removed. If any trace is left you won't get a good edge on the polish, it will peel and overlays will lift as they don't bond with skin, only nail.

Once the nail fold has been lifted and eased back if necessary, the cuticle can be rubbed off. (I find it quite surprising how much is on the nail plate and quite invisible until you get to work on it.) Remove the layer of dead skin from the nail up to the nail fold, but do not dig around under it, you could inadvertently break the seal. Any part of the cuticle that does not rub off can be cut with nippers and this is quite distinct from the nail fold.

Correct use of nippers

Nippers must be sharp and disinfected. (Replace them when they begin to feel a little blunt, they don't last forever.)
Hold firmly and place over the area to be cut, open, squeeze firmly and release – do not pull! (I've seen many manicurists do this without thinking and it tears the skin.)
When you've finished, brush away any debris, wash with soap, water and disinfect them.

Cuticle grows quite fast and even just a week later there'll be more on the nail. At a first appointment with a new client make sure you find the edge of the cuticle. It can be a lot higher up the nail than you expect.

One last piece of information: it's perfectly safe to remove the spikes of nail plate that are found along the sides of the nail. In fact it's recommended, as your client will find them annoying and probably bite them off. If they're pulled it will be painful and probably result in inflammation and possible infection. **S**

I strongly recommend reading Doug Schoon's article *'Where's the cuticle'* at www.dougschoon.com

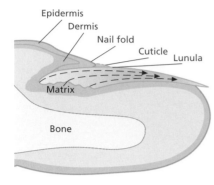

Growth of the nail plate from the matrix

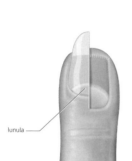

Lunula

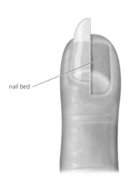

The nail bed

Evaporation of water soaked up by the nails can be quite damaging as it breaks down the bonds that hold the cells together and causes weak and peeling nails. In fact, water is one of the most damaging substances for nails.

The uppermost layer of nail is formed in the deepest part of the matrix, while the lower layers are formed nearer the cuticle. This results in a very hard surface and much softer lower layer of the nail plate. Different parts of the matrix form slightly different variations of keratin.

The layers of keratinized cells form themselves into three main layers of nail plate. The upper and lower layers are the thinnest with the middle layer making up approximately 75 per cent of the nail plate. The upper layer is dense and hard, but thin. This is the layer that often peels, due to the damage caused to the bonds between it and the middle layer, exposing the slightly softer but thicker middle layer. The break in these bonds allows more water to seep between the layers and causes further peeling. The lower layer of the nail plate is very thin and contains some soft keratin. This layer bonds strongly to the **nail bed**.

When nails become too dry and peel, not only are they thinner, but also the hard upper layer has been lost, leaving the pliable and weaker lower layers. Nails must be protected from this condition and that is why wearing gloves for washing up, etc. is always recommended. **Nail varnish** can also help protect the nails, as can massaging oils or cream into the cuticle area.

As the nail plate leaves the end of the finger, it forms a projection called the **free edge**. This appears whiter than the main body of the nail as it is not attached to the nail bed where light reflects off the coloured nail bed.

The nail plate has a proximal and **distal** area and the free edge could be described as the distal edge.

Lunula   The **lunula** is also known as the half moon, an area of the nail by or under the proximal nail fold, and the front end of the matrix.

It appears whiter because the cells are not yet completely keratinized, slightly plumper and not totally transparent. Not every person has an exposed lunula and it is a misconception that the lunula (or half moon) should be visible. The nail is still slightly soft in this area and easily damaged so, if anything, it is better that the lunula is protected by the nail fold. People who have a large exposed lunula often have very ridged nails which is often more noticeable on the thumbs. This is due to continual trauma to the soft nail from everyday living. During a manicure or any work done in the cuticle area, care must be taken not to press too hard on the lunula, as it will cause a ridge in the nail that will need to grow up and off the end before it disappears.

The nail bed   This lies directly under the nail plate. It is skin just like on the rest of the body and has many things in common with the facial skin. It has a very rich supply of blood and lymph vessels in the dermis to keep the nail healthy. There are many different types of epidermis in the body and that which is the nail bed closely resembles the lining of the mouth. The type on the nail bed is called **bed epithelium**. This is extremely sticky and it sticks very tightly to the underside of the nail plate. The dermis of the nail bed has a series of ridges from the lunula to the free edge. As the nail grows forward the bed epithelium separates from the dermis and slides along on these ridges like a railway track that keeps the train in place while allowing it to move. This is what holds the nail onto the nail bed. If the ridges are disturbed or if the nail plate becomes too thin and flexible, this 'hold' is broken and causes the nail plate to separate from the nail bed. This is a dangerous situation as it allows bacteria in under the nail that could cause severe problems. Nail technicians must

take extreme care not to over-buff the nail, as this will cause the nail to become too thin. If this thinning occurs anywhere on the nail, it will eventually grow up to the end of the nail bed where it is most likely to result in separation. Over-buffing that causes heat acts like a friction burn on the nail bed and the bed epithelium will 'let go' of the dermis causing separation. The bed epithelium grows along with the nail and will appear under the free edge of the nail. This will slough off naturally or can be removed during a manicure. This now useless part of the epidermis is sometimes referred to as the **solehorn**.

The hyponychium This is the area of skin at the very end of the nail bed under the beginning of the free edge. It forms a very tight seal that prevents bacteria entering. There are many nerve endings in this area that act as a warning to this seal being broken.

The onychodermal band This is the area of the **hyponychium** where a slight change of colour in the skin can be seen. This is where the bed epithelium leaves the underlying dermis and is part of the seal protecting the nail bed from infection. When applying a **French manicure** or artificial nails using a **white-tip powder** or gel, it is referred to as the **'smile line'** and its ideal shape should mirror the shape at the base of the nail to create a symmetrical 'top and bottom'.

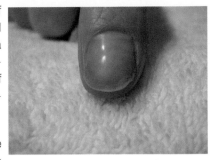

Thinned (over-buffed) nail plate showing ridges on nail bed. Seen as red stripes on the nail bed near the free edge.

The process of nail growth

Rates of growth

Like hair, nails grow at different rates in individuals and at different times of the year but, unlike hair, grow continually. Fingernails grow faster than toenails. As an average guide, nails grow at the rate of between 3mm per month and it takes approximately 5–6 months for a fingernail to grow from the matrix to the free edge and up to a year for a toenail. The growth rate is faster in the summer and during pregnancy and usually slows down with age. It can be speeded up or slowed down by illness. This slow growth rate complicates the treatment of nail conditions as damage caused to the nail plate takes a long time to grow out.

The speed or strength of nail growth is not linked specifically to diet, vitamin or mineral intake but can be improved, along with the condition of skin and hair, if a well-balanced diet is followed.

It is quite common to be able to see the effects of systemic trauma on the nails. For example, a general anaesthetic, major emotional trauma, illness, etc. will often show up as a line or ridge on the nail plate where the growth has been affected.

Technicians and their clients will often notice an increased growth rate immediately after artificial nails have been applied. This is due to the stimulation produced by buffing during application. The nail matrix and nail bed have a concentrated supply of blood and lymph vessels that supply the area with **nutrients** and remove waste products. Stimulation of the circulation in this area will improve this function and assist growth.

Buffing the natural nail during a manicure is a valuable treatment, but care must be taken not to thin the nail or create too much heat through friction, as this can cause splitting.

The effect of stimulation to the circulation can be seen in the general growth of nails: nails on the dominant hand grow faster, as does the forefinger. Nail biters have faster growing nails owing to the continual nibbling.

As a technician, the growth rate of an individual's nails will affect maintenance treatments (see Chapter 5). Artificial nails must be maintained to compensate for this growth. The majority of clients will need to return every 2–3 weeks, but some clients need to return only every 4–5 weeks, as their growth rate is slower.

TOP TIP
An excellent stimulation for nails to encourage faster and healthier growth is to place the hands together, like praying, then curl the fingers in so the nails touch each other. Then rub them back and forward to produce a clicking sound.

Nail composition and strength

Keratin and amino acids The skin cells that are formed in the matrix have, in their nucleus, the 'instructions' needed to keratinize but, unlike the keratinized skin cells of the stratum corneum that form a barrier and then are lost, these cells form together to create the hard nail plate layers.

Keratin is a type of **protein** that is made in the body and the body has many different proteins that are essential to its functioning. Proteins are made up of certain sequences of **amino acids**. Amino acids are chemicals created by the body that, when linked together in various specific sequences, make the necessary proteins. The linked amino acids form long 'strands' and these strands are then linked together at intervals with another amino acid, bonding the strands together and creating a strong structure. The keratin of the nail has many more of these bonds than that of the skin and hair.

Hard and soft nails The progression of cells from the matrix to the nail plate is very similar to those making the journey in the epidermis of the skin. The cells are created by cell division deep in the matrix and, as they are pushed forward, lose the cellular fluid and become flatter. The lunular is an area where this process has not quite finished, hence its whiter appearance. As the cells are pushed forward by the reproducing cells behind, they become completely keratinized, flat and hard. Therefore the nail plate nearest to the nail fold is softer than the distal edge, and can be easily damaged.

- A strong nail is one that can withstand breakage. This does not necessarily mean hard as 'hard' could suggest **brittleness** and the nail could easily snap. Many products on the market are nail 'strengtheners', and that can mean nail 'hardeners'. If a weak nail is hardened too much, it will become brittle. If a hard or brittle nail becomes too soft and flexible, it will tear. The spaces between keratinized cells are full of moisture from the nail bed beneath and from external sources. The right amount of moisture will keep the nail flexible and help absorb shocks. Too much, and the nail bends, too little and the nail becomes dry and brittle.

- The nail plate is very absorbent and too much water can cause splitting and peeling. Excessive water can cause the nail plate to soften and swell. Repeated softening and swelling can cause surface peeling.

- The only truly effective moisturiser for skin and nails is water (and natural lipids), but in the right amount. Using creams and oils is beneficial as they can seal natural moisture in and keep too much out. **Solvents**, such as acetone and nail varnish removers, can remove natural oils and water and can be the cause of dryness if overused.

- The perfect nail is a combination of **strength** and **flexibility**.

A nail specialist should be able to diagnose the exact condition of a client's nails and be able to recommend the ideal treatment and products. It may be that a weak nail needs a hardening treatment for a period of time followed by a moisturising treatment. A brittle nail may need moisturising then hardening. An understanding of nail growth and structure brings with it the ability to correctly diagnose conditions.

Protein, calcium and nails As mentioned before, nails are keratinized skin cells. Keratin is a protein composed of amino acids formed together in long chains and linked by an amino acid bond. The vast number of these strong bonds is specific to nails and is what makes them so much harder than skin and hair. The protein, keratin, is mostly composed of

> **TOP TIP**
>
> Nails that are naturally thick or thin are hereditary. A longer matrix will produce a thicker nail. Conversely, a short matrix can produce only a thinner nail.

carbon, oxygen, nitrogen, sulphur and hydrogen. The nail plate also has traces of many other chemicals, e.g. **iron**, zinc, sodium, calcium, titanium, even aluminium, copper, gold and silver.

There are many myths about calcium and nails. The body's intake and absorption of calcium is essential for teeth and bones, but as calcium is only 0.07 per cent of the nail (and most of this comes from external sources picked up by the fingers), it does not play a large part. The body needs vitamin D in order to absorb calcium and that is obtained from the sun and diet. If this vitamin is lacking, conditions such as rickets can occur. White spots on the nail are often blamed on a lack of calcium, but this is incorrect (see Chapter 9). They are usually caused by trauma to the matrix causing a slight distortion of the cells. Calcium painted on the nail will not have any effect on the condition of the nail neither will taking calcium supplements.

The artificial nail and the natural nail The strength of the nail can be influenced, even during the wearing of artificial nails or varnish. The nail plate is at its softest in the area of the cuticle and there should be a narrow margin of nail that is not covered. A nourishing oil massaged into this area daily will affect the new nail growing, so weak or brittle nails can be improved while artificial nails are worn. The massaging will stimulate the area and the oil will help to reduce the moisture loss from the new nail. If the artificial nails are correctly maintained, the natural nails should be stronger when they are removed.

Can artificial nails damage natural nails? They certainly can if they are incorrectly applied or the wearer does not understand how to look after them properly. It is usually an inexperienced or unprofessional technician or an uneducated client who causes damage to natural nails. It is really important that technicians explain what the wearer needs to do (or not do) in between treatments.

Summary

This chapter has explained the basic anatomy and physiology of skin, muscles, bones, blood circulation, the lymphatic system, the nervous system and nails, nail structure and growth and the potential problems a technician may encounter in treating a client if nail trauma or past illness has occurred.

ASSESSMENT OF KNOWLEDGE AND UNDERSTANDING

1 Explain eight functions of the skin.

2 Name the layers found in the epidermis.

3 What are the main structures found in the skin?

4 Describe four functions of blood.

5 Explain how blood is circulated around the body.

6 What are the main purposes of the lymphatic system?

7 Name the bones of the hand and foot.

8 What are the three different types of muscle and where are they in the body?

9 How do muscles work in pairs and what are the terms used to describe the groups?

10 Describe the nervous system in general terms.

11 What part does the matrix play in the process of nail growth?

12 Why is it important to understand the process of nail growth and factors that affect it?

13 Why should special care be taken when working in the area of the lunula?

14 Describe the cuticle in detail.

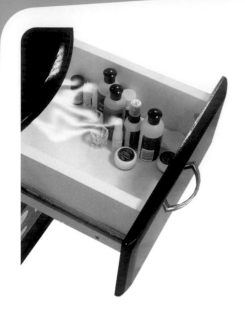

3
Preparing the work area

Learning objectives

In this chapter you will learn about:

- the equipment and furniture required by a nail technician
- how to create a comfortable and safe working environment
- how to work with potentially hazardous chemicals
- how to protect yourself, your clients and colleagues
- hygiene procedures
- the legislation affecting technicians and salons
- the information and correct usage of all tools and equipment
- pricing treatments and services.

Introduction

The only way to provide professional nail treatments is in a suitable, comfortable and safe environment with the right tools, correctly used. This chapter will show how to create that environment, make it safe for both technician and client and how to keep it that way while abiding by the relevant legislation.

Starting with the general environment, we need to think about what sort of area is needed for a nail technician to work in, what is required within the salon or a client's home and what problems need addressing that are specific to nail services.

Equipment

Whether the technician is working in a nail salon, a client's home, a beauty salon or a hair salon, a minimum amount of space is needed. In comparison to the other services, however, the space needed is very small. This industry has a great many mobile technicians, but virtually all of the requirements that make a salon a safe, hygienic and comfortable place also apply to working as a mobile technician. The only difference is that tools, equipment and products need to be portable for a mobile technician. As clients are always central to the work, all the safety rules must still apply.

The desk

When thinking about the minimum space required for a nail technician in a salon, a desk is the first consideration. There are many nail desks available from wholesalers that have been specifically designed for the job. If space is at a premium, the minimum worktop would need to be approximately 75 cm wide and approximately 35 cm deep. Ideally, the desk should have a couple of drawers, and be very stable in construction. The width of the desk should be not so wide that the technician needs to stretch to reach the client's hands if the client is sitting back in the chair, nor should it be so narrow that it causes the technician to bend their neck down too far. Before buying a ready-made desk, make sure the measurements are right for the space in the salon; sit in the chairs that are going to be used for both the technician and the client. Think about storage of all the equipment needed and, if necessary, the space required for any additional storage needs. Most ready-made desks usually have a suitable worktop that can easily be kept clean, but remember to take that into consideration.

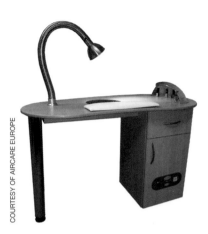

COURTESY OF AIRCARE EUROPE

Beech table

Many salons have their desks made specially to match the image of the salon. It is possible to make a functional desk fit in with any décor, but remember that the suitability and safety of the desk and chairs must take priority over image. Think of the essential requirements first and design the desk around them, rather than thinking of the design first and trying to make it work.

Dust is one of the most important issues in health and safety for nail technicians. It is potentially more hazardous than any of the volatile products that are used. Dealing with the control of dust at the source, i.e. at the desk, is the best method. Many desks are available at reasonable cost that have efficient dust extraction. For a busy nail technician that has a lot of nail enhancement clients this should be considered an essential piece of equipment.

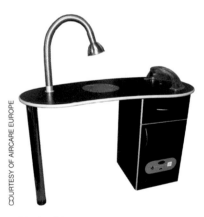

COURTESY OF AIRCARE EUROPE

Black table

When using a desk with dust extraction, keep the fan on during the whole service so a good flow of air is generated. Also make sure that the filter is cleaned (according to manufacturer's instructions) very frequently. If it is an efficient extractor the filter will be full at the end of each day. The best situation is a fan that removes dust that drops into it but also a fan that takes the finer airborne dust (that is the most hazardous) from above the working area.

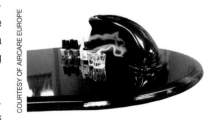

COURTESY OF AIRCARE EUROPE

Good working practices will minimize vapours generated from working with nail products. However, it is always worth the investment in a system that helps remove these vapours from the atmosphere, again, at the source.

The technician's chair

There should be sufficient space around the desk for a comfortable seat for both technician and client. Care should be taken when choosing the technician's chair, as there are several factors to take into account:

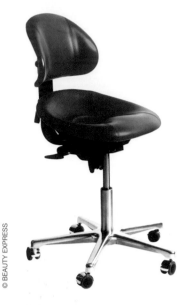

© BEAUTY EXPRESS

Nail Technician's chair

HEALTH & SAFETY

Always sit square to the desk without crossing your legs or leaning on one arm.

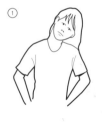

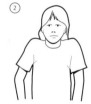
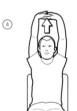

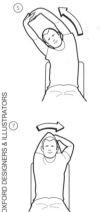

OXFORD DESIGNERS & ILLUSTRATORS

- A busy technician can be sitting in the same place for, sometimes, up to 12 hours a day with very few breaks. This is far from an ideal situation, but most salons have at least one late night.

- As with any work equipment, safety must come first. A chair must have the correct support for the user. The seat should be padded and of a depth that supports the legs. The tilt of the seat also affects how we sit. The backrest should give support to the back and the combination of the back and seat should encourage the user to sit upright with a slight hollow in the lower back. Technicians are forced to work in a very unnatural position, leaning forward and with the head looking down. This puts great strain on the back and neck. Every technician should be aware that this position causes stress in the neck and shoulders and could lead to severe problems in later years.

- Many technicians work by leaning one elbow on the desk and having their body twisted. This is obviously very dangerous. The upper body needs to be square to the desk with the back straight and only a slight tilt forward. The shoulders should be kept relaxed and the neck should not be held bent too much. There are 'posture' chairs available, on wheels and incorporating a rocking motion, that are designed to help those working at a desk. These chairs have a tilted seat and a padded support for the knees to rest on. They are ideal for the person who sits upright all the time, such as a typist, or a person who needs to lean forward slightly, as they will keep the curvature of the back in the correct position. However, owing to the nature of the technician's work, a lot of pressure is put on the knees in this position, which can be quite painful by the end of a day and may cause problems later.

- There are several exercises that a technician can do at various times throughout the day, but, at all times sitting in the safest position and staying relaxed is essential advice.

Exercises

1 Sit comfortably, relax shoulders and breathe in. While breathing out, drop chin onto chest. Relax. Breathe in again and, while breathing out, drop head to one side. Relax. Repeat for the other side then drop head back. Drop chin back to chest while breathing normally.

2 Breathe in and lift shoulders towards ears, breathe out and let shoulders drop. Relax. Repeat several times. Rotate one shoulder several times, then the other while breathing normally.

3 Interlace your fingers and stretch your arms out in front of you with palms facing out. Feel the stretch in your upper arms and upper back.

4 Move your arms up above your head with fingers still interlaced and push up. Feel the stretch on the outer edge of your arms and ribs.

5 With your arms still extended, lean from the waist, first one side then the other.

6 Clasp your hands behind your head, push your elbows back and pull your shoulder blades together.

7 Put one arm over the opposite shoulder, hold just above the elbow and push elbow towards the shoulder while looking the other way. Repeat with the other arm.

ACTIVITY

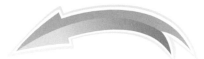

Research the market to find some suggestions of suitable furniture for a salon. Look at whole-salers but also other possible sources such as Ikea. Collect the information as if you are planning your salon (or home salon). This could also include suitable storage units and retail display.

Collect information on portable dust and vapour extraction that will provide the safety aspect of using a plain desk without internal extraction. Suggest how these can be used to maximum effect.

The client's chair

The chair for the client is almost as important as the one for the technician.

- The client must feel comfortable, but must also be in the right position for the technician. A client could spend up to 2 hours in the same chair, so comfort is important. A fabric-covered chair with a soft seat is preferable (plastic can get uncomfortable). The height of the seat should be such that the client can rest their arms on the desk easily while keeping them and their shoulders in a relaxed position. They should also be able to get close enough to the desk so that their arm is still supported if they lean back into the chair.

- When seating a client, and during the whole treatment, make sure they are sitting straight in front of the desk. This is important for the treatment because if a client is sitting sideways, their hand will not be in the centre and not held straight to the technician. This could result in artificial nails being applied unevenly on the finger.

It is worth acquiring the very best furniture that you can afford at the time. It is often a false economy to buy things cheaply thinking that they can be replaced soon. What usually happens is that the cheap items wear out and start looking shabby very quickly, but there is always some other priority that requires the money. If space in the salon is not at a premium, it is often worth having a much larger desk than necessary (as long as it is not used as extra room to make untidy!) as small displays can be put on the extra top space. There are many inventive technicians who have designed wonderful desks with display areas, built-in waste disposal and multiple desks.

The desk lamp

Desk lamps play a very important part in the work of the technician and their desk set-up. It is essential to have excellent light when providing any nail treatment, so a lamp of the right design is important. Good light will help prevent eye strain while carrying out close work; direct light, which casts no shadows, is needed to examine artificial nails for imperfections; applying varnish and nail art needs bright light to ensure accuracy and neatness.

Lamps are visually very obvious on a desk, so they must look pleasing and fit in with the décor of the salon. More importantly, there a number of factors that need to be taken into account when choosing a lamp.

Heat One of the most important factors is heat. Commonly used tungsten bulbs give off a great deal of heat. 'Daylight' bulbs, useful for keeping colours looking true, also get very hot. This is far from ideal for the technician. The lamp needs to be quite close for the best effect, but the working temperature for the technician can get very uncomfortable. The heat will also affect many artificial nail products and make working with them difficult, for example volatile products, such as nail varnish remover and liquid monomers will evaporate faster, creating a potentially high concentration of vapour in the air space around the

TOP TIP

Make sure there is plenty for the client to look at while they are sitting at your desk, especially retail lines. It will be something interesting for them and should encourage questions that could lead to sales.

HEALTH & SAFETY

Make sure all electrical equipment is subject to regular certified checks.

technician and client. Halogen or low energy bulbs do not get too hot and are a good choice.

Shape   The shape of the lamp needs to be such that the light does not glare into the eyes of the technician or the client; it must be close enough to be effective but not in the way; it also needs to be stable on the desk.

Electricity supply   Thought must be given to the electricity supply for the lamp. Trailing wires in a workplace are a safety hazard and should be avoided. A socket close enough to avoid trailing wires is the most suitable, but there are many alternatives. Some manicure tables have a plug socket attached to them for electrical equipment. This, of course, needs to be connected to an electricity supply and, again, wires across the floor must be avoided. If there is no alternative to a wire on the floor by a desk or any area where people could walk, then it must be covered with a rubber conduit that draws attention to it and has sloping sides to prevent tripping while protecting the cable from damage. There should be no wires on the floor under the desk as the wheels of the chair could run over them, damage them or pull the equipment off the table. Wherever possible, wires and cables should be attached to the desk, floor or wall using special clips designed for the job that are readily available from any DIY shop.

TOP TIP

If wires along the floor are unavoidable, make sure they are covered with a rubber flex cover or taped to the floor so that no one can trip over them.

Remember, 'nails' are part of the image industries, so make sure you always present the right image to your clients.

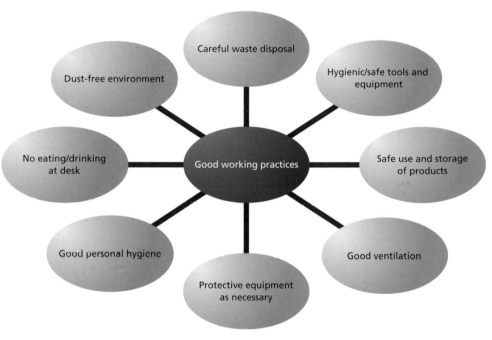

Good working practices

Using nail products safely

Problems with irritants and corrosive materials

The majority of nail products come under the category of **hazardous** chemicals and many of them are classed as **irritants**. Care must be taken when using these types of products. There are some irritants that are also classified as **corrosive** and these will cause a bad reaction with everyone. A day-to-day example of this is household bleach that stings and itches when in contact with skin.

● A common example of this type of chemical in the nail industry is an acid-based primer. This is a product commonly used in artificial nail systems and, as the name suggests, is an acid that will sting and itch on contact with skin. Washing in running water will remove the chemical, but it is likely that the skin will be temporarily damaged.

● Many other commonly used products are irritants – for example, nail adhesive is an irritant, and every bottle and tube should carry a warning. Obviously the adhesive will bond to skin very easily, but a drop of it spilled onto skin can also cause a chemical burn. (Water will stop the burning and acetone will debond the skin.) If adhesive is spilt onto clothing and penetrates through to the skin, very severe burns can be caused. The chemicals in the adhesive react with man-made fibres in the clothing and burns requiring cosmetic surgery have been known as a result of this accident.

● It is a legal requirement for there to be warnings on many labels, but the absence of a warning does not necessarily mean a product is safe. All products should be treated with respect and all potentially hazardous products should have a document called the Material Safety Data Sheet (**MSDS**) available from the supplier (see Chapter 4).

> **TOP TIP**
>
> Make sure adhesive container lids are on securely and that there are no air pockets in the application nozzle that could cause the adhesive to spurt out. Clean the nozzle with remover before replacing the lid.

Allergies and sensitivity

All chemicals are potentially harmful but the dividing line between a safe and harmful chemical is often the *quantity* of it. This dividing line varies from person to person. When a harmful chemical touches the body in any way, the body reacts to it. This reaction can take many different forms, but the most common is an allergic reaction.

● People develop an allergy or sensitivity to a substance by coming into contact with too much of it. It is this level of 'too much' that is so variable. One individual may become sensitive to a particular ingredient in a hand cream after two uses; another may take years before a reaction occurs, if one occurs at all.

● As many nail products are classed as irritants, it is very likely that most individuals will develop a sensitivity to them at some time. As no one can tell how long this will take or how much of a specific product needs to come into contact with a person, it is important to take measures to avoid the possibility of a sensitivity building up. It is also just as important to be able to recognize the first signs of this in both the technician and their clients (see Chapter 4).

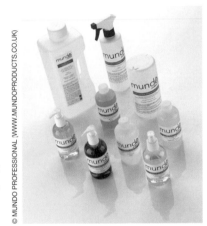

© MUNDO PROFESSIONAL (WWW.MUNDOPRODUCTS.CO.UK)

Absorption, ingestion and inhalation

There are three ways that potentially harmful chemicals can enter the body and if each of these **'routes of entry'** is prevented as far as possible, all hazards are avoided. The 'routes' are:

1 **Inhalation**: that is, *breathing in* vapours or dusts. This one is not so easy to control, but by following strict working practices and hygiene rules, the problem can be solved.

2 **Ingestion**: that is, *through the mouth*. Avoidance of this is even easier! Wash hands frequently, especially before eating; do not eat or drink at a desk; and follow reasonable salon hygiene rules.

3 **Absorption**: that is, chemicals can enter *through the skin*. This is probably the most common cause of problems for technicians and their clients and can be easily avoided.

We will look at all three in more detail.

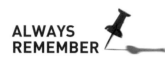

ALWAYS REMEMBER

Reducing the risk of evaporation while working is the BEST method to avoid vapours. There is no system that can completely purify the air that will suit a salons' commercial budget.

ALWAYS REMEMBER

'Low odour' products means that they do not smell as much as others. This does not mean they do not produce vapours!

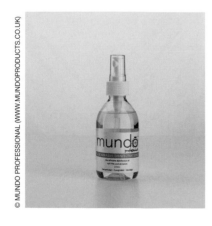

Inhalation

If you think about the salon environment and what type of salon it is, you will realize there are certain requirements to ensure the safety and comfort of staff and clients.

Vapours

- Many nail products involve *volatile chemicals* and even the tidiest technician cannot totally prevent some of the **vapours** escaping into the air. Adequate ventilation is therefore essential. In a very busy nail salon a sophisticated **ventilation** system is ideal, but this can be costly and is not always necessary for smaller establishments with a few nail desks. If a larger salon decides that suitable ventilation is needed, expert advice should be sought as there are complicated calculations involved in determining the type of ventilation equipment required to change the air in the salon several times an hour.

- Chapter 7, will discuss this in more detail, but vapours are **molecules** of actual chemicals *in the air* and, although most nail products have strong odours, if there is no obvious smell it does not mean the vapour is not there. Not all hazardous chemicals have odours that can be detected. A fan in a salon is no substitute for a ventilator, all it does is move the air around. The salon needs the air to be changed regularly, and this can only be achieved by proper ventilation. There are vapour extractors on the market that sit on or inside a desk that remove vapours at the source, i.e. where you are working. Vapours are not removed by dust extraction units. There needs to be efficient filtration of the air through several specific filters, usually activated carbon or charcoal.

- The vapours that need to be eliminated are *always heavier than air* so the molecules will collect nearer the floor. High-level extractors, if of a sufficient size for the room, will in theory lift the vapours up and expel them. However, in doing that, the air is brought up past the breathing spaces of those in the salon so some of the vapours will be inhaled. Some vapours will also be left at the lower levels. Extractors that are set lower down will remove the vapours without having to lift them up.

- Some nail products are used as a *spray.* This is an obvious potential hazard as the chemical vapour is actually being put into the air. Pump sprays are less harmful than atomizers or aerosols as they produce larger droplets rather than a fine **mist**. Keep the use of sprays to a minimum, but if they are used, good ventilation is essential.

- Wearing a disposable dust mask will not protect anyone from vapours. Chemical molecules that are present in the air are much smaller than dust particles and the mask is not a barrier to them. There are vapour masks available, but these are much larger pieces of equipment and are costly to buy. They are also very off-putting to clients!

- Safe, hygienic and correct working procedures will avoid almost all vapours escaping into the air and, in a smal-to-medium salon, this, together with adequate ventilation from an open window or door, should be sufficient to ensure safety.

Vapours and eyes

- *Contact lenses*: Never wear contact lenses when working with nail products. It is possible that vapours can be absorbed by soft lenses and seriously affect the eye. Safety glasses worn with lenses will not protect your eyes from vapours when wearing contact lenses.

- *Safety glasses*: Wearing plain safety glasses is highly recommended. It is a practice with some technicians to nip off old overlay, a practice that is very strongly discouraged as it severely damages the nail plate; however chips from this can fly and enter the eye. But eye accidents can also happen to the most careful technician, by clipping a plastic tip or nail, or opening a bottle of adhesive that has an air bubble in the nozzle, for example. A busy technician spends many hours very close to a number of hazards and eyes are very precious!

Keeping vapours to a minimum There are a few simple rules that can be followed to keep vapours to a minimum:

- Keep all bottles and jars closed.
- Keep any dishes covered at all times other than for the few seconds you are using them.
- Do not wipe your liquid and powder brush on a tissue. If you need to wipe your brush have a small wipe dampened with an alcohol-based liquid on the desk for this purpose.
- Clean your brush in monomer after every use, wipe it dry with a pad and discard this pad in a metal bin with a lid.
- Store your brushes flat in a closed container in a drawer. Not open on the desk.
- Have a metal waste bin with a lid at every nail desk.
- Put all nail wipes/cotton wool straight into the bin after use.
- Change the paper towel under client's hands after each stage and put into the bin.
- Wipe up spills immediately with absorbent paper and put paper in an outside waste bin.
- When using a solvent to remove artificial nails, keep the bowl covered with a towel and remove directly after use.
- Keep the use of sprays to a minimum.
- Discard all unwanted solvents and nail monomers immediately by soaking in absorbent paper and placing in a covered waste bin; larger quantities should be placed in a safe place in the open and allowed to evaporate – do not pour down sinks or lavatories.
- Maintain adequate ventilation at all times, and make sure the salon is not too hot.
- Follow all these rules if working in a client's home and have several windows open.

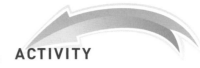

ACTIVITY

Make a chart listing all the products you are using. Create a column for:

- safe storage
- safe and correct usage (e.g. methods of decanting, personal protective equipment (PPE) if required, etc.)
- spillage removal from hard surfaces
- any specific health hazard
- comments.

HEALTH & SAFETY

If you cannot smell a chemical in the atmosphere it does not mean it is not there! Good working practices are the best safeguard.

HEALTH & SAFETY

Always have an eye bath with several small bottles of distilled water available in case of accidents involving eyes.

ANECDOTE

A client of mine always kept a small bottle of nail adhesive in her bag in case of accidents. One night she was on her way to dinner with her husband; they were in the car, it was dark and she was in the passenger seat. She felt a bit tired and her eyes were 'gritty'. She knew she had some eye drops with her, so rummaged in her bag to find the bottle. She opened it and tipped her head back to use the eye drops. Out came a drop but … she had mistaken the eye drop bottle for the nail adhesive bottle. She didn't go to dinner, but spent the night in casualty! Luckily although her eye was sore for a few days, there was no permanent damage done.

TOP TIP

In larger salons it may be worth having a large glass jar with wire mesh across the top. This can be placed in the open air but not anywhere near a designated smoking area. Volatile liquids can be put in the jar to evaporate safely. This is only suitable for small quantities as larger amounts need specialist disposal.

Dust Dust is a major problem in the salon. Although the amount of dust can be minimized by correct working procedures, it is impossible to avoid the production of quantities of dust.

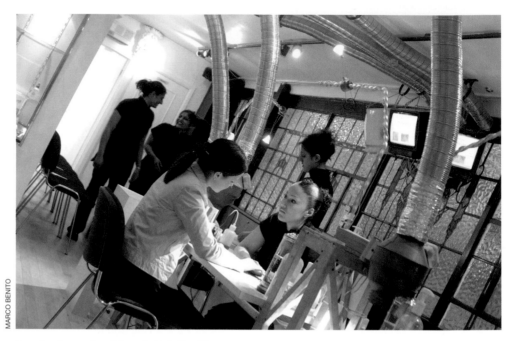

MARCO BENITO

An extraction system integrated into the décor

- Dust falls into two categories: the dust you can see and the dust you cannot see. All dust is potentially harmful, but the dust you can see is slightly less harmful than the dust you cannot see. Larger dust particles will settle on surfaces and not float around in the air to be breathed in. The body has some very clever mechanisms to prevent unwanted 'foreign matter' entering it. Our respiratory system is designed to take air in through the nose and out through the mouth. The nose has thousands of hairs inside it and is lined with a mucous membrane, which act together to trap particles that must not be breathed into the lungs.

- This safety mechanism is very efficient in catching the dust particles that can be seen. It is not as efficient at catching the particles that cannot be seen, as they can be so small that they can be inhaled right into the lungs. There are more mucous membranes in the lungs that will catch a great deal of the inhaled dust but it is an irritant and excess dust can cause respiratory problems.

Avoiding excess dust Like any potential risk situation, it is far better to try to avoid it than correct or treat any problems that arise. There are a number of ways that excess dust can be avoided.

- The ideal arrangement is to have a dust extractor fitted into the desk. These units, like extractor fans, create a light suction that draws the dust being generated from filing through a grille in the desk top and into a collection bag or unit, rather like a vacuum bag. The collected dust can then be regularly disposed of; an efficient unit can remove almost all the dust before it disperses in the air. The grille need only be exposed during the stages that generate dust; otherwise it can be covered with a manicure mat and towels for the comfort of the client and hygiene of the salon.

- If this type of extractor is not possible, the following suggestions should help to cut down on dust:

  - Lay several sheets of disposable towels over a terry towel before each client arrives. After each stage of treatment that generates any dust, fold the top layer and discard. This ensures that dust is not left lying under your hands and being continually disturbed.

  - Wipe the desk surface after each client with a damp cloth to collect any dust. This is also the ideal time to use a hard-surface disinfectant to dampen the cloth.

  - Wipe all surfaces in the salon with a damp cloth every day. Dusting with a dry cloth will just 'rearrange' the dust.

  - Keep air moving with adequate ventilation via windows and doors, which will help remove fine airborne dust.

  - Brushing reusable files and buffers to remove dust will lengthen their life. Brush them under running water before disinfecting them.

  - Buffers and files should not be used for more than one client without disinfecting. Put used files in a covered box until the cleaning process as they will 'shed' dust wherever they are put down.

Dust masks   For those technicians who feel susceptible to dust, a *disposable mask* can be worn. They are comfortable to wear and should be changed very frequently. Dust masks need to fit correctly in order to be effective. They should be the right size for your face and should have an adjustable nose band. Breathing through the mask for any length of time causes it to become damp. This dampness will trap dust and this could be a problem in itself. Change a mask often and follow the manufacturer's guidelines. It is unlikely that a client would need to wear a mask, as they are exposed to the dust for a much shorter length of time. A technician, however, is working in the same environment all day. A technician who wears a mask should explain this to all clients in case they feel at risk.

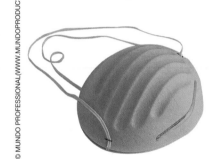

© MUNDO PROFESSIONAL(WWW.MUNDOPRODUCTS.CO.UK)

Disposable dust mask

Electric files   Modern products and techniques do not require the use of e-files, unlike the old, thick and brittle dental acrylics that took hours to buff. Good application techniques should negate the effectiveness of e-files. If a technician chooses to use a drill, a course of practical tuition must be undertaken to fully understand the correct use of the equipment. It should also be understood that drills create huge quantities of very fine dust. Anyone using a drill must wear a dust mask for their own safety and follow stringent rules for the management of the dust. The use of correct bits and slower speeds will help lower the creation of dust. Carbide bits create less dust than diamond bits as the abrasive on them scoops rather than grinds.

Ingestion

Obviously, technicians do not make a habit of eating or drinking any of their nail products! It is, however, exactly what does happen in a great number of salons by hundreds of technicians. Every time there is a coffee cup on the desk, every time a technician grabs a quick bite of their lunchtime sandwich or the sandwich is left open in the salon, small amounts of dust and vapours are getting into the food and are being ingested.

It is unlikely that this will affect a client as they will drink a coffee or eat a sandwich in the salon so infrequently. A technician, however, could be doing this every day and several times a day. The levels will soon build up.

Simple rules to follow would be:

- Do not drink hot liquids at the desk; it is possible for them to absorb vapours from the air.

- Avoid placing any drinks on the desk, as the container could collect dust.

- It is possible for uncovered food to absorb vapours or dust; keep all food away from the salon.

- Wash your hands before eating anything, even a small piece of chocolate.

Absorption

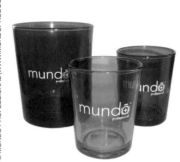

Every time a chemical, even water, touches the skin or nails, some of it will be absorbed into the skin. The body is quite happy to have thousands of different chemicals enter the upper levels of the skin. Specific cells within the blood maintain total vigilance and investigate anything 'foreign'; most of these 'foreigners' are recognized as being friends and are left alone. However, there will also be many 'foreigners' that are not recognized as friends, and they will be removed and destroyed. These cells will recognize any non-friendly chemicals if they appear again and may just remove and destroy them without any fuss. However, if these foes continue to appear, the blood will develop a substance that will fight them and this is when a reaction is noticed.

- The most obvious reaction is irritated skin in the area of absorption. If the irritant is not immediately removed, this can develop into a very painful skin condition that will take a very long time to clear up.

- Local irritation is not always the first sign of an allergic reaction. Puffy or itchy eyes could be a reaction to a product on the nails. Headaches, tiredness, mood swings, nosebleeds, dizziness, coughs, or a sore throat can also be signs of a reaction to chemicals via any of the routes of entry.

- If the irritating chemical is removed, the symptoms should also disappear. They will, however, reappear if the chemical is reintroduced, as once the body is sensitized it will always be sensitized to that substance. From the point of view of a technician, if this sort of sensitivity is created to a commonly used product it may be difficult to find an alternative. This could mean that the technician can no longer work, which is a very drastic result of what amounts to laziness or lack of understanding. For a client, it can be very distressing and they may be lost as a client or, worse, take legal action against the salon or technician.

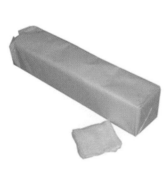

As these potential problems can all be avoided with a little extra care and a real understanding of the work, it is not worth taking any risks.

Ways to avoid **sensitization**:

- Nail products are designed for the nail therefore keep them OFF the skin.

- Do not touch the skin with your brush. If you find this difficult when applying a liquid and powder overlay, use a smaller brush.

- Do not wipe your brush on the towel your hand is resting on.

- When removing the sticky inhibition layer (which is uncured monomer, one of the most active allergens in nail products) on a **UV light cured** material start with the smallest nail up to the largest nail to avoid putting the residue on the skin.

- Wipe the nail away from the cuticle area towards the free edge.

● Make sure ALL the inhibition layer is removed as this will fall into your hand as you are shaping the overlay.

● Wear protective gloves if you are susceptible to allergic reactions and always wear gloves if you notice any redness or itching of your skin.

Decontamination

What is this and why do nail technicians need to know and understand about it? Decontamination or hygiene is essential to prevent the spread of infection and disease. Technicians need to understand how this happens and the most efficient methods to prevent it. It is also very useful to understand measures that are unnecessary now that a greater understanding of how infection is spread.

The most common problems faced by nail technicians and salons are:

1 Bacterial infections: these are probably the most common and can be caused by nail services. They can affect the nail and skin. On the nail an infection shows as a discoloration (often seen between the nail plate and artificial overlay) and on the skin can be a soreness, swelling and often heat.

2 Fungal infections: these can also affect both skin and nails. Nails usually appear thickened and crumbly. Skin can be red, inflamed and scaly. Examples are athletes foot and ringworm. The infection has probably come from outside the salon but technicians must take care to avoid any possibility of spreading the condition.

3 Viral infections: this type of infection is common as it includes common diseases such as colds, flu, chickenpox, etc. Conditions such as verrucae and warts are viral infections and are very easily spread.

In the past, HIV/AIDS, hepatitis and tuberculosis were considered to be concerns for the salon. However, these life threatening diseases are not spread by nail services or salon environments.

'Between 1983 and 2004 over 6 billion salon services were preformed in professional nail salons without a single case of transmission of either HIV or tuberculosis by these services. Not even one! Why? These illnesses are not spread by salon services. It's never happened and probably never will. But even if it did we'd know the odds are more than 1 in 5 billion! So why would some people claim that we need disinfectants to prevent HIV and tuberculosis in the salon? They argue that because it hasn't happened doesn't mean it won't happen someday. They've been making this same argument for over 20 years and it still hasn't happened. Why should a salon protect against something that has never happened? HIV, hepatitis or tuberculosis cannot be spread by manicures, pedicures or other nail services.'

Nail Structure and Product Chemistry, Douglas D Schoon.

Sterilization, disinfection and sanitization

Hygiene in the salon can be divided into three categories:

1 **Sterilization**: this process kills all living organisms.

2 **Disinfection**: this will kill all **pathogens** with the exception of spores.

3 **Cleaning**: this will inhibit the growth of certain living organisms and must be used to clean hands and prepare nails for treatment.

We will look at each of these in more detail.

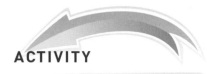

ACTIVITY

Would you like to see how much dust is generated during an artificial nail service?
Start with a clean nail desk and equipment. Provide an artificial nail service, such as apply tips and overlays or a maintenance service without using any local dust extraction and just a towel on the desk.

When you have finished, get a vacuum cleaner and 1–3 sheets of kitchen roll. Layer the sheets and push the centre down inside the hose, then attach the small flat attachment of the vacuum (the number of sheets will depend on their thickness and the size of the hose and its attachment). Make sure the corners of the sheet are outside the hose and held firmly in place. Vacuum your desk and towel. Then remove the vacuum attachment very carefully and tip out the contents of the sheets!

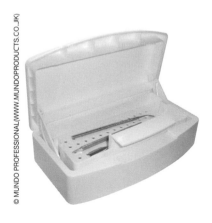

HEALTH & SAFETY

ALWAYS read the manufacturer's instructions carefully and follow them exactly. For tools, it is usual that a fresh disinfectant solution must be made every day. When dealing with any disinfectant solution you should wear protective equipment as they are always irritants.

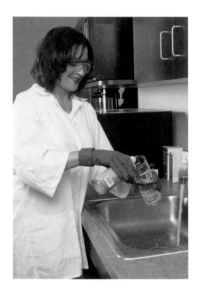

Wear gloves and saflety goggles while handling disinfectant

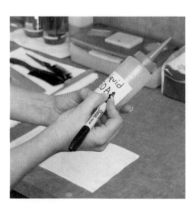

All containers should be labelled

Sterilization

This level of hygiene is only necessary in operating theatres and surgical wards in a hospital. Adequate and effective disinfection methods are needed even if tools have come into contact with blood.

Disinfection

There are many disinfectants on the market specifically formulated for salons and nail services. The solutions are at different strengths depending on the job they are designed to do. The stronger concentrations are for metal tools; the slightly weaker concentrations for hard surfaces and the very low concentrations are for hand washes etc.

The commonly used tools that will need to be disinfected are cuticle nippers, nail clippers and cuticle knives—that is, anything with a sharp edge or blade.

Tools that are not so easily disinfected and can sometimes carry the same risk are files and buffers. Occasionally, a technician may break the skin with a file or buffer around the nail plate or sometimes clients have very delicate skin at the side of the nail or a hangnail so that rough handling breaks the skin. If this happens the only safe procedure is to discard any file and buffer that has been used.

Discard files and buffers if they have been used on a nail with a bacterial infection.

Disinfection methods

Metal tools In preparation for disinfection, tools should be scrubbed with soapy water to remove any grease or debris as these will create a barrier to the disinfectant. Then they should be immersed in the disinfectant solution following the manufacturer's instructions.

Ideally this should be after every client. However, realistically, if you are confident that they have not been in contact with any broken skin they can be wiped with an alcohol solution (or a wipe designed for the purpose). They should be thoroughly disinfected after every few clients so it is worth having several sets.

TOP TIP Have a clean, covered container for clean tools and another for used tools. Then the disinfecting process can be carried out at the end of the day.

When tools are removed from the disinfectant follow the manufacturer's instructions then pat dry and store in the 'clean container' ready for use.

NB: UV cabinets do NOT disinfect tools. They maintain a clean environment for the storage of disinfected tools.

Work surfaces There are many areas that require regular disinfection. This process will destroy many bacteria, viruses and fungi and is essential for general salon hygiene.

All hard surfaces should be cleaned on a regular basis with a disinfectant solution. For example, desks should be wiped over after every client, preferably with a weak disinfectant; they should have a thorough clean at the end of every day. Floors, light switches, sinks and basins should all be cleaned with disinfectant on a regular basis.

Towels Terry towels used during treatments and those used to dry hands should be washed in a washing machine with the addition of a suitable disinfectant solution.

Commercial disinfectants are often available at beauty wholesalers or cleaning-product wholesalers that are suitable for all these jobs. Some beauty and nail product companies also supply products designed for this use.

Files and buffers
Files and buffers should either be disposable, personal to specific clients only, or be of a quality that can be submersed in water.

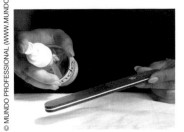

Used files and buffers should be stored in a covered container until they can be cleaned of dust and then placed in the disinfecting solution. The most efficient method is to use a stiff brush to clean away the dust in the abrasive. Do this under running water to prevent the spread of the dust then immerse in the disinfectant solution. After the minimum time period, they can be removed, rinsed to remove the solution and left on paper towels to dry.

Cleaning

This is a process that is essential for the cleansing of hands and the preparation of nails. Skin cannot be sterilized or disinfected as the chemicals that can do this are irritants and sometimes corrosive. Cleaning is the lowest level of **decontamination**, but it is necessary to avoid the spread of diseases and, in the case of nail preparation, is essential to maintain healthy nails.

Technicians
Technicians' hands should be washed before and after every treatment for the safety of themselves and their clients. It not only limits the spread of bacteria and viruses, it also removes traces of artificial nail products and dust.

Washing the hands in soap and water is not always enough. Ideally, an antibacterial soap should be used that contains moisturisers to prevent the skin becoming dry. Hands should be dried with paper towels, as terry towels can become an efficient breeding ground for bacteria and there is some proof that hot air driers can also cause problems with bacteria.

Do not use a moisturising hand cream immediately before providing a nail enhancement service as the dust will stick to the cream.

TOP TIP

If an antibacterial wash is used, there could be a build-up of some of the ingredients on the skin. Thorough rinsing is needed to prevent this and this regular immersion in water must be counteracted with the regular application of moisturisers.

Clients
Clients should also have clean hands and nails. A huge amount of debris can collect under the free edge and on the surface of the nail. Ask the client to wash their hands with soap and water. To ensure that under the nails are clean, ask the client to use a nail brush that is provided at the sink. Have a dish with clean nail brushes for this purpose plus a dish for used brushes. Disinfect these brushes at the end of the day.

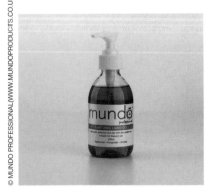

As an extra precaution, both the technician and the client should use a hand sanitizer at the desk.

Legislation for salons and equipment

There are many acts of parliament and other pieces of local and national legislation that refer to salons with five or more employees. However, every technician should be aware of all of these. All the necessary information and ready-made forms are available in the Habia Health & Safety Implementation Pack that is strongly recommended for all salons. Use of this pack also provides valuable evidence in the gaining of qualifications. There is additional useful information on the Habia website: www.habia.org.

Habia Health & Safety
Implementation Pack

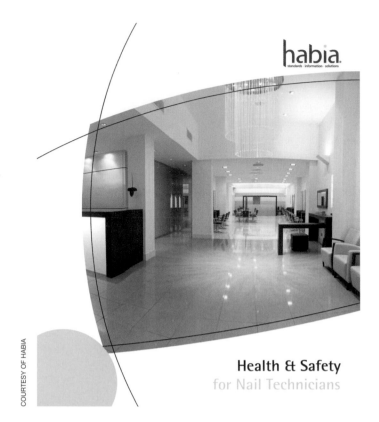

COURTESY OF HABIA

habia.
standards information solutions

Health & Safety
for Nail Technicians

There are actually 20 Acts and Regulations that affect salons:

- Health & Safety at Work Act 1974 **(HASAWA)**
- Workplace (Health, Safety and Welfare) Regulations 1992
- Working Time Regulations 1998
- Management of Health & Safety at Work Regulations 1999
- Control of Substances Hazardous to Health Regulations 2002 **(COSHH)**
- Health & Safety (Training for Employment) Regulations 1990
- Employers' Liability (Compulsory Insurance) Regulations 1998
- Electricity at Work Regulations 1989
- Health & Safety (First Aid) Regulations 1981
- Reporting of Injuries, Diseases and Dangerous Occurrences Regulations 1995 **(RIDDOR)**
- Health & Safety (Information for Employees) Regulations 1989
- Health & Safety (Consultation with Employees) Regulations 1996
- Regulatory Reform (Fire Safety) Order 2005
- Environmental Protection Act 1990
- Provisions and Use of Work Equipment Regulations 1998
- Personal Protective Equipment at Work Regulations 1992
- Health & Safety (Display Screen Equipment) Regulations 1992

- Manual Handling Operations Regulations 1992

- Work at Height Regulations 2005

- Disability Discrimination Act 1995.

Fortunately, not all of these need be fully understood in order to gain a relevant qualification! Some of them, however, are essential and they are covered in some detail in this chapter. Others apply to employers but employees need to know they exist so a brief explanation is included. The rest are listed for information but must be dealt with by employers.

Health & Safety at Work Act 1974 (HASAWA)

This Act relates to an employer but its requirements make for good working practices. Also, employees have a duty to work following these rules to ensure their safety, that of their colleagues and clients. The Act requires that an employer must:

- Provide safe equipment and safe systems of work.

- Ensure that all substances are handled safely, stored and transported correctly.

- Provide a safe place of work with safe access and exit routes.

- Provide a workplace that is safe with regard to fire, first aid and the recording of accidents.

- Provide all the necessary information, instruction, training and supervision and ensure that all staff are aware of all the relevant safety issues, for example of where fire fighting equipment is and its correct use.

- Supply all necessary personal protective equipment free of charge.

Every establishment of five or more employees must have a written Health & Safety Policy. Employees include part-timers, trainees and those working in different locations. All salons should have a written list of good housekeeping rules. The policy, the housekeeping rules and any amendments must be brought to the attention of all employees.

HEALTH & SAFETY

What are the Housekeeping Rules in your establishment?

There must be a person who has designated responsibility for:

- overall health and safety

- health and safety on a day-to-day basis, plus a deputy

- healthy and safety training

- general housekeeping

- fire safety

- first aid

- keeping the accident book up-to-date and reporting accidents

- carrying out, updating and monitoring COSHH assessments

- inspecting electrical equipment and arrange for annual checking.

An employer must ensure all these requirements are met and every employee must be aware of them and work in such a way that they ensure their own safety and that of their colleagues and clients.

TOP TIP

Your 'establishment' refers to your place of work, your training establishment or your place of assessment.

HEALTH & SAFETY

Do you know who is responsible for each of these items in your salon or training establishment?

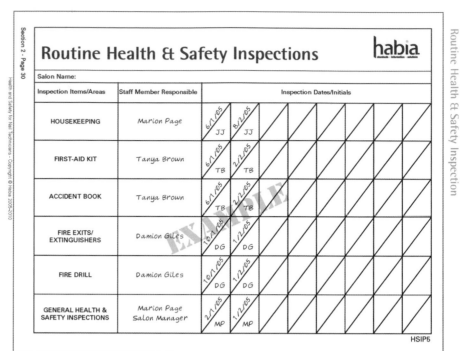

Routine Health & Safety Inspections

Salon Name:

Inspection Items/Areas	Staff Member Responsible	Inspection Dates/Initials								
HOUSEKEEPING	Marion Page	6/1/05 JJ	8/1/05 JJ							
FIRST-AID KIT	Tanya Brown	6/1/05 TB	2/1/05 TB							
ACCIDENT BOOK	Tanya Brown	6/1/05 TB	2/1/05 TB							
FIRE EXITS/ EXTINGUISHERS	Damion Giles	10/1/05 DG	1/2/05 DG							
FIRE DRILL	Damion Giles	10/1/05 DG	1/2/05 DG							
GENERAL HEALTH & SAFETY INSPECTIONS	Marion Page Salon Manager	2/1/05 MP	1/2/05 MP							

Section 2 · Page 30   Health and Safety for Nail Technicians – Copyright © Habia 2005–2010

HSIP5

HEALTH & SAFETY

What ventilation system is being used in your establishment?

Workplace (Health, Safety and Welfare) Regulations 1992

This addresses specific areas within the workplace, such as ventilation and temperature, sanitary and washing facilities, eating and changing facilities.

Working Time Regulations 1998

This covers obligations relating to working hours, rest periods and holidays.

Management of Health & Safety at Work Regulations 1999

This is legislation that requires employers to appoint a person or persons to make regular assessments of the risks to health and safety to employees, clients and any other visitor. This means regular **risk assessments** must be carried out on the entire salon. (A young person, aged under 18, has special requirements in terms of risk assessments.)

HEALTH & SAFETY

Who is responsible for risk assessments in your establishment?

There are steps that need to be followed and records to be kept concerning these assessments. See the Habia Health & Safety Implementation Pack. An employer must follow these steps and an employee must be aware of who is appointed to be responsible for the various issues.

Control of Substances Hazardous to Health Regulations 2002 (COSHH) (as amended 2004)

This set of Regulations is particularly relevant to all nail technicians. Many of the products used in nail treatments fall into the category of hazardous substances and every technician must be aware of these hazards, how to manage them and how to protect themselves and their clients from being harmed by them.

Employers have very specific obligations under the Regulations. Hazardous substances must be identified and the risk to health from exposure to these must be assessed.

Different people will pose different levels of risk (for example, a receptionist is at less risk of skin contact with acrylic liquid than a technician; a person who suffers from asthma is more at risk from dust irritation than someone who does not have the condition). When a complete assessment has been made, substitutes of less hazardous products are made where possible, precautions must be taken to prevent or control the exposure to any potential risks.

Employers must:

1 Identify substances in the workplace which are potentially hazardous.

2 Assess the risk to health from exposure to the hazardous substances and record the results.

3 Make an assessment as to which members of staff are at risk.

4 Look for alternative, less hazardous substances and substitute if possible.

5 Decide what precautions are required, noting that the use of PPE should always be the last resort.

6 Introduce effective measures to prevent or control exposure.

7 Inform, instruct and train all members of staff.

8 Review the assessment on a regular basis.

Product companies are obliged to supply a product data sheet for each product that details any risk associated with using an individual product and precautions that should be taken for its safe use.

Steps for a COSHH assessment:

1 Read the manufacturer's instructions and data sheet for every product.

2 If the product is potentially hazardous, record it on an assessment form (see example).

3 Decide what the risk is, the degree of that risk and who is at risk.

4 Decide how that risk is going to be minimized and controlled.

5 If further action needs to be taken, such as replacing a product with a safer version, or finding and providing protective equipment, a COSHH action plan should be made and carried out.

6 All details of the COSHH assessment, results and action plan must be made very clear to all members of staff and any relevant training provided and recorded.

7 The assessment should be regularly reviewed and any new products added.

These steps do not just apply to salons. A mobile technician is well advised to carry out this procedure to protect themselves, their clients and their clients' homes.

A general list of the products likely to fall into the 'hazardous' category will include:

- cleaning materials (e.g. bleach)
- sterilizing and disinfecting solutions
- detergents
- solvents
- cuticle removers
- nail varnishes

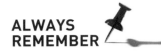

ALWAYS REMEMBER

PPE should always be the last resort. COSHH assessments must be carried out, precautions taken, all information recorded and the situation reviewed on a regular basis.

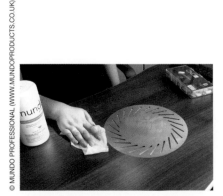

© MUNDO PROFESSIONAL (WWW.MUNDOPRODUCTS.CO.UK)

HEALTH & SAFETY

Carry out a risk assessment on all your personal products. Record and file your assessments.

- nail treatments
- hand creams
- adhesives
- acrylic liquids
- accelerators
- nail primers
- nail preparation products.

COSHH Risk Assessment habia

Updated May 2010

Health and Safety for Nail Technicians · Copyright © Habia 2005-2010

Section 5 · Page 9

COURTESY OF HABIA

COSHH Risk Assessment

Company Name: Beauty Spot   **Compiled By:** Natasha Smith   **Date:** 1st Sept 2008   **Review Date:** 10th January 2009

What are the hazards?	Who might be harmed?	What are you already doing?	What further action is necessary?	Action by whom and when?	Done
Young persons – may be inexperienced, immature, reluctant to ask for help	May put themselves or others at risk	• Young persons are supervised at all times. • Young persons do not handle, mix or use any chemicals that pose a special risk eg: acetone, acrylic etc, unless assisting a technician whilst being trained and thus under constant supervision • Skin checks are undertaken on a weekly basis • Must follow the extra precautions highlighted in this risk assessment in bold. • Young persons under the school leaving age are registered with the Local Authority Education Welfare Officer	• Copy of risk assessment to be provided to parent or guardian of young person	• Manager During each young person first week	
Aerosols – can contain flammable gases and irritant chemicals. Risk of fire, explosion and intoxication. (List aerosols used in your salon)	Everyone in the salon, but in particular the user of the aerosol and the client.	• Do not expose to temperatures above 50 C. • Do not pierce or burn containers. • Do not inhale. • Do not store in direct sunlight or close to any heat source	Look for aerosols with non-flammable gases.	• Manager • 10/01/09	10/01/09

HSIP2

Section 5 · Page 10

Health and Safety for Nail Technicians · Copyright © Habia 2005-2010

Updated May 2010

COURTESY OF HABIA

COSHH Risk Assessment habia

What are the hazards?	Who might be harmed?	What are you already doing?	What further action is necessary?	Action by whom and when?	Done
Acetone– Irritant to the skin and eyes. Moderately toxic if swallowed or inhaled. (List specific products used in your salon)	Technicians, juniors, trainees and clients Staff may suffer skin irritations, dermatitis or asthma Clients may suffer skin allergies Splashing injuries to the eyes	• Store in a cool place. • Reseal after use. • Do not use on damaged or sensitive skin. • Avoid breathing in. • Report any sign of breathlessness to supervisor • Never place in an unlabelled container. • Staff consult with client to determine history of allergies, skin damage etc	• Skin checks are to be carried out at 3 month intervals • Use the Habia guidance booklet for training staff • Purchase an eye bath for use in case of splashing injuries	• Manager 1st Dec 08 and quarterly after that • Manager 14/09/08	5/12/08 14/09/08
Cyanoacrylate	Staff may suffer skin irritations,	• Wear appropriate gloves – Non latex gloves are provided for use by all salon staff, in a range of sizes and materials • Manager to observe staff (especially young persons) to ensure gloves are worn • Staff are trained to adopt good hand care routines, including, washing, drying thoroughly and moisturising regularly			
Spillage of chemicals –Slips/trips; irritant to skin	Anyone with access to immediate area	• Clear area around spillage. • Warn anyone in surrounding area. • Take details of product from another sample and go to a safe area to read the instructions on the label or the COSHH assessment sheet. • Clean the area using the correct cloths, mops and ppe where required			

HSIP2

Health & Safety (Training for Employment) Regulations 1990

These Regulations state that any person carrying out work experience or any form of training that is not an employee must receive the same health, safety and welfare protection as those employed. Remember a young person must have closer supervision.

Employers' Liability (Compulsory Insurance) Regulations 1998

Every employer must insure all their employees against any injury sustained or disease developed during the course of their employment for a minimum of £5 million. This insurance certificate must be displayed for the information of all employees. If any person is working in the salon that is not an employee (e.g. work experience or agency worker) the insurer should be informed.

HEALTH & SAFETY

Where is the certificate displayed in your establishment?

Electricity at Work Regulations 1989

Every piece of electrical equipment used is covered by these Regulations. There must be a person responsible for ensuring that all electrical equipment, including wall plugs, light switches, fuse boxes, etc. is safe and regularly inspected. All equipment must be tested by a certified electrician each year and all records kept. See the Electrical Equipment Register and Electrical Test Records.

Health & Safety (First Aid) Regulations 1981

This Regulation requires that every employer provides adequate supplies of first aid equipment and products. First aid boxes can be easily purchased from high street chemists and beauty wholesalers and the size will depend on the number of employees. This information is given on the first aid boxes. An eyewash bottle should also be provided in a salon, preferably

Section 8 - Page 6

Health and Safety for Nail Technicians - Copyright © Habia 2005-2010

Electrical Test Records

Electrical Test Records

habia

Salon Name: Top to Toe		Test Date:							
Names and Addresses	Phone Number	TARGET	ACTUAL	TARGET	ACTUAL	TARGET	ACTUAL	TARGET	ACTUAL
ELECTRICAL CONTRACTOR									
Goldman Bros. 22 Cantley Terrace Smithton GG7 1FY	324-6690	4/3/02	10/3/02	4/9/02	22/10/02	4/3/03			

EXAMPLE

HSIP6

HEALTH & SAFETY

Where is the first aid box in your establishment?

with a bottle of distilled water for washing the eye if necessary. No medication of any kind (e.g. aspirin) should be kept in a first aid box and should never be given to staff or clients.

In salons of over 5 (but under 50) staff there should be a qualified 'first aider' who is responsible for this role. There is a new course available (Emergency First Aid at Work) that only takes 1 day instead of the First Aid at Work that takes 3 days. These courses are available form the local Red Cross or St John's Ambulance.

Electrical Equipment Register   habia

Salon Name: *Top to Toe*

No.	Description	SERIAL NUMBER	DATE OF PURCHASE	DATE OF DISPOSAL
1	Waxing Machine	SN002456733	20/1/95	26/2/02
2	Cash Register	XXM-666743A	2/3/97	
3	Microwave	ZNA0098235561	3/9/01	
4				
5				
6				
7				
8				
9				
10				

EXAMPLE

HSIP7

Reporting of Injuries, Diseases and Dangerous Occurrences Regulations 1995 (RIDDOR)

Again, this applies to employers, but all employees should be aware of the requirements and who is responsible for them.

This Act requires that any personal injury suffered at work is recorded in the accident book that all salons should have, even if the injury is very minor. A more serious injury must be recorded and reported to the Incident Contact Centre (ICC) (for example an injury that results in incapacity for more that 3 calendar days). Also, if any client is injured and taken to hospital, a report must be made to the ICC.

Any accident involving a learner must be reported to the training provider or managing agent.

Certain diseases are reportable. Two that are especially relevant in a salon are occupational asthma and dermatitis. These should be reported only when a doctor's letter has been received.

The ICC must also be contacted if a visitor to the salon is taken to hospital.

HEALTH & SAFETY

Where is the accident book in your establishment?

Accident Report Form

Salon Name _The Nail Bar_   **Number** _4_

Details of the person who had the accident
Name _Julie Harpen_
Address _2 Miles Walk, Guildford, Surrey_
    Postcode _GU16 1BZ_
Job Title _Nail Technician_

Details of the person who filled in this accident form
Name _Mary Murphy_
Address _Hilltop, West Lane, Farnham, Surrey_
    Postcode _FN12 7QR_
Job Title _Manager_

Details of witness
Name _None_
Address
    Postcode
Job Title

Accident Details
Date of accident _27/08/03_   Time _10.30_   Place _Staff Room_
How did the accident happen:
Hot water splashed out of kettle when making client a cup of tea

Details of any injuries (be specific e.g. cut little finger on right hand above first joint)
Slight scald on back of left hand below middle finger.
Did not form blister.

Details of any treatment
Rinsed in cold water for five minutes

Is the accident reportable under RIDDOR?   Yes ☐   No ☑

If yes, how was it reported (by phone, by fax etc)
Who reported it?

Signature of person who had the accident: _Julie Harper_   Date _27/08/03_

Signature of person completing the form: _Mary Murphy_   Date _27/08/03_

Health and Safety for Nail Technicians - Copyright © Habia 2005-2010

Health & Safety (Information for Employees) Regulations 1989

These require that employees are provided with approved information on health and safety by means of posters or pocket cards. A new poster was published by the Health & Safety Executive (HSE) in 2009 that must replace the previous version by 2014.

Health & Safety (Consultation with Employees) Regulations 1996

These require an employee to discuss any health and safety issues with staff. This can be carried out on a personal basis or in staff meetings. Records of these two-way discussions should be recorded.

Regulatory Reform (Fire Safety) Order 2005

The need for fire certification under the Fire Precautions Act 1971 have been rendered superfluous by this Order (It is no longer necessary to have a fire certificate).

This Order requires a responsible person (usually the employer) to ensure the safety of all people on the premises. The responsible person can appoint a competent person who is most suitable to:

- carry out a fire risk assessment

- develop fire evacuation procedures

- provide and maintain clear means of escape, signs and notices

- provide emergency lighting

- provide fire detection and alarm systems

- provide adequate means of fighting fires

- train staff

- consult with staff on fair arrangements.

Guidance on fire risk assessments and checklists are available in the Habia Health & Safety for Nail Salons.

Fire Equipment Test Records										
Salon Name:										
Names and Address	**Phone Number**	**TARGET**	**ACTUAL**	**TARGET**	**ACTUAL**	**TARGET**	**ACTUAL**	**TARGET**	**ACTUAL**	
FIRE EQUIPMENT CONTRACTOR										

HSIP11

Health and Safety for Nail Technicians - Copyright © Habia 2005-2010

COURTESY OF HABIA

Fire Equipment Test Records

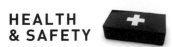

HEALTH & SAFETY

Where are the extinguishers in your establishment?

Classes of fire and types of extinguisher There are five classes of fire:

A. Fire involving solids such as paper, wood, hair, etc.

B. Fire involving liquids such as solvents.

C. Fire involving gasses such as propane or butane.

D. Fire involving metals.

E. Fire involving hot oil such as cooking oil.

There are five main types of extinguisher:

1 Water
   These are red and are only appropriate for Class A fires. They must NEVER be used on electrical fires.

2 Foam
   These are red with a cream/buff label and used for Class B and small Class A fires.

3 Carbon dioxide (CO_2)
   These are red with a black label and appropriate for all classes of fire and are particularly suitable for Class B (solvents) and electrical fires.

4 Dry powder
   These are red with a blue label and suitable for all fires.

5 Wet Chemical Extinguisher
   These are red with a yellow patch and are suitable for oil/fat fires in kitchens and replace the fire blanket.

> **ANECDOTE**
>
> Accidental fires can happen in the safest of environments and are usually due to human error! In the salon I shared with a partner, there was one such incident that by happy coincidence happened on my day off. A junior staff member put a technician's lunch (a jacket potato in a polystyrene box) in the oven to keep warm. For some reason she turned the heat up to maximum and forgot about it. A much later visit to the kitchen by the junior due to the smell of burning resulted in the discovery of a fire started by the incineration of a polystyrene box and jacket potato.
>
> The senior member of staff was alerted and a 999 call made. The staff tried to evacuate everyone, as black smoke was now issuing from the back of the premises into the salon at the front of the building. It was a Saturday and most of the clients present were going to a social event later in the day. The staff tried extremely hard to get everyone out, but clients were reluctant to go saying: 'Couldn't you just finish painting my nails?', 'But I need these done for tonight!' The fire brigade arrived in minutes and were deliberately deaf to the pleas for finished nails. They were amazed that the clients waited as close as possible to the salon and rushed back in as soon as they were told it was safe! Obviously nothing comes between a woman and her nails!

Environmental Protection Act 1990

Under this Act, every technician has a duty to dispose of waste safely (see earlier in this chapter).

Provisions and Use of Work Equipment Regulations 1998

All equipment used must be suitable for the purpose it is being used for, properly maintained and all relevant staff trained in its correct use. There are several pieces of equipment that fall into this category. For example:

- UV lamps
- heated mitts and bootees
- foot spas
- airbrushing equipment
- paraffin wax baths
- electric files.

As with most of the Regulations, written records of this equipment should be kept, who is trained to use it and its safety check record.

General guidelines for safe working practices In general, every employee has legal duties under all the health and safety legislations to:

- Take reasonable care of your own health and safety and that of colleagues and clients
- Cooperate with your employer on all health and safety issues
- Use all equipment correctly, including personal protective equipment, by following your training instructions
- Never interfere with or misuse anything provided for health and safety purposes
- Be aware of what your employer is required to do or provide with regards to your health and safety and that of others.

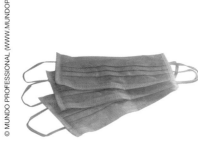

Personal Protective Equipment at Work Regulations 1992

Every employer must provide suitable PPE for every employee. These would normally include gloves (nitrile are recommended as these avoid possible allergies to latex), dust masks (fitted correctly), eye shields, aprons (for use when decanting liquids).

Health & Safety (Display Screen Equipment) Regulations 1992

As so many salons now use computerized salon systems these Regulations now apply:

- Manual Handling Operations Regulations 1992

These apply to members of staff handling stock. It can also apply to staff who are sent to collect stock. (The employer must check that the person has suitable car insurance.) Correct lifting techniques must be taught and enforced.

Work at Height Regulations 2005

Risk assessments must be carried out if staff are required to reach areas beyond their reach. This could be during cleaning, getting stock, putting up Christmas decorations, etc. Chairs must not be used.

In addition to the vast array of health and safety legislation the following Act also affects salons.

Disability Discrimination Act 1995

The Disability Discrimination Act (DDA) gives disabled people important rights of access to everyday services. Service providers have an obligation to make reasonable adjustments to premises or to the way they provide a service. Sometimes it just takes minor changes to make a service accessible. Disabled people can have a wide range of disabilities that do not all involve wheelchairs. They may be registered blind or hard of hearing for example.

It may be just a simple adjustment such as providing a ramp. However, 'reasonable adjustment' is what is required. This means the adjustments must be practical and within the resources of the business. If a salon can make some minor adjustments that will make it easier for any disabled person to use the services, they must be carried out.

Safety

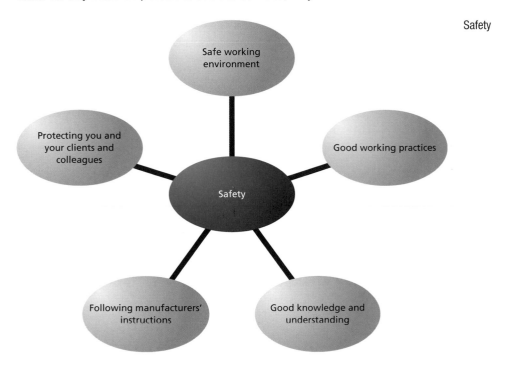

Tools of the trade: their correct use and cleaning

The following section lists and explains the correct use of the various tools used during nail treatments and the methods for keeping them hygienic.

Files and buffers

There are many, many files and buffers available. In some cases their use is specific and, in other cases, personal choice is relevant. In general a file (sometimes called an emery board) is used to shape natural and artificial nails, remove length from a natural or artificial nail and remove and shape product on an artificial overlay. A buffer, on the other hand is used to refine, smooth and polish natural and artificial nails. Files are usually long and flat with an abrasive on both sides and buffers are usually chunkier, cushioned and can be either long and thin or in a block form.

Before understanding the various uses of files and buffers, it is important to understand their abrasive qualities. An abrasive is able to grind down by rubbing and it is measured

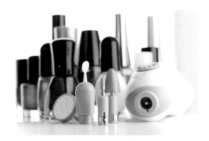

by the amount of **grit**, that makes the abrasive, on an area of 1 square inch. Therefore, low numbers describe an abrasive that has fewer, larger pieces of grit per square inch. This makes it harsher. The higher numbers have more, smaller pieces of grit, so the abrasive is finer. The most common grit sizes used in the nail industry are:

- 80 grit: very coarse. Only used for hard, old fashioned powder/liquid overlays or those using methyl methacrylate (MMA) as the liquid (see Chapter 7). Unnecessarily harsh for any modern artificial product.

- 100 grit: coarse. Can be used for removing old and bulky overlays.

- 180 grit: medium. Can be used for shaping or removing overlays and length of artificial nails.

- 240 grit: fine. This is the lowest grit that should be used on the natural nail, either the free edge or nail plate. Any lower number grit size will cause damage that is easily avoidable.

- 360 grit: very fine. Used as a natural nail file for delicate nails but excellent as a general file for manicure treatments.

- 400–900 grit. This is usually the grit used in block buffers that are designed to refine the shape and smooth the surface of artificial nails prior to shining. Can be used gently on a ridged big toenail before buffing.

- 900–12000 grit. Usually used on a three-way buffer where the roughest side is used first to smooth, then the next to refine and remove any scratches followed by the smooth side to bring surface to a high shine. Used on natural and artificial nails.

When carrying out manicures, it is unnecessary to have files harsher than a 240 grit. Pedicures may need a file of 180 grit, as the big toenail can be quite tough.

A good file to use for all artificial nails is a combination of 180/240. This means that when the natural nail is touched (free edge or nail plate during blending the tip or during maintenance) the finer side can be used. The slightly rougher side can be used for all artificial products, such as the tip and overlay.

When choosing a file there are several things to take into account. Can it be washed? Can it be immersed in water? How long will it last? What is the price? As with most tools, the longer-lasting files are usually more expensive. It is worth having a basic understanding of the components of a file in order to help you decide which ones to use.

There are three parts to a file: the core, the backing and the abrasive, all of which can be made from a number of different materials.

1   The core:

a.   Wood – the old traditional method of making a file. It is inexpensive but cannot even be washed. It is also very brittle and prone to breaking.

b.   Plastic – usually a polystyrene that is slightly flexible. This type of core reduces the vibration felt during filing. A good plastic core has a balance of rigidity and flexibility so pressure can be exerted without it snapping or bending.

c.   Foam – cushions the file and increases its efficiency. The foam could be an open-celled foam that is soft but porous so cannot be put into water or a closed-cell foam that is waterproof.

d.   Many files have a combination of a plastic core for strength covered by foam for efficiency.

2 The backing. This is the material that the abrasive is put onto:

   a. Paper – has a short life and cannot be made wet.

   b. Waterproof paper – has an oil-based resin coating that lengthens its life and allows it to be immersed for short periods, but it will soon break down.

   c. Mylar – a trade name for a specific polyester material. It is washable, can be immersed and is durable.

   d. Cloth – usually cotton, this has a cost implication but is long lasting.

   e. Foam – quite expensive but durable and immersible. The abrasive is sprayed directly onto the foam.

3 The abrasive. This comprises the particles that are glued to the backing:

   a. Garnet – a common gemstone that is inexpensive and long lasting. The old, traditional files, still available today, are made from wood, paper and garnet but are very harsh and should not be used on a natural nail.

   b. Silicon carbide – the black grit file in common use today. It is a synthetic crystal composition. It is very hard and very jagged. It also has the characteristic of losing little bits that leave behind a fresh jagged edge. This is annoying for the user but does prolong its life and efficiency.

   c. Silicon carbide with zinc stearate coating – the coating acts as a lubricant to make filing smoother and quicker. It also prevents dust from building up between the particles and blunting the file.

   d. Aluminium oxide – this abrasive can be coloured. It is less jagged so therefore less harsh.

The ability of a file to be immersed in water is not only dependent on the materials used in its construction, but also on the glue used to assemble it. Files are usually labelled as washable or submersible. Washable files cannot be submersed in water so cannot be disinfected, they can only be sanitized with an antiseptic spray. If there is no labelling, they cannot be washed.

Ideally, a file should be used on one customer only and then either thrown away (or kept for their exclusive use) or disinfected. The cleaning method for files that can be immersed in water is:

- Using a stiff brush, clean away all dust from the file under running water. This will avoid the spread of dust.

- Rinse the file and place it in **disinfectant** for the manufacturer's recommended time.

- Remove the file, rinse, blot dry, and place between paper towels to dry thoroughly.

- When dry, keep in a closed container ready for use.

A tip when using a new file is to remove the sharp edges with another file. It is very easy to cut the soft tissue around the nail with a brand new file.

When using a file on a natural nail it is important to file in one direction only (see Chapter 5). When using a file on top of the nail during artificial nail treatments, the whole length of the file should be used without too much pressure. Although everyone has their own way of holding a file when more practised, a good way to start, that will ensure efficient filing without causing too much damage to the nail plate, is the following:

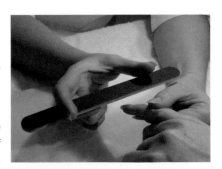

The correct way to hold a file for buffing

- Place the end of the file between the forefinger and middle finger with most of the file pointing towards the thumb.

- Place the thumb near the other end of the file.

- By holding the file in this way, the whole length can be used during use, the wrist can be kept flexible so the curve of the nail can be followed and it is difficult to exert too much pressure on the surface of the nail.

Cuticle knife

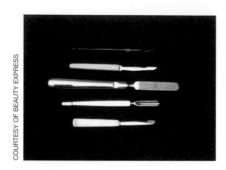

COURTESY OF BEAUTY EXPRESS

Examples of cuticle tools

For an experienced technician, a correctly used cuticle knife is the most efficient method of removing softened cuticle. There are many shapes and sizes available and personal preference plays a large part in choosing the right one. It is a metal tool and, as such, can be easily cleaned and disinfected. It is also capable of causing damage with incorrect use.

General guidelines:

- Cuticle should be softened before removal otherwise the nail plate can be damaged.

- Whatever the shape of the tool, it should be used quite flat against the nail plate to avoid damaging the nail.

- Cuticle cannot always be seen and can have grown quite far up the nail plate. With experience, cuticle can be distinguished from nail by the feel of the surface when using the cuticle knife.

- Care must be taken not to mistake nail for cuticle. A sharp knife is quite capable of scraping off a layer of nail.

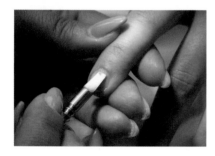

Remove cuticle

- Force should never be used. If the cuticle does not come away easily it must be softened more or left until the next treatment when home care by the client has helped.

- A cuticle knife is not to be used for pushing back the eponychium. This can be gently lifted off the nail plate but not forced.

After use, the knife should be wiped with a solvent or antiseptic solution using a disposable wipe to remove any debris and product. If there is any possibility it has come into contact with any areas of skin that is broken it should be disinfected for the appropriate length of time. If the tool is doubl-ended, remember to turn it around to disinfect both ends.

Cuticle nippers

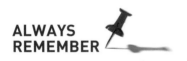

ALWAYS REMEMBER

Do NOT cut the skin of the eponychium. This is living skin.

It is important, when buying nippers, that a good quality pair is chosen. It is worth paying a little extra to get better quality. The blades of nippers need to be very sharp as otherwise they can tear the skin. Nippers that have become blunt or where the ends of the blades have become bent must never be used. Consider having several pairs of nippers as they need regular disinfection.

Cuticle nippers are not to be used to cut away the lifted skin of the nail fold. They are for removing cuticle that has been lifted by a cuticle knife and is still attached to the nail plate. They are also used for removing hangnails.

The correct use is by closing the blades over the skin to be removed, squeezing and releasing the blades. The tool should never pull the skin as this will tear it. A good, sharp pair of nippers will efficiently remove the unwanted skin without causing damage.

After use, the blades should be wiped with a solvent or antiseptic solution on a disposable wipe, then immersed in a disinfectant solution for the appropriate length of time.

Nail clippers

Clippers, as opposed to scissors, are tools that have blades that meet together in a pincer movement. The blades are usually curved but the cutting edge is flat (see picture). They are used for removing the excess length of a nail, either a finger or toe-nail.

As with all blades, they must be very sharp so the nail is efficiently and cleanly cut through. Blunt blades will cause **trauma** to the nail and cause splitting and splintering. This will lead to peeling.

When cutting a nail, several cuts must be made following the curve of the nail. The nail must never be cut in one movement. As the cutting edge is flat, the blade would flatten the nail and pressure would be put on the sides. This could not only cause some damage, it is also uncomfortable for the client.

Clipping nails leaves a rough edge. Always file the nail after cutting to smooth and seal the edge and therefore prevent peeling.

When cutting toenails, always use the larger, heavy-duty clippers as toenails can be very hard. Never make one cut on a nail for the reasons given above and also to prevent the nail flying up into your eyes.

Clippers can also be used to remove the length of a plastic tip once it has been applied to the nail. As with natural nail cutting, make several small cuts following the curve and never one big cut.

After use, follow the cleaning procedure for all metal tools.

Hoof stick

These are usually made from plastic with a rubber end. They are not designed to remove cuticle but are used to make the skin of the nail fold neat following treatment. The rubber end is used to gently ease the skin into a neat oval at the base of the nail as it can be left untidy after the cuticle treatment.

The other end is often pointed and is for cleaning under the free edge. It can be used for this purpose, but disposable orange sticks are more hygienic.

After use, wipe with solvent or antiseptic solution and disinfect if it has come into contact with a wound.

Orange sticks

These are inexpensive wooden sticks that can be used in a variety of ways. Some manicurists use them in place of a cuticle knife but, not being a blade, they are not very efficient for this use.

They usually have an angled shape at one end and a point at the other. They also come in different lengths. The longer length is probably more useful to a technician but the shorter ones can easily be used. They have a number of uses and should be discarded after each use:

● Use the pointed end to clean under the free edge towards the end of any treatment. They can then be discarded to avoid any contamination.

● The angled end can be used instead of a hoof stick to neaten the cuticle.

TOP TIP If small glass disinfecting jars are being used for this tool, place a disc of cotton wool in the bottom to prevent damage to the tip of the nippers. Replace the cotton wool each time a new solution is made.

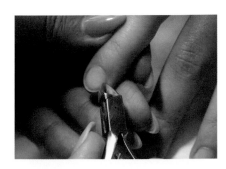
Hangnails

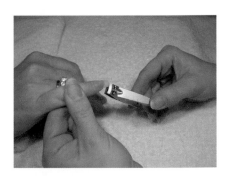
When using clippers, several cuts must me made following the curve of the nail.

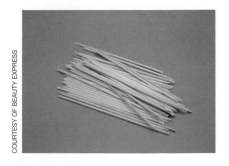
Orange sticks

TOP TIP

Wrap a little cotton wool around the angled end of an orange stick, wet with remover and use to clean up around the edge of the nail after painting. Or saturate cotton wool with cuticle oil and sweep it around the cuticle area for an instant tidy.

- They can be used to clean up the skin if it is touched with polish. Use dry if the polish is still wet and dipped in remover if dry.

- When practising overlay applications, stick a plastic tip on the end with either Blu-Tack or adhesive, then hold the stick while applying the overlay to the tip.

- Use in the same way when creating or practising nail art designs.

- When applying polish secures, dip the pointed end into water and pick up the polish secure. It can then be accurately placed on the nail. Alternatively, mould a small piece of Blu-Tack on the end to form a point. This will easily pick up polish secures.

- In an emergency, a stick can be used to apply adhesive to a tip. When the nozzle comes off with the lid or becomes too blocked to use and there is no other bottle to hand, dip the stick into the bottle and apply the adhesive onto the tip. Discard the stick safely.

Skin abrasives (foot files, pumice)

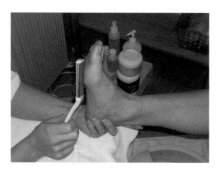

Remove hard skin with an abrasive file

During a pedicure treatment, the hard skin is removed using an abrasive. Its method of use will depend on the type being used. Following the treatment it needs to be dealt with in much the same way as files and buffers. It should be washed under running water using a stiff brush to dislodge any debris, then with soapy water in case there are any creams or oils remaining and then immersed in a disinfecting solution.

Scissors

There are many different types of scissors. They are not necessarily the best tool for cutting natural nails. The action of scissors can traumatize the nail plate and cause peeling unless they are very, very sharp and large enough to cut through thick nails easily. However, the various types of scissors have many other uses.

- Cutting fabric: scissors with long thin blades are ideal for cutting the fabric used in some overlay systems. The fabric is very thin and delicate and needs very sharp blades. The long thin blades are also good if the fabric needs trimming after it has been applied to the nail.

- Pre-tailoring tips: very often the contact area of a tip needs removing or shortening before application and occasionally the sides of a tip need removing. A curved blade is useful for this.

- Nail art: there are many, many uses for small sharp scissors when creating images using various materials.

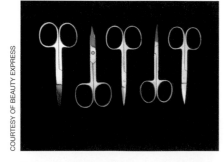

Variety of scissors used for cuticle removal, cutting nails and fibre

As the above uses of scissors do not bring them into contact with skin they do not need disinfecting, but must be kept clean and free from any products. If they are used for cutting nails, the usual procedure for metal tools must be followed.

Tip cutters

When applying artificial tips, it is very useful to have tools designed for specific jobs. Clippers can easily be used for cutting tips but a 'one cut' tip cutter is especially useful. They are designed like the clippers vets use for claws and have a guillotine action. They efficiently cut the tip without putting any stress or pressure on the nail bed (see Chapter 8 on ways of cutting tips).

Wiping them with a solvent is sufficient cleaning. Occasionally the spring mechanism will need some oil to keep it working smoothly.

Brushes

There are several different types of brushes for the wide variety of nail treatments. This section will deal with them generally in specific groups, but there are many available on the market.

- Liquid and powder brushes. These are almost always made from natural hairs of varying quality. Personal preference and budget are the main factors when choosing a brush for this purpose. They do need careful treatment if they are to work efficiently and last a long time. General guidelines for care include:

  - Only use the liquid monomer on them. Do not clean them with anything else as some of the chemical you use will remain in the brush and contaminate your monomer.

  - When using a new brush for the first time, the 'dressing' in the hairs must be thoroughly removed. Pour a little monomer into a clean dappen dish. Dislodge the dressing by rubbing the brush between your fingers then dip the brush into the monomer. Lift the brush out and wipe on a disposable towel. Do this several times until the brush is completely clean. Discard the remaining monomer and wipe out the dish. Shape the brush on a tissue while wet into a point.

  - Store brushes flat in a covered container. Do not store upright in a pot as monomer will run down the brush into the ferrule (metal collar) where it will stay until the brush is dipped in fresh monomer. The old monomer will then contaminate the dish and cause discoloration in the overlay.

  - Never put the brush down during or after use without cleaning it on a disposable towel and shaping it to a point. If this is not done cured acrylic will stay in the brush and the brush will be clogged and unusable.

  - Never shape the brush with your fingers as the monomer should not touch your skin.

  - If the brush does get clogged with acrylic, soak it in a little monomer. The acrylic may soften enough to remove. Discard the monomer.

  - The brush should never touch any skin and the monomer is strong enough to prevent any bacteria from growing on the hairs. No additional cleaning is required.

- Gel brush. These are usually, but not always, made from synthetic hairs. These must be cleaned after every use. Use a specific brush cleaner as recommended by the Gel manufacturer or use acetone on a disposable wipe. Wipe the brush thoroughly with the wet wipe and store in a covered container.

- Nail art brushes. There are many shapes and sizes of brushes used in nail art. All of them can be cleaned in water if wate-based paints are being used or remover if oil based or varnish is being used. They should be stored in a covered container with their bristles protected from damage.

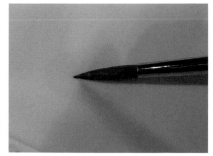

Shaping a powder/liquid brush to a point

Dappen dishes

There are several types of containers available for the liquid and powder system as small amounts of each need to be decanted for use with each treatment. They should all have lids fitted to prevent contamination and evaporation. Only the amount you expect to use for each treatment should be placed in the dishes as product must not be returned to the bottle of monomer or container of powder. The monomer is contaminated with powder every time a brush is dipped into it, so larger quantities of monomer just get more contaminated as the day goes on. Keep the lids closed when not in use.

When the treatment is completed, discard unused monomer into a disposable towel and put that into the covered waste bin. Throw any remaining powder into the bin. Then wipe out each dish with a clean disposable towel. Wash occasionally with soapy water, but make sure all the soap is rinsed away and the dishes are left to dry thoroughly overnight.

Pricing structures in the salon

One of the most difficult challenges when first starting out, either as a mobile technician, working freelance in a salon or opening a salon, is deciding a pricing structure. A good way to start is to research the local area to see what other salons are charging for specific services. Also look through the local paper, especially if you are planning to work as a mobile technician.

When you have a good idea on the level of prices in the area, you need to decide whether you want to be cheaper or more expensive than your competitors. There are benefits to both ways: lower prices may attract some of their clients who want to try a less expensive service, it may also attract new clients who call several salons to compare prices; higher prices may encourage potential clients to try your services in the belief that more expensive should mean better. Most technicians opt for the safer, cheaper route but, if you truly believe the service you are offering is the best, then charge a little bit more and make local standards higher rather than lower.

After you have done your research and decided where you want to price yourself, you must do your sums to make sure you will be covering all your costs and make a profit. This is difficult when opening a salon, as definite costs are not known until it has been open for a few months. However, if you want to succeed in your new venture or career, planning is very important. It is not sufficient to base your prices entirely on someone else's. What makes a good enough profit for them may not work at all for you.

Most product suppliers will be able to give you a rough idea of the cost of products used in specific treatments, particularly if you are using a complete branded range. If you buy your supplies from a wholesaler, this information is not always available so you will have to work it out yourself by estimating how many treatments can be given using each item. For example:

- A tub of hand cream at £10 (incl. VAT) will be sufficient for 20 manicures (or similar), therefore each manicure will cost 50p in hand cream.

Complete this exercise for each product you are going to use. Then make a list of all the products you use for each treatment, including all disposable items. This will give you a cost per treatment.

When you are still learning and need plenty of practice, it is a good idea to work out these costs to you and then offer to give treatments to all your friends and family. Ask them to pay for the products used, which will be a very small amount, and you will give your time for free. In this way everyone wins: they receive a treatment that is enjoyable and, hopefully, has good results, you get some practice at estimating quantities of products used and giving treatments without it costing you in products.

There are many other costs or overheads you need to take into account and these will depend on how you are planning to work. If you work as a mobile technician, then the cost of your car (petrol, tax, special insurance, servicing, wear and tear), professional insurance, wear and tear on your equipment, promotional material, etc. must be covered by the income you make. These costs would be similar if you work freelance from a salon without the travelling costs, but with the additional costs of rent (or equivalent) paid to the salon.

To make sure you have everything covered, add up all your costs or overheads for a year, then divide this figure by 12 to bring the overall costs down to an amount for each month. Divide this figure by the number of days you intend to work each month. This will give you a figure that you need to earn each day before you make any profit. If this is added to the approximate cost of products you can expect to use in a day, you will have a good idea of the total overheads you will incur by working.

If you are opening a salon, seeking professional advice to create a proper business plan is really essential. The principles are the same as above, but many more things need to be taken into account.

After you have carefully worked out your cost and pricing structure in this way, you will have a good idea of the cost of products plus the additional costs that need to be met and how they relate to your income from charges. It does seem an awful lot of work but it will be worth it, as it will ensure that you will earn a living from the skills you have worked to acquire.

TOP TIP

Remember that as a self-employed person, you are responsible for your own tax and National Insurance. This means that any profit you make will immediately be decreased by at least 30 per cent.

TOP TIP

Essential reading

- *Habia Code of Practice Nail Services*
- *Habia Health & Safety Nail Salons*
- *Nail Structure and Product Chemistry By Douglas Schoon*

Summary

This chapter has demonstrated how a safe and comfortable environment may be created and maintained by the technician to comply with all local and national legislative provisions on workplace health and safety in self- or salon employment. It has provided the necessary information on the use of tools and equipment and guided a technician towards appropriate service pricing structures.

ASSESSMENT OF KNOWLEDGE AND UNDERSTANDING

1. Why is it important to have suitable desks and chairs for treatments?

2. How do the Health & Safety at Work Act and the Control of Substances Hazardous to Health Regulations relate to the products being used?

3. What are the main 'routes of entry' of a chemical into the body?

4. How can potentially harmful chemicals be prevented from entering the body?

5. What are the three levels of decontamination?

6. Why is effective decontamination essential before, during and after each treatment?

7. Give one example of the type of products that could be used for disinfection and **sanitization**.

8. How should solvents be disposed of?

9. What is an allergic reaction?

10. How are metal tools effectively cleaned?

11. What does the term 'good working practices' mean?

12. What is the purpose of an accident book?

13. What is the Health & Safety Policy in a salon that relates to you?

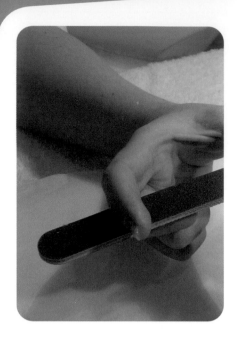

4

Preparing you and your client

Learning objectives

In this chapter you will learn about:

- how to prepare a safe working environment for you and your client

- how to recognize the skin and nail conditions that could restrict treatments

- how to recognize the skin and nail conditions that could prevent treatment

- the importance of a good client consultation

- how to provide suitable treatment advice

- what aftercare advice should be given.

Introduction

As discussed in Chapter 3, the preparation of the working area is very important for the comfort and safety of both the technician and their clients and in order to comply with the legal requirements that ensure the working environment is a safe place for all. From a technician's point of view, it is important that every client is safe, but clients are in the environment for only a short period of time while technicians are exposed to many hazards during all their working hours, and this chapter builds on Chapter 3 to detail how correct client preparation can be a crucial factor in workplace hygiene and sanitization. A thorough client consultation will also help you to provide the best possible service for your client.

'Making a remedy into a poison'

There are two quotations from a very useful textbook that are relevant to this issue and are always worth remembering:

- 'The Overexposure Principle'. This rule says, 'Every chemical substance has a safe and unsafe level of exposure. Simply touching, inhaling or smelling a potentially hazardous substance can't harm you. Exceeding the safe level of exposure is the danger you must learn to avoid.'

- 'Paracelus, a famous 14th-century physician, was the first to study and understand **toxic** substances. He said, "All substances are poisons; there is none which is not a poison. Only the right dose differentiates a poison from a remedy." Over the last 500 years, the public has forgotten what Paracelus discovered. The Overexposure Principle is the modern day interpretation of what he learned.' (Douglas D. Schoon, *Milady's Nail Structure and Product Chemistry,* Delmar Learning (Milady), 1996.)

Paracelus is correct; everything is potentially a poison, therefore we must avoid the dose that makes the remedy into a poison. All products should have a MSDS, available from the manufacturer or distributor. An **MSDS** provides the information on things such as how to store the product, any specific hazardous ingredients, emergency first aid advice, possible routes of entry, how to deal with large spills, and similar advice. It is obvious that the chemicals that are considered a potential hazard on any MSDS, or those that require a warning on their labels, are more likely to have a much lower 'poison' dose than any others. But technicians are not in the position to know what the 'poison' dose for each individual is for each of the chemicals. It is therefore far safer to assume that any dose is a potential 'poison' dose to prevent any problems.

Following all the simple rules for safety in Chapter 3 will ensure maximum protection. Further protection will be gained by following correct working practices, as described in this book, and also following the manufacturer's instructions on the use of the various products.

HEALTH & SAFETY

Water is essential to life but exceed the safety limit or be exposed to incorrect use and you can drown in it!

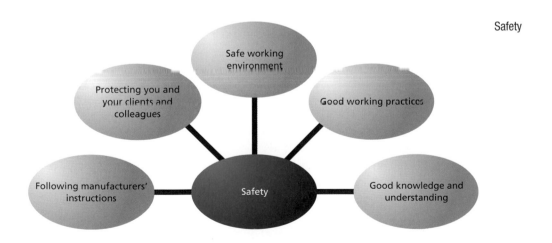

Safety

Allergies and overexposure

There are two frequent queries or worries that tend to be expressed by both experienced and new nail technicians. One of them concerns allergic reactions and the other is health and safety in the salon. There are some general rules that should be followed.

Allergies

Allergic reactions and sensitivities can occur to anyone at any time. Unfortunately, this is a very common problem in an industry that uses a variety of chemicals every day. However, it need not be such a problem if good working practices are adhered to, such as practising strict hygiene and not letting artificial nail products touch any soft tissue.

- Any individual, at any time, can become allergic to a particular product or food. It may be something that has been used for years or a few days but there is usually a warning that an allergy has developed, e.g. itchy skin, rash, headaches, etc. This happens when an individual has been exposed to too much of the product but every person's level of 'overexposure' is different.

- If a technician or client develops an unusual symptom, the most common one being an itchy rash on the hands or fingers, there is a likelihood that an allergy is starting. In the case of a technician, they must stop using the product or start wearing gloves and, in the case of a client all the products must be removed immediately. Do not wait to see if it gets worse: it will!

- If a client telephones you to tell you of a problem they have noticed ask them to come in to you as soon as possible. It is impossible to have a good idea of what the problem is without seeing it.

- If these actions are taken quickly enough, the symptoms may go fairly rapidly. If not, the condition will worsen and the hands could become swollen and bleed, with the nail plate lifted and distorted. Obviously, the chance of infection at this stage is very high and will make the whole condition even worse. It is really not worth taking the chance of reaching this stage.

- Once the product has been removed, the condition may go. If the client is willing, a different system could be tried which may be successful. If the initial reaction is severe, however, it would be a good idea to do a patch test in the same way as for lash tinting. There are a few products that are the most likely to cause an adverse reaction in any system. Top of the list is the liquid monomer in any acrylic system (or unreacted monomer that may be found as a sticky layer in a UV-cured system); an acid-based primer is corrosive so that could be the culprit if it has touched the skin; or sometimes it could be the nail adhesive. It is unlikely (but not impossible) that the dust from a cured acrylic will have any effect nor will the dust from a light-cured material as long as there is no trace of the 'sticky layer'. (Excess dust, however, can cause other problems, so it should not be considered safe.)

- If the condition does not go within a few days or if it should seem worse after the removal of all products, the client or technician should get medical advice. It is important to remember that technicians are not medically qualified and should never diagnose any condition. Instant removal of products as soon as any reaction is noticed is the only safe course of action; leaving it to see if it gets better is unacceptable and could result in legal action being taken against the technician and salon for negligence. To leave a product on a client knowing that it could be the cause of a reaction is negligent.

- There is little point in blaming the manufacturer or seeking recourse if things go wrong. Correct labelling should have all necessary warnings and a professional technician should be aware of how to use all products correctly and safely. We all know household bleach is corrosive and will burn skin and bleach clothes; whose fault is it when this happens with correctly labelled bottles?

ALWAYS REMEMBER

If a client should develop the signs of an allergic reaction it should be noted on the client record card. The steps as outlined above should be followed and these also noted. If you do not deal with this in a responsible manner you could be liable! All the advice available recommends these actions. There have been cases reported in the media of horrific results of an extreme allergic reaction. When discovering more about the situation it is almost always because the technician did not act quickly enough or failed to recognize the signs.

'Safe' levels of exposure

A little story that should raise a smile: it is not always easy to explain to some people about safe levels of exposure and how everyone is different. Some just cannot grasp such intangible concepts. I heard a comment recently, about a trainer who was running a course for beginners who, while struggling to explain this to one particular blankly-faced student, used an analogy of how products with peanuts seem to have been in the news in recent years as some people have developed an allergy to them. The light suddenly came on behind the student's eyes and a delighted voice said: 'Oh right, I see now. So which of these products have peanuts in them?'

Avoiding allergic reactions

Although allergies can be caused by just about any product, they are more common when providing nail enhancement services. Following simple working procedures will minimize the possibility for both the technician and their clients.

- Keep the nail desk clean and free from dust.

- Change the disposable towel between clients and several times during the service when dust is created.

- Do NOT touch the liquid monomer on any skin:

    - Avoid the skin surrounding the nail during application.

    - Do not touch the brush with your fingers.

    - Do not have a patch wet with monomer where you have wiped your brush and then lean in it.

- If using 'low odour' or UV-cured liquid and powder systems be aware of the dust on the client's fingers, your fingers and in the palm of your hand that is holding the client's finger. This usually has some unreacted monomer in it and can cause problems.

- When wiping away the inhibition layer on light-cured gels, start with the smallest finger and wipe from the cuticle to the free edge to avoid smearing uncured monomer onto the skin.

TOP TIP

If a technician develops a rash on the fingers of the hand using the file and the palm of the other hand it usually means that there is an amount of unreacted monomer on the surface of the overlay that is buffed off during the refining stage. The monomer is touching the fingers holding the file and dropping into the palm of the other hand. If this is happening often, an allergic reaction starts. More care at the removal of the sticky layer is needed or a longer **cure** time if the product is a light-cured liquid and powder system.

Treatable conditions and untreatable conditions

As nail specialists, it is important to be able to recognize various nail and skin conditions. There are many common conditions that do not prevent manicures or application of nail enhancements, others which need special care and, less commonly, some which prevent any treatment altogether.

ALWAYS REMEMBER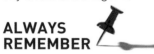

Always remember the two key rules:

1. Professional technicians are not doctors or dermatologists and therefore should not diagnose a medical condition.

2. If there is any doubt about a condition, do not continue, but suggest the client sees a specialist.

It is worth pointing out that if a client has an obvious medical condition of the skin or nails and is treated by a technician without an agreement from their GP or specialist, the technician's insurance can be void and he or she would be directly responsible for any claim against them should problems arise. It is often not practical to get an agreement from a doctor. If this is the case then the condition must be noted on the client record card and the client should sign it to say that they take responsibility for the nail service to go ahead.

Treatable nail conditions

These are conditions of the hands, feet and nails that do not prevent treatment, but an understanding of the condition is important as suitable care needs to be taken.

1 **Leukonychia:** white spots on the nail plate. Some people are more prone to these than others and it can depend on the client's occupation. If white spots are prevalent on most nails, there may be a systemic cause but, more commonly they are caused by minor trauma injuries to the matrix such as knocking. The spot is where the nail plate cell are distorted or not fully keratinized in a small area. The spot will grow out but is likely to be a slight problem when it reaches the end of the nail, as it may peel.

2 **Splinter haemorrhage:** tiny black streaks under the nail. Usually due to minor trauma and occasionally due to illness. They are splinter shaped due to the forward growth of the nail plate. They will grow out.

3 **Beau's lines:** horizontal ridges across the nail plate. This is where the natural nail growth has been interrupted within the matrix. Usually caused by an illness they can be hardly noticeable through to very deep indentations that could cause the nail to shed. The minor versions will grow out but should not be buffed to smooth them.

4 **Beaded ridges:** longitudinal lines with little bumps are usually associated with circulatory problems. Buffing them will thin the nail plate so should be avoided.

5 **Age related ridges:** longitudinal lines on some or all nails are quite normal and usually noticed in older clients. Again, buffing could thin the nail plate.

6 **Onychorrhexis associated with a furrow:** these are usually prone to splitting down from the free edge. This occurs when the matrix is permanently damaged at some stage. The nail plate grows slightly deformed and thinner in this area. If the damage is recent it may cure itself within a year. If the damaged part of the nail is prone to splitting extreme care should be taken at the free edge as it is very easy for infection to get into the nail bed. The nail should either be kept very short with no free edge or it could be protected from splitting by a thin, light overlay.

7 **Lamellar dystrophy:** peeling or flaking nails. Usually caused by dryness. Use gentle filing with a very fine emery board, moisturise nails and cuticles and advise client to avoid too much water, detergents, etc., apply a nail oil at least daily and perhaps keep a clear polish on the nails to seal the edges against more water damage.

8 **Onychophagy:** nail biting. Frequent manicures will help stop this problem, as the cuticle can be treated immediately to improve appearance and condition and that is often enough encouragement to stop the habit. Artificial nails can be applied but must be kept very short (to the end of the finger) and the client must return weekly until the natural nail has grown enough to support the artificial one.

9 **Furrows:** longitudinal lines from matrix to free edge. A single furrow may be congenital or caused by injury to the matrix (see above). Multiple furrows are usually

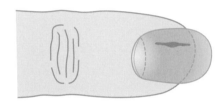

Splinter haemorrhage

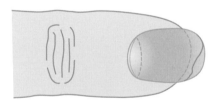

Beau's lines

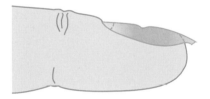

Lamellar dystrophy

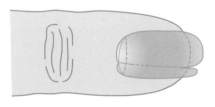

Onychorrhexis

caused systemically. Treat with care, as the furrow may be very thin. Do not over-buff to try to smooth the ridge as this will cause splitting.

10 **Blue nails:** nails with a bluish tinge. Usually due to poor circulation or sometimes illness. The nails are often weak and thin. Hand massage and careful buffing will stimulate the circulation in the area. Artificial nails are not recommended if the nails are very thin, as the treatment will cause too much trauma to the nail.

11 **Hangnail:** small tear in the cuticle or sharp point on the side of the nail, usually due to neglect of cuticles or dryness. The nail fold, if neglected, will often stick to the nail plate and, as the nail grows, is pulled with it. If this happens and the skin is over-stretched, it will split at the sides leaving a ragged corner. The lateral folds (side walls) can often produce sharp points of skin. Both of these may be carefully removed with a clean pair of nippers. This condition can be prevented by gently lifting the nail fold, when softened, from the nail bed and keeping it moisturised.

12 **Bruised nails:** dark spots of blood under the nail plate. Avoid the area if painful, if there is pressure under the nail or the bruise covers more than a quarter of the nail. Otherwise treat gently. The blood will eventually grow out.

13 **Eggshell nails:** thin, pale and fragile nails, usually curving under. Can be hereditary but can also be indicative of illness or medication. Treat very gently.

14 **Habit tic:** a series of horizontal ridges down the centre of the nail. Caused by picking at the nail fold. Usually associated with a very large and exposed lunula. Advise the client of the damage being done, but do not try to buff out.

15 **Koilonychia:** flat or spoon-shaped nails, which are thin and soft. Can be caused by an iron deficiency or excessive exposure to oils or soaps. Treat gently.

16 **Pitting:** small pits over the surface of the nail, usually due to psoriasis or dermatitis. Can also be caused by applying a cortisone cream to another area of the body. Treat gently.

17 **Pterygium:** this is an abnormal condition where the skin adheres to the nail plate and is stretched by the nail growth. This usually happens as a result of damage to the area at the base of the nail and can also be seen under the free edge. Warm oil manicures and gently massaging oil into the area will help but never try to remove it. Avoid using any solvent-based product.

18 **Psoriasis** of the nail: a mild case of this condition is seen as pitting on the nail. The nail will be delicate and must be treated with care. A more sever condition can result in the destruction of the nail plate and should not be treated.

Common and avoidable nail conditions

1 **Bacterial infection ('Greenies')** This is, unfortunately, a common condition seen during nail services. This is caused by an overlay lifting from the nail plate and bacteria entering. The warm moist environment is a perfect condition for the bacteria to grow. It is seen as an area that is discoloured. This starts as a faint yellow and can progress, if left untreated, to a very dark green. This colour is a by-product of the bacteria and not the bacteria itself. It will remain as a stain on the nail plate even after the bacteria has gone. If this is treated early it will not cause any long-lasting problem. But, if left, can, eventually destroy the nail plate!

This is virtually always associated with an area of lifted overlay and can be treated by a technician if caught early. To do this, remove all the existing overlay by gently

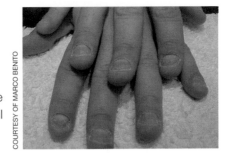

Severe nail biter

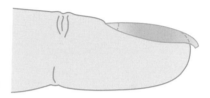

Eggshell nails

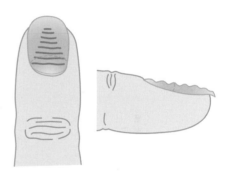

Habit tic

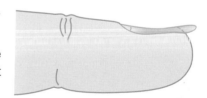

Koilonychia

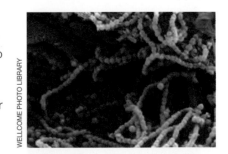

Example of a microscopic bacteria - streptococcus bacteria on the tongue

buffing or soaking in **acetone** depending on the type of overlay. Throw away the buffer used and the disposable towel that has caught the dust. Then dehydrate the nail. Now the environment does not support the bacterial life. The stain will remain until it grows out but should not change in colour or size. It is safe to reapply the overlay.

As this is caused by lifting, the technician should take care with the nail preparation and application procedures. Also the client should be advised to return if they notice any lifting of the overlays. It is possible to have a bacterial infection after just a few days of lifting!

Skin conditions where restricted services can be offered

1 **Hyperidrosis:** this is over-activity of the sweat glands on the feet. If the condition is severe, then the client should be referred to a GP or chiropodist. It can be quite mild and is sometimes detected by the very soft skin and even 'pulpy' skin between the toes (not to be confused with athlete's foot). The client should keep the feet clean and dry at all times and the use of a fungicidal foot powder may be helpful.

2 **Corns:** this is a patch of hard skin often found on the side or top of the toes and usually caused by pressure from ill-fitting shoes. The surface of this can be removed during the hard skin removal stage but, if the corn is big, the client should be referred to a chiropodist.

3 **Callus:** similar to a corn, but over a larger area such as the heel or under the foot.

4 **Bunion:** a misaligned toe joint. This can be very painful so care must be taken when working in the area.

Other common skin conditions

1 **Dermatitis:** this is a general term that describes a non-specific inflammation of the skin. This is common with nail technicians and often due to overexposure! The subject has been extensively covered in Chapters 3 and 4. this type is called allergic contact dermatitis. This is not necessarily localized and can be anywhere on the skin. There is another type commonly seen in salons. That is irritant contact dermatitis. This is caused where the skin has been irritated by contact with some substances. Frequent hand washing can sometimes be the cause and products such as disinfectants. This type of skin condition is localized to the area of skin that has been in contact with the irritant.

If a technician develops allergic dermatitis then gloves are essential! If a client already has dermatitis then any nail services will need some restrictions. The client will probably be aware of what products affect their skin so these should be avoided. If they do not know what causes their condition all skin products should be avoided.

If the skin around the nail is unaffected, services that treat just the nail can be provided but extra care must be taken to avoid touching the skin.

Recommended additional reading: *Nail Structure and Product Chemistry*, Doug Schoon.

2 **Eczema and psoriasis:** these are common skin conditions. They are both red inflamed skin and are usually seen in specific areas of the body. Psoriasis is usually characterized by scaly plaques on the skin. Neither of them are transmitted but both need careful treatment. If there is any sign of them on the hands then water and

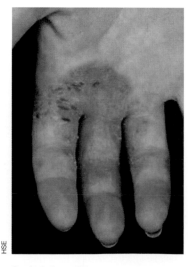

HSE

Contact dermatitis

perfumed creams should be avoided. Most sufferers of these conditions know what is best for them but, remember one of the important rules: if in doubt, don't!

Untreatable conditions

These are conditions where the technician must not give any treatment. If you are unsure whether you may treat, refer your client to their GP for permission.

1   **Infections/inflammation:** if there is any noticeable infection or inflammation, treatment should be avoided. Not only is there the possibility of aggravating the condition, there is also, in the case of infection, a risk of the technician becoming infected. Examples of this are:

- Infected **hangnail**.

- **Whitlow** – localized painful, swollen area at the side or base of the nail plate.

- **Paronychia** – inflammation of the soft tissue surrounding the nail. This can be painful and is caused by the same bacteria as causes the green stain seen on the surface of the nail between the nail plate and overlay. The area should be avoided and the client advised to use a mild antiseptic, asking a pharmacist or, if severe, going to their doctor.

- **Warts** – raised lumps of horny tissue, caused by a contagious viral infection. These are highly contagious. Avoid the area and advise seeing the pharmacist.

- **Verruca** – found on the foot. This is similar to a wart but is in-growing. It can often be identified by a black spot in the centre. A chiropodist should treat this or a pharmacist can advise on the appropriate product to use.

2   **Onychocryptosis:** ingrown nail. More often seen on toes but can occur on the fingers. Often associated with inflammation and pain. Suggest that the client sees a chiropodist. It can be avoided by rounding the corner of the toenails to avoid a sharp corner that can embed itself into the soft tissue.

3   **Onycholysis:** separation of the nail plate from nail bed. Seen as a white area. This can be an allergic reaction and is often associated with a fungal or bacterial infection. If a narrow white area is noticed on several nails, it is usually the beginning of an allergic reaction. All products, including nail varnish must be removed from the nails. If the condition does not improve quickly, the client should see their GP. If the seal is broken under the free edge, fungal or bacterial infections can enter and grow on the nail bed. A GP's or pharmacist's advice should be sought. Sometimes, psoriasis can cause separation, but this is usually associated with pitting or other evidence of the disorder. This can also happen if the nail plate is thinned by over-buffing or improper use of an electric file. The bond between the nail plate and the nail bed can be disrupted if the nail is too thin and flexible. This is one of the important reasons why a nail plate must not be damaged during nail services.

4   **Onychomadesis:** the nail becomes loose at the cuticle and the new nail pushes the old one off. This is usually caused by a severe trauma in the cuticle area. The base of the nail separates from the nail bed but the new growth will continue to push the old nail plate forward. This is quite common on the big toe and often with clients who play a lot of sport. If the toenail has any free edge, tight-fitting shoes put pressure on the nail and acts as a lever, lifting it up in the matrix area. It will eventually grow off the finger or toe. It is very easy to get an infection under the departing nail so it must be kept clean and dry. If there is no sign of any infection it may be possible to apply a thin overlay to the toe to stop it being ripped off by accident.

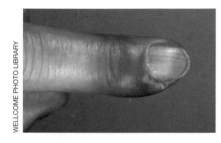

WELLCOME PHOTO LIBRARY

Paronychia

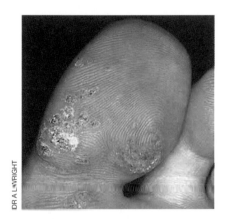

DR A L WRIGHT

Verruca

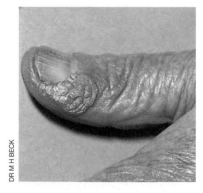

DR M H BECK

A wart

5   **Onychomycosis:** lifting, discoloration or rotting of the nail plate. A fungal or bacterial infection. Some fungi feed on the non-living keratin of the nail, others on living tissue. Any infection must be avoided and the client referred to a GP.

6   **Fungal infections** of the skin or nails: This is sometimes noticed as white areas under the nail plate. An example of a fungal infection of the skin of the feet is athlete's foot. This is usually noticed between the toes as flaky, cracking skin that can look quite wet. This is contagious and should be treated by the client before any pedicure can take place.

The professional technician and communication

When meeting someone for the first time, a person has only one chance to make a 'first impression', but this impression can have enormous implications for the future of the relationship. As a professional person, the first, second and every impression the technician has on the client is important.

A technician can be an amazingly good practitioner when it comes to applying nails or providing manicures, but will not be taken seriously if their appearance and manner towards their client is inappropriate.

When dealing with the public, personal hygiene and dress requires certain standards. Just think how you would expect a professional person to be when you are paying for their services and hoping to be confident in their advice and skills. You would expect them to be clean, neat and tidy and following an acceptable dress code for the environment in which they work.

There is a large aspect of 'nails' that is connected with image and a professional working within that type of industry should promote a good image. It is not always necessary for a technician to wear a clinical white uniform, unless the establishment has such a dress code, but a technician should be suitably dressed in clean and pressed clothes that are of a style that cannot cause any offence to anyone. A technician's nails should be well cared for and immaculate. Jewellery on the hands should be kept to a minimum for the safety of the technician (products could get trapped under jewellery and cause a skin reaction) and hair should be worn in a way that does not impede working.

A professional approach in manner is also very important. Clients should not be kept waiting but, as this is sometimes unavoidable, it helps if it is dealt with rather than ignored. If a technician is running late with a previous client, acknowledgement of the situation must be made with apologies. The waiting client must be comfortable and made to feel that they are important, their custom is valued and their patience in waiting appreciated. If waiting is unacceptable to a client who has arrived on time for an appointment, remember it is not their fault and they may be pressed for time. Everything must be done for that client's convenience; for example, another technician (or junior) could start to prepare the client for their treatment or someone else might finish the late running client.

Those dealing with the public, especially in the service industries, must have good communication skills. Their approach, while professional, should also be friendly and interested. They should make the client feel at ease and comfortable, and genuinely important.

A common mistake of those working in this type of industry, and one often parodied, is the technician who continually talks about themselves, their relationships, their social life, their clothes, etc. More often than not, clients are not actually interested in their technician but are much more interested in themselves, their nails and what their technician is doing in the

TOP TIP

Hair that is continually being tucked behind the ears could create an allergic reaction on the face Tie or clip it back.

treatment. Use the time during a treatment usefully and educate your client in understanding what they need to do with their nails, hands and feet. You have a captive audience so use the time wisely. The education of clients is essential so they understand the service you have provided for them. They need to take care of their nails when they have left you and retailing suitable products should be a routine part of the service without making them uncomfortable in a 'hard sell' situation.

Client consultation and assessment

Initial information

Assessing the client for treatment is a very important part of every client's appointment. It is a requirement of the NOS and the keeping of records is a requirement for insurance purposes. It is widely accepted that the first appointment with a new client warrants a client consultation; what is very often missed is the importance of a consultation before every treatment. A full client consultation should provide a great deal of important information:

- **Name, address and telephone number:** this is obvious, but it is a very useful tool for the professional technician. The address can allow you to do mail shots, send invitations to special events, greetings cards, etc. A record of a daytime and evening telephone number can also be essential if a problem arises with an appointment, such as a technician who is unwell. A timely call to the client can avoid unnecessary travel or upset schedules.

- **Date of birth:** this is a recognized part of an individual's identification, although it is not necessary information for a nail technician. Some clients are not forthcoming with their date of birth and it can be an optional element. One use would be to send a regular client a birthday card as a good PR exercise. If a technician suspects a client is under 16 years, then the question of age must be asked, as it is necessary for under 16s to have a letter of consent for any treatment from a parent or guardian. A minor should also be accompanied by an adult for the whole service.

- **Name of GP:** this is another piece of information that could be considered to be intrusive. There are not many circumstances when a technician would need to contact a client's GP. If medical assistance is sought or approval is needed from a GP, it is the responsibility of the client to get it and the technician to keep that approval on record in case of later problems. There are some advanced beauty treatments where a GP's information would be useful, but there is no reason why this should apply to nail treatments.

- **Occupation:** a useful piece of information, not only for conversational reasons but also to give an idea of the type of nails a client could cope with. It could also offer clues to any nail and skin problems.

- **Medical history:** with nail treatments, it is unnecessary to go into any medical history in any depth. A client may be quite willing to tell their technician all manner of medical details but what, as a technician, can be done with that information? Without medical training, the implications of the many illnesses and conditions cannot be known. There are some that are relevant in a general way and the main questions that should be asked are:

    - **Allergies:** If a client is prone to allergies, there is a good chance that they may be allergic to some of the products that will be used. If this is the case, it would be a good idea to carry out a skin test on a test nail.

- **Diabetes:** if a client suffers from this condition great care must be taken with all treatments. Circulation is often poor and consequently diabetics are slow to heal. Any injury sustained during a treatment could therefore result in a problem. Diabetics who do not have their condition under control and are unwell should really have approval from their doctor before embarking on any course of treatment.

- **Other:** a general enquiry of the client should be made to ascertain whether there is any other condition that may be relevant to nail treatment, for example any loss of sensation in the hands or fingers, past nail or skin conditions that may reoccur and heart conditions that may affect circulation in the extremities.

- **Previous nail treatments:** it is worth finding out if the client has received nail treatments in the past. Results from these treatments would be useful to know, as a sensitivity to products may have occurred or the client may be unable to keep on artificial nails owing to lifestyle or habits (like nail biting or picking).

- **The condition of the skin and nails:** this should be noted on the client's record card at this early stage. If everything looks healthy and in good condition, it should be noted in case something changes at a later stage. If there is any indication of a skin or nail condition, whether it restricts treatment or not, *it must be noted*. Obviously any condition that prevents treatment should be noted, together with the recommendations made by the technician. On occasions when medical approval is necessary, the letter should be attached to the card. Sometimes doctors are not prepared to give a letter. If this is the case, but the client has seen a doctor who has verbally agreed to the treatment, this should be noted on the card and the client sign to say that this is true. The technician has then done everything possible to safeguard both the client and themselves.

If there is any condition, however minor, that is noticed on hands, fingers or nails, it should be noted with a full description. The reason for this is to make sure that the condition does not get worse. Examples could be minor nail separation or a minor skin condition on the hands. This is an area where great care must be taken. The technician must be confident that any treatment will be safe. If there is any doubt, all treatments should be avoided especially where irritating chemicals are involved.

Treatment advice

The initial information-gathering part of the consultation should provide the technician with lots of preliminary ideas as to potential treatments. This information should be gathered in an area of the salon where other clients and technicians cannot overhear, as some people do not want others to know their personal details. The client can be asked to complete a questionnaire on their own.

The next questions that need to be asked concern the treatment that the client expects during the appointment. An important piece of information would be to find out exactly what the client *expects from the treatment*. It can often be the case that, owing to a lack of knowledge or understanding, the client may expect the most amazing results. A common expectation is for the client to think that a set of artificial nails will stay on forever and never need any maintenance. Another commonly held belief is that artificial nails damage natural nails. This could mean that the client thinks that they can never have artificial nails as they are not prepared to accept the damage or it could mean that they are ready to accept the damage for the sake of beautiful nails. Obviously this is wrong and the technician needs to thoroughly explain that damage will not occur if the nails are correctly applied and maintained and if homecare advice is followed.

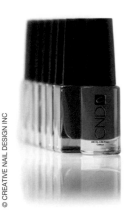

© CREATIVE NAIL DESIGN INC

The treatment booked is not always the best one for the client and another treatment may be more appropriate. The reasons for this are varied but three common situations are when:

- The client has nails and surrounding skin in poor condition and expects one manicure to put it right immediately. This will not happen. Several manicures may be necessary and they will need to support the improvement you are trying to achieve by following careful homecare advice.

- The client has reasonably long nails but they are in poor condition or a bad shape. The client may be unaware that natural nails can be overlaid to strengthen them and correct the shape and has assumed that artificial nails are the only option.

- The client does not realize that a full set of artificial nails requires a commitment of both time and finances. They may be prepared to wait a little longer for long nails and start a course of manicures that still involves time but does not cost as much. If they are not prepared to commit to either the time or the financial aspects, it may be better to suggest that they should not have artificial nails as neglecting them will result in damage.

Once this discussion has taken place it is worth reminding the client of all the options available in order that both parties are sure the correct choice is being made. The technician should note down on the record card what the treatment is and what the client's expectations are. This can be referred to later to see if the expectations were fulfilled and it is also useful if another technician treats the client.

Data Protection Act 1998

This Act affects any establishment or person that processes personal data and a client record card is classed as personal data. The previous Act was concerned with data that was to be stored electronically, that is on a computer and therefore only affected salons that used an automated record and booking system. The Act has been updated to include any relevant filing system or accessible system.

The general principles of the Act are:

- Personal information is fairly and lawfully processed. It is reasonable to assume that a certain amount of information about clients must be collected and stored.

- The information is processed for the relevant purpose and will not be processed for any other reason. For example, it will not be passed on to any third party or used for any purpose other than efficient and effective salon business.

- Personal data shall be adequate, relevant and not excessive in relation to the purpose. Therefore, there is no need to go into in-depth medical history that cannot be used by a technician. This may be appropriate for more advanced beauty treatments but not nail treatments.

- The information will be accurate and kept up-to-date.

- The record will not be kept longer than necessary. So if a client has not returned for a considerable time, their record is destroyed.

- Data subjects have rights and these must be observed.

- All reasonable measures will be taken to avoid unauthorized or unlawful processing or accidental loss or destruction. Client records should be kept in a safe and secure place and should not be removed from the salon.

BEST PRACTICE

At the end of the consultation and discussion on treatments, the information should be recorded in writing on the client's record card. This should include all the information about the client and the condition of their nails and skin, their expectations of the treatment, the recommendations of the technician and the treatment that has been agreed. The client should then sign this and a note made of which technician carried out the treatment.

There is a new category that involves 'sensitive' personal data and this has additional safeguards. There is no reason why any data of this nature would be kept on a record card. It involves areas such as racial or ethnic origin (skin type is relevant, but this has no real bearing on ethnic origin), political opinions or religious beliefs, physical or mental health.

The additional safeguards require the person to give their explicit consent to these data being processed. This means that if any reference to racial origin or physical health is made, the client must read it, understand and sign to say that this has been read and is approved. Therefore a signature will cover this requirement.

There is no need to be overly concerned by this Act, if reasonable and professional procedures are followed with regard to record cards.

Products and aftercare

Details of products used should be noted, if there are options, and some technicians, especially during training, like to make a note of the size of tips used. The importance of **aftercare** or homecare advice cannot be stressed enough. The easiest way of ensuring this happens is to provide every client with a pre-typed list of aftercare points with space to add any extra ones. If this list is given to the client, it should be noted on the record card. Then, if a client returns with a problem and insists that they were not told what to do, there is a record that this is not the case.

All of this information forms the full treatment plan for the individual client and it should be kept in the salon in a secure place. On subsequent appointments, the record card should be available and read through before any treatment begins (see Chapter 9).

Client preparation

After the client consultation has finished, the technician and the client must be prepared.

Cleansing the hands

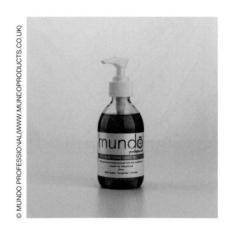

The first step is to ensure that the hands of both the technician and client are clean and that any protective equipment required is in place (such as a mask or a plaster for cuts on the client's or technician's hands).

- The most common form of hand cleaning is soap, preferably antibacterial, and water. If this method is used, great care must be taken to dry the nails and surrounding area. It is better if disposable towels are used for this to avoid the spread of any bacteria from unclean terry towels or hot air dryers.

- The free edge of the nail should be cleaned using a nail brush (see Chapter 3).

- There are many antibacterial **gels** and sprays available on the market today that can make the use of water unnecessary. These can be used by both the technician and the client at the desk and can often be a much more efficient method of decontaminating the hands. Some branded products will state which bacteria and viruses will be eliminated and many will be much more effective than antibacterial soap and water. There is also the additional benefit of not having to leave the desk. (NB: this method does not clean under the nails.)

- The technician should be aware that hand washes and antibacterial soaps can build up on the skin if not thoroughly rinsed and frequent hand washing will dry out the hands. Regular applications of a moisturising hand cream or barrier cream will benefit the hands of the technician.

The technician and the client are now ready to begin the agreed treatment.

Client Record Card

Summary

This chapter has explained how to conduct a good client consultation while being able to recognize treatable and non-treatable nail and skin conditions. It has shown how to create a safe and comfortable environment for both technician and client and has provided the necessary information for suitable treatment and homecare advice.

ASSESSMENT OF KNOWLEDGE AND UNDERSTANDING

1 What is 'overexposure'?

2 How can overexposure be avoided?

3 Why is effective communication with clients so important at the consultation stage?

4 What treatment alternatives should clients be aware of?

5 Why is it important that clients understand all aspects of the treatment, homecare and subsequent treatment requirements?

6 Why are client record cards necessary?

7 How does the Data Protection Act affect you?

8 How are the correct methods of correct product usage discovered?

9 Name four treatable conditions of the nails.

10 Name four untreatable conditions of the nails.

11 Name four treatable conditions of the skin.

12 Name four untreatable conditions of the skin.

13 Why should a technician be able to recognize nail and skin conditions?

14 How would you avoid an allergic reaction?

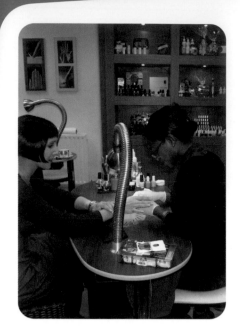

5

Providing a manicure treatment

Learning objectives

In this chapter you will learn about:

- **what a manicure is**

- **all the techniques used in a treatment and their purpose**

- **painting techniques**

- **the purpose of products used**

- **additional treatments, their procedure and purpose**

- **various treatment alternatives and their timings**

- **aftercare advice.**

Introduction

There are many variations to treatments that improve the hands and natural nails. This chapter explains in detail the various techniques that may be used during these treatments, their purpose and value and procedural steps for a variety of treatments.

Why a manicure?

Our hands are obviously very important parts of our body and should be kept in good condition. For centuries, both men and women have decorated their hands to make them more interesting and attractive or to demonstrate their class or standing in society. Today the reason for looking after your hands is probably a little simpler: appearance is important to most people and good looking hands and nails are a part of good grooming, plus the decoration of the hands with jewellery and paint on the nails is very much part of today's fashion culture.

A **manicure** is becoming a more commonplace treatment for both sexes. The importance of appearance continues to grow and the availability of disposable income increases with every generation. Another reason for the importance of this treatment is the fact that their owner sees the hands all the time! A 'bad hair day' or a blemish on the face can usually be forgotten until someone looks in a mirror. Dry skin on the hands, short or broken nails, chipped or old polish usually makes a person want to hide their hands and not use them where they will become too noticeable. However, good looking hands and nails can be displayed and used more in emphasizing a glass or pointing to an object. In fact, they can make the person feel better and more confident and are in evidence to their owner every moment of the day.

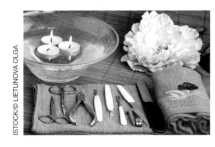

ISTOCK/© LIETUNOVA OLGA

Hand and nail treatments

There are several levels of treatment that are relevant to the hands and nails. The manicurist can carry out some of them and others will require a medical practitioner.

- The simplest treatment (other than good homecare) would be a short manicure that temporarily improve the appearance of the hands and/or nails. This would be appropriate for a client whose hands and nails are in excellent condition and wants this to be maintained with perhaps the addition of having the nails painted. Alternatively, it would suit a client who has time or financial restrictions and needs a fast or inexpensive treatment maybe in the form of an application of hand cream or a reshape of the nails plus paint or it might concentrate on improving the nails.

- The next level would be a manicure that was part of a treatment plan that improved the condition of the skin and nails suffering from common conditions such as dry, rough skin or weak, peeling, dry, brittle or bitten nails. The condition of the hands and nails cannot be dramatically improved immediately, so this type of treatment would be part of a plan for the client that was working towards permanently improving these type of conditions. It could also be a one-off treat for a client who wanted a bit of pampering.

- A manicurist cannot diagnose or treat more serious hand or nail conditions and the client should, initially, see their GP who may be able to recommend and prescribe a course of treatment. A pharmacist can treat some conditions, such as minor eczema or dermatitis and minor fungal or bacterial infections.

- If a condition is difficult to diagnose or treat by a GP then referral will be made to a dermatologist who may recognize the condition or conduct various tests in order to accurately diagnose and treat the condition.

The following section takes each stage of a manicure treatment, explains its purpose and benefits and how the procedure is carried out. Although the stages are in a logical order they do not necessarily relate to a complete treatment. The next section discusses the various manicure options and lists the stages in the order they should be carried out.

Manicure treatments

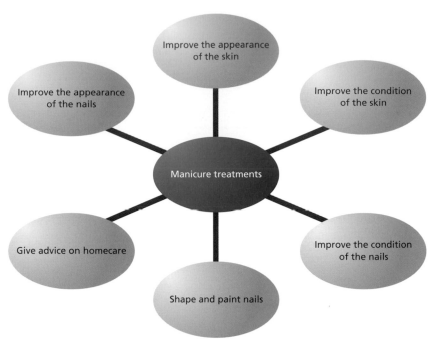

ALWAYS REMEMBER

A manicurist must never diagnose a skin or nail condition that has a medical or systemic basis. Simple environmental damage, such as dry skin or peeling nails, are part of the manicurist's remit, together with individual characteristics that result in similar, common conditions such as weak, thin nails or delicate skin. The manicurist will come across many different conditions on many different clients and must be able to recognize all the more common ones and know when a manicure can continue and improve the condition (e.g. peeling nails, dehydrated skin), when a manicure can continue but with certain restrictions (e.g. when bruising or minor eczema are present) or when a manicure treatment cannot be carried out and a client should be referred to a pharmacist or GP (e.g. severe eczema, fungal or bacterial infections).

Manicure techniques
Filing

It is easier to file a nail into a good shape when it is at it hardest (that is before it is put into water or soaked with oils). This is because an over-hydrated nail will have a tendency to bend and it will be difficult to achieve a smooth and even edge. Also, the moisture may disturb the natural bonds between the nail plate layers and filing could cause the layers to separate.

For all natural nails, a very fine file or emery board must be used. The edge of the nail is easily damaged by causing trauma to the layers and a harsh **abrasive** will splinter the layers and cause them to part.

If you imagine the nail plate as being similar to a piece of plywood, layers of the wood can be seen when looking at the edge. This is how the nail plate layers are at the free edge. Now imagine using a heavy rasp on that edge; the thin wood layers would splinter leaving a ragged edge, especially if the rasp were used in a backwards and forwards motion. Think of using sandpaper on the edge of the plywood; the edge would be smooth and

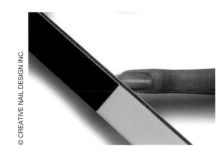

not splintered and the **glue** between the layers would still be intact holding them tightly together to form a solid piece of wood. This is exactly what happens to the nail plate when a rough file is used in comparison to a very fine file.

Thinking of the same piece of wood, again, imagine a large pair of pincers cutting into the extreme edge to make the piece of wood shorter. The layers would be squashed between the blades and the thin layers would splinter. Now imagine the wood being cut with very fine and very sharp blades that slice through the wood with very little pressure, leaving behind only minimal damage and splintering, which a fine sandpaper could smooth away. This is what happens when any tool other than one with extremely sharp blades is used to cut nails.

When removing length, it is important to file from the side of the nail into the middle and then from the other side into the middle. Again, reference can be made to our piece of plywood: working against the grain of the wood or against a curve causes trauma and more splintering, whereas filing with the grain or in the direction of the curve is smooth. Filing downwards towards the side of the nail can not only damage the layers, but also feels most uncomfortable for the client.

When shortening the nail, the file should be held at right angles to the edge of the nail as this will efficiently remove the edge. When the right length has been achieved, first of all bevel the top of the nail to help 'seal' the nail plate against water invasion, then angle the file slightly under the edge to refine the shape and help to seal the edge of the layers.

The top layer of nail is slightly harder than lower layers so, by making this slightly longer it will help to protect the end-on layers from the trauma of knocks (e.g. typing, tapping nails on a hard surface), which can cause the layers to peel.

It is very important to the condition of the nail that the layers are kept sealed. The slightest break in the bonds between the layers allows water to seep between them and cause more bonds to break down. This is the main cause of peeling nails and therefore weak nails. Day-to-day living causes trauma to the nail plate and the bonds between the layers. Knocking the nails, using the ends of the fingers, washing the hands, putting hands in cleaning chemicals, etc. are likely to cause minor (or major) layer separation. Without attention, this situation can become a vicious circle with water seepage, layer separation, top layer peeling so the seal cannot be repaired and therefore more water seepage occurs.

A client, following the manicurist's advice, should remove the extreme edge of the nail at least once a week either during a regular manicure or once a week following a weekly home maintenance routine. The ends of hair become dry and split with day-to-day living and these are removed during a trim in order to keep the hair healthy looking and prevent the hair breaking off. This is exactly the same as nails but the 'trim' needs to be more frequent as nails suffer more abuse.

The shape of the filed nail should be to the preference of the client who may follow the current fashion or have a personal preference. If client has no real preference and leaves the decision to the manicurist, the shape that best suits the finger is the one that mirrors the shape of the cuticle.

Other shape options would be **oval**, **square**, **'squoval'**, or **tapered**. It is important with all shapes to maintain the strength of the nail. The weakest part of the nail is on the sides where it leaves the protection of the lateral nail folds. This is one of the most common places for breakages to occur. The edge of the nail plate where it leaves this part of the finger is quite thick but if it is filed away a thinner, weaker nail plate is exposed. This part

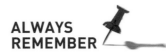
ALWAYS REMEMBER

If nails need to be severely shortened, cutting with a sharp pair of scissors of clippers followed by filing with a fine emery board is safe. For minor length reduction, a file is all that is needed.

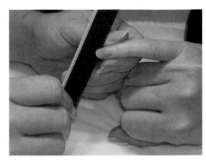
Filing from sides to middle

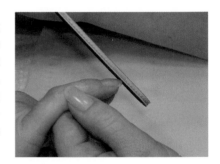
Bevelling the nail

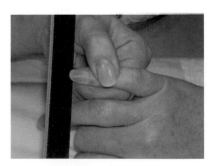
Finishing with the file – file is angled slightly under the edge

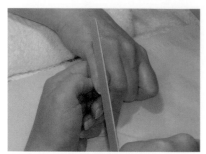

File down finger for even free edge

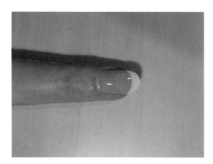

Oval nail

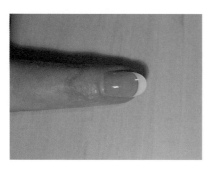

Tapered nail

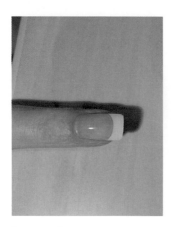

Square nail

of the nail must be allowed to grow straight before any curve is created. Even on an oval or tapered shape, the edge of the nail plate must not be filed for the first 1–2 mm.

The nail shape should be even and not longer one side and all the fingers should be the same shape. A client comes to a manicurist because this may be a difficult effect to achieve on themselves and expects a manicurist to be experienced and skilled at creating the finished results. However, not everyone has a natural eye for form, shape and balance and many less experienced manicurists and technicians file a shape that leans to one side. This is not acceptable and there are ways of checking that the shape is even and in line with the finger.

Take an emery board (not a buffer or thick file) and place it, upright down the centre of the finger and nail. Few fingers are straight so an overall middle line should be found. Then look at the shape of the free edge, first one side of the file and then the other. They should match each other and be perfectly even. The most common fault, and one to look out for, is the shape of the free edge on either side of the file. One side can be very different from the other but, without the help of the file, they can look the same.

This technique can also be very helpful when creating a perfect free edge shape.

- For an oval or tapered shape, place the file along the centre line of the finger. Look at the placement of the file on the extreme edge of the nail. This is where the centre of the oval should be: central to the finger. Sometimes the shape of the **eponychium**, that may be uneven on the finger, disguises the centre of the finger. This is not so important if the nails remain unpainted, but if the nails are painted, the free edge will look uneven. When the 'middle' has been clearly identified, the nail can be shaped using the sides-to-middle movement.

- For square or 'squoval' shapes, the 'squareness' of the nail needs to be at right angles to the finger. Place the file as before and look at the free edge. The extreme edge of the nail on one side of the file should be at right angles to the file. If necessary, place another file on top of the first and at right angles to it to see where the straight edge of the nail needs to be.

  For an extreme square, file this straight edge and leave the sharp corners of the nail intact or, for a less extreme square, create this straight edge and then slightly angle the file under the free edge to remove the sharpness of the corners. For 'squoval', create the straight edge first and then round it off to make a slight curve on the extreme edge.

Obviously the length of the nail is another element of the shape to take into account. This should be dictated by either the preference of the client or the condition of the nails.

A longer nail is weaker than a short one and it would be difficult to grow a long nail if the condition is very weak or peeling. Although client preference is important, as a general rule a natural nail is reasonably strong and looks very good if the free edge is no longer than one-third of the length of the nail bed. This can be thought of as the 'pink and white' parts. If the white is too long the nail is weaker and does not look naturally attractive. However, if a client likes a longer white and is prepared to look after a weaker nail, that is their prerogative.

Cuticle removal

This is often an area of some confusion for manicurists and consumers and it is very important that a good manicurist fully understands this area and how to deal with it.

Return to Chapter 2 where the nail unit is described and make sure you have a good understanding of the difference between the **lateral nail fold**, the **eponychium** and the **cuticle**.

Where the skin of the finger folds back to create a seal with the nail plate (eponychium), it is the extreme upper layers of the epidermis that forms the frame in this area of the nail plate. There are no dermal layers on the edge of this fold and no supply of nerves and blood capillaries. It is literally a fold in the epidermis and appears as a pale, almost clear, margin around the nail. This is *not the cuticle* and should not be removed.

The cuticle (as its name implies: a thin layer on the surface) is a layer of epidermal skin that is shed from under the nail fold and sticks to the nail plate. It is this that can be removed but not as far back as the seal of the eponychium.

The effects of not removing cuticle are:

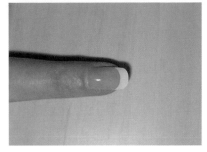

Squoval nail

- The skin of the nail fold sticks to the cuticle and the cuticle sticks to the nail plate. The nail grows and so does the cuticle. The nail fold gets pulled along with this growth and the depth of the fold of the epidermis increases as it is pulled up the nail. This results in an unsightly margin of skin around the nail that, when pulled beyond its elasticity will split at the sides. This split can be sore and become infected. It always becomes dry and annoying.

- Nail polish does not bond with skin; it peels off. If the cuticle is left on the nail plate then any polish applied will probably peel off in this area.

When the cuticle is softened with water, oil or proprietary removers, it is very easy to remove it from the surface of the nail. Usually, the correct use of a good cuticle knife will make an efficient job of this with the very occasional use of a pair of clean, sharp cuticle nippers.

When the cuticle is removed in this way, the nail fold has nothing to stick to and is therefore lifted from the surface of the nail. This lifted area of skin should not be cut off! Cutting it may result in a very neat frame to the nail but this is living skin and part of the skin of the finger. The body has excellent mechanisms to protect itself and cutting living skin stimulates the body to grow stronger skin in that area. Hence, continual cutting in this area results in thick, rough skin that grows back quicker and quicker.

The nail fold only grows in depth because it is being pulled by nail growth. If the cuticle is removed and the lifted nail fold kept moisturised and healthy, it will shrink back to a small neat margin around the base of the nail.

Therefore, cuticle nippers may be used to remove cuticle *not* the skin of the nail fold. They may also be used to nip off spikes of nail or skin (hangnails) that sometimes appear tucked inside the lateral nail folds. These can sometimes become very hard and dry and annoying. Pulling at them or biting them can sometimes break the skin and a painful infection can result.

> **TOP TIP**
>
> Advise the client to massage the cuticle area with nail oil daily. This will condition the skin and minimize the growth of the nail fold by preventing it from sticking to the cuticle and therefore shrinking.

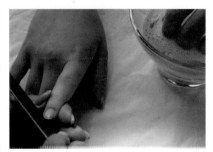

Soak

Good client education and homecare advice is necessary during this part of the treatment. Clients should be encouraged not to request excessive nipping and, if the process is explained to them, should understand the reasons and outcomes. If the nail fold is very overgrown, it will not look very neat after the first treatment and it is essential that the client understands why this is. It is also essential that the client understands that this area must be kept moisturised several times a day as it will become dehydrated very quickly and become annoying and hard. The skin will quickly shrink and, with continued care, will stop being a problem.

Some clients may insist that the skin is cut off. This is really not recommended and it becomes even more important to make sure the client understands what the results will be. However, it may, *on occasion*, be unreasonable to refuse, for example, if this is a first treatment on a severely overgrown area of skin, it will look extremely unsightly when lifted from the nail plate and it will be almost impossible to prevent it dehydrating. Alternatively, it may be that the client is having the treatment for a special occasion and wants their hands and nails to look their best. When this happens, the emphasis must be placed on subsequent manicures that must *not* include removal of this skin.

The actual procedure of cuticle removal requires that the cuticle is softened. This may be achieved in four ways.

1   Soaking the client's nails in softened warm water placed in a manicure bowl (most brands have a softening product for this purpose, otherwise use a small drop of fabric softener). There are many ingredients included in brand-name hand/cuticle soaks. Sometimes there will be an ingredient that will help to remove staining on nails; this may be lemon or a very mild bleach (for example 20 per cent volume hydrogen peroxide) or even oxygen bubbles from a tablet used to clean false teeth! This process needs only a couple of minutes as the cuticle softens very quickly. A long soak in water is not good for the nail, as it soaks up a great deal of water that will eventually evaporate taking with it some of the natural oils and moisture. After a couple of minutes in the water, ask the client to remove their fingers from the bowl and place into a clean dry towel you have waiting. Thoroughly dry the fingers, nails and around the edges of the nails.

2   A branded product to remove cuticles. These are usually alkaline-based (for example potassium hydroxide) and often have moisturisers in them too. Alpha hydroxy acids (AHAs) are a popular ingredient, as they soften the layer of skin, help exfoliate and aid cell renewal. The manufacturer's instructions must be followed, but the usual procedure is to apply a small amount to the cuticle area and leave for 2 minutes before washing off. This can easily be done during a manicure and the product washed off in a bowl of water and dried as above, or it could be removed using a disposable wet towel.

3   Nail oil. An application of nail oil to the cuticle area will soften the cuticle sufficiently to remove. This does not need removing, as it is nourishing for the area.

4   Following a hot oil treatment, or heated mitts treatment when the area has had a good application of creams. As before, the cream or oil does not need removing before cuticle work can begin.

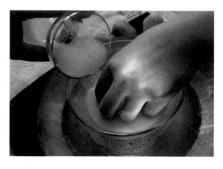

Luxury soak

The methods used during any kind of manicure will depend on salon procedure or the brand of manicure products being used. It is always advisable to closely follow manufacturer's instructions.

Once the cuticle is soft, a clean cuticle knife can be used (see Chapter 3) to remove the cuticle on the nail plate. The nail fold will be gently lifted during this process. An orange stick covered in cotton wool or a hoof stick can be used to neaten the nail fold after this process, but these tools are not sharp enough to remove all of the cuticle. Explain to your client what you are doing and advise against them using a cuticle knife of any kind at home. They can use a covered orange stick dipped in oil to moisturise and neaten the area between visits.

When this has been completed, check the sides of the nails for hangnails and nip these off.

Buffing

This is a useful procedure for several reasons:

- the stimulation to the nail plate increases blood circulation in the area
- it can remove superficial staining caused by polish
- it produces a very healthy looking shine that will last several weeks
- it will minimize ridges

- it helps to make the nail plate less porous

- polish bonds better and is therefore less prone to chipping

- when used on the free edge, it will help to seal the layers and make the edge smooth and rounded.

An old fashioned way of buffing the nails for stimulation and some shine involved a chamois leather buffer and buffing cream that had a slightly abrasive quality. This can be used if pre-ferred, but the easier method by far is to use a three-way buffer or a two-sided glosser, a tool that has progressively finer abrasives on its two or three surfaces. Usually they are coloured for the first and most abrasive side, then white for a finer abrasive, and finally grey for a smooth surface.

The abrasives must be used in the correct sequence. The first side must be used gently to buff over the surface of each nail and then on the free edge. Only a few buffs are necessary to just remove the natural shine on the nail plate. The finer abrasive follows this and slightly more buffing can be used, including on the free edge. Finally, buff each nail with the smooth side. It is not necessary to build up any heat while buffing, in fact excess heat can have an adverse affect on the nail plate and cause the layers to part.

Care must be taken not to over-buff as this can thin the nail, particularly over ridges. The full three-side buffing should only be done about once a month as any more could thin the nail. The last two sides can be done more often to bring up the shine.

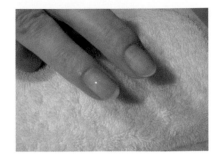

A buffed and unbuffed nail

Massage

Clients often say that the massage is the best part of the manicure as it is so relaxing. It is also definitely the only stage that they cannot carry out effectively at home and it can turn a manicure into a real treat and luxury treatment.

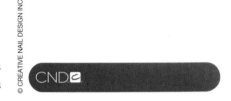

© CREATIVE NAIL DESIGN INC

Nail File

Apart from keeping the client happy, there are many reasons why a massage of the hand or, time allowing, hand and lower arm, is beneficial. The hands and feet are the extremities of the body and are often the first to feel the cold or suffer from sluggish or poor circulation.

Benefits

- Blood circulation is stimulated and, therefore, during the period of the increase, becomes more efficient at delivering nutrients and oxygen to the cells of the area and removing cellular waste.

- The improved circulation will also help with muscle tone, skin tone and colour,

- Lymphatic drainage is improved by the manual friction, so waste from the tissues is removed and the body's mechanism for dealing with infection has a period of increased efficiency.

- Absorption of the nourishing cream used during the massage is improved so its nutrients reach deeper tissues.

- A good massage can relieve tension in the muscles and joints.

- It is relaxing and soothing for the client.

Restrictions Avoid massage entirely:

- over open cuts or wounds as cross-infection could occur or bacteria could be introduced to the open skin

- over recent scars as they could be stretched

- in any inflamed or infected areas
- over areas of bruising.

Restrict massage:

- over painful, inflamed joints, for example in clients with arthritis whose joints should be avoided during the massage
- at any joint that is painful.

Movements   There are four main massage movements but only three of them are relevant to hand and lower arm massage. Once you understand the effects of the movements it is best to create a routine of your own.

1   **Effleurage**. This is the movement that usually starts and finishes a massage sequence, as it is used to spread the massage medium, prepares the client and then, at the end of the sequence, slows down to physically show the client that the massage is coming to an end.

It is a stroking movement, either lightly or with deeper pressure, applied by the flat of a relaxed hand. The pressure should be slightly increased in the direction of the circulation towards the heart and pressure lifted on the return stroke while keeping contact with the skin.

Quick movements in this way will stimulate the circulation while long, slow movements aid lymphatic flow and also relax the client.

2   **Petrissage**. This is a more active movement that has a stronger effect on the blood circulation, often resulting in a reddening of the area. Work is concentrated on the muscles in a rhythmic way that is both soothing and stimulating for the client. The hands pick up the skin and underlying muscle in a kneading motion. Absorption is increased from the tissues and the skin as the lymphatic vessels are squeezed and released.

3   **Frictions**. For this movement the thumb is used to massage tissue below the skin in small areas. This is excellent for releasing tension in muscles. Small circular movements are made by the thumb, reaching down under the skin to underlying areas of muscle.

4   **Tapotement**. This movement is not appropriate during a hand and arm massage. It is suitable for the larger muscle areas of the body where maximum stimulation is needed, or for certain areas of the face to encourage drainage. As the name suggests, it involves tapping.

A massage routine

- Make sure you have sufficient massage medium in your hands for the complete massage of one hand and arm. Knowing how much to use will only come from experience with the specific product and your client's skin. As a general guide, pour the medium into your palm – about the size of a ten-pence piece – and rub your palms together to spread the medium and warm it.

- Make sure both you and your client are in the most comfortable position and the hand and arm can be manoeuvred without knocking anything over.

- Have a clean, soft pad covered with a disposable towel under your client's arm for comfort and support.

- Once you have started the massage, do not take both hands away from the area at the same time. This can be disconcerting for the client. One hand may be removed to move position but never both.

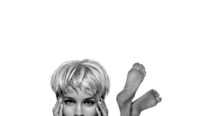

- When the massage is coming to an end, slow the movements down and finish by placing the client's hand down on the desk. Make the final stroke down the hand and off at the fingers.

- The client will need to roll up her sleeves and remove any jewellery. If necessary, tuck a tissue around the edge of the sleeve to protect it from the cream.

- Encourage the client to keep her hands very relaxed and remind her if the hand starts to tense.

The best response a manicurist can get is a client who is very relaxed and truly thinks that the massage is the best part of the manicure. Ideally, the skin will have absorbed the massage medium by the end of the treatment. If not, use a clean towel or soft disposable towel to remove any excess cream. At the completion of this stage, ask your client to replace her jewellery.

Hand creams

If a manicure system is being used, there will be specific creams for different skin conditions. Hands usually need a heavy duty moisturising cream as they are so abused and least protected. Detergents and soaps destroy the natural moisture, even deep in the skin.

Step-by-step: massage routine

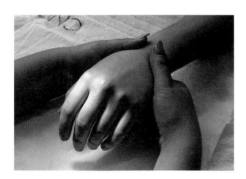 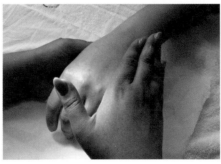 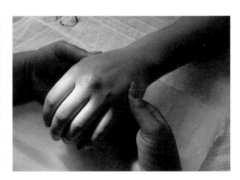

1 With firm petrissage movements massage the back of the hand and arm

- With the chosen massage medium on both hands, take your client's hand with one of yours to support the hand and arm and, with the other, spread the massage medium up the arm to the elbow. Repeat with the other hand so the area to be massaged has been spread with sufficient medium for the treatment. Repeat these actions 2 or 3 times as a relaxing start to the massage.

2 Supporting the hand, use firm petrissage movements up both sides of the hand and arm, lifting the skin occasionally.

- Continuing to support the hand and arm with one hand, and using the fingers and thumb of the other, gently squeeze and release the muscle near the wrist on one side and repeat this up the arm to just below the elbow (petrissage). Slide your hand back down to the wrist. Repeat this once or twice more then repeat with the other side of the arm.

3 Using small circular movements massage hand and arm

- Holding the client's hand, palm down, in both your hands, use your thumbs to apply effleurage movements over the back of the hand in a rhythmic movement. Apply more pressure on the stroke towards the wrist.

- Supporting the client's hand in one of yours, use your thumb to apply small friction movements between each metacarpal on the back of the hand from the fingers to the wrist.

- Repeat but use a deep sliding movement with firm pressure on the upward stroke. This is a lymph drainage movement.

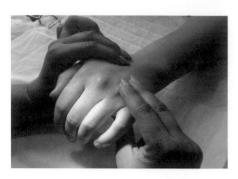

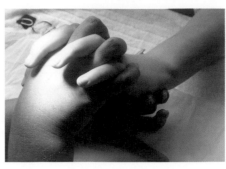

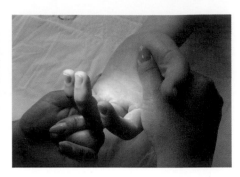

4 Massage the palm of the hand with firm circular movements of your thumb

- Turn the client's hand over and use your thumbs to apply deep friction movements all over the palm of the hand. Pay special attention to the pad at the base of the thumb as this can often release tension in the area.

5 Interlock your fingers and rotate the wrist while supporting the arm

- Grasp the client's wrist, palm down with one of your hands and interlock the fingers of your other hand with those of your clients. Rotate the hand from the wrist a few times in each direction. Finish with a gentle pull to stretch the wrist joint.

6 With palm facing upwards, spread the fingers to release any tension

- With both your hands, spread the client's palm by hooking your little fingers between her little and ring fingers and forefinger and thumb and smoothing the palm with your thumbs.

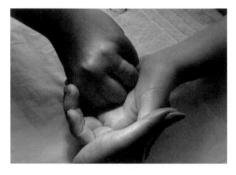

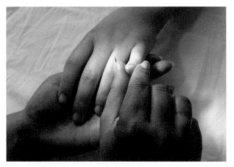

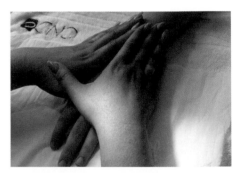

7 Firmly massage the palm of the hand using your knuckles

8 Rotate each finger in both directions

- Still supporting the hand, start at the little finger and with your free hand, grasp and gently rotate the finger once or twice in each direction and finish off with a gentle pull, sliding up the length of the finger. Repeat for the other fingers and thumb.

9 Finish off massage with gentle effleurage movements over hand and arm. Gently place hand on table. Repeat steps for the other hand

- Apply a few gentle effleurage movements to the hand and arm becoming slower, and finish off with the last down stroke coming off at the fingers as you place your client's hand down on the pad. Repeat for the other hand and arm.

Ideally a moisturiser (or emollient) that has skin softening properties but does not leave the skin too greasy should be used. They all have quite a high water content with emollient and fragrance.

Another type of treatment for hands is a barrier cream. This is not necessarily used in salon treatments, but it is a useful homecare product as application of this cream will help protect damage to skin from detergents and soaps. It works by leaving a layer of a type of wax on the skin that prevents the absorption of chemicals and the loss of natural moisture.

Painting

Nail varnishes (or **nail enamels**) are clear or pigmented layers. (See Chapter 7 for more information on **nail polishes**). They all have basically a similar formulation in that they are a film-forming plastic in a solvent. The solvent evaporates leaving behind a film of clear glossy plastic, with or without pigment (colour).

The plastic is usually a nitrocellulose with a plastic resin for the gloss, a plasticizer for flexibility, a solvent for quicker drying and pigments. Nitrocellulose and solvents are highly flammable, so bottles must be kept away from flames or heat (e.g. a window in the sun).

There has been a great deal of debate in recent years about some of the ingredients in varnish, mainly centred on formaldehyde and toluene. Formaldehyde has now been banned in the USA and many varnishes sold in Europe no longer have it in their formulations. Formaldehyde in its natural state is harmful to the body, but it was used in varnishes in the form of a resin with other chemicals to give a good, hard wearing gloss. Some people are allergic to this but a good alternative has been found. Toluene is another debated ingredient. It is commonly used as a solvent in varnishes, but some people may be allergic to it.

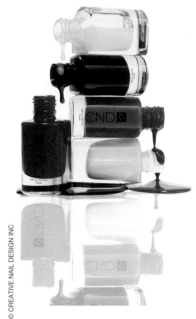

Not every client will want painted nails, but those who do should be delighted with the result and the colour or effect achieved. A beautiful, professionally painted set of nails should be better than most clients can do for themselves. The paint should last longer and the finish should be perfect.

© CREATIVE NAIL DESIGN INC

Clients can see the result of your painting skills long after they have forgotten the lovely massage or the comfort of the salon and their beautiful nails are what they will show their friends and, hopefully, receive plenty of compliments.

Colour collection for 'grooming'

Some clients know exactly what colour or effect they want. This may be because they have a favourite or because they want it to match a specific outfit or lipstick. Many clients, however, like a bit of help and guidance in choosing a colour as too much choice can often be confusing.

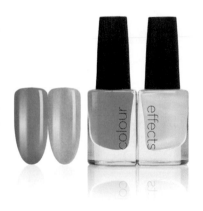

It can sometimes be difficult to help a client choose a colour that they will like during the manicure and then continue to like for the next few days. I believe that there is an easy way to help you decide where to start with your recommendations. All clients who want their nails painted fall into one of three categories:

1   This group of clients likes their nails to be part of good *grooming* in the same way as they like a good hairstyle, clean, neat clothes and nice make-up. They do not necessarily want their nails to be dictated by fashion trends, but are looking to complement their general style with a colour that they can wear for several days without it clashing. These clients will like a colour that is from a range that will complement all of the colours in their wardrobe. They may like a 'French' as it looks clean and healthy and will not clash with anything or they may like a colour that is very neutral and complements their skin tone. It is unlikely that they will be happy with a strong colour in any colour range (unless they have one predominant strong colour in their wardrobe).

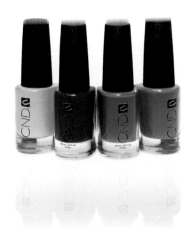

2   For these clients, their nails are a *fashion* accessory. They will like the seasonal trend colours that perfectly complement or match their clothes or make-up. They will also like the current thinking on length and shape and will be happy with any bold colour (as long as it is 'in'), or 'French', or pale or neutral. In fact any colour or effect that gives them more opportunities (i.e. their nails) to accessorize their current 'look'.

3   The third group of clients like to make a *statement* with their image. This usually accompanies a total image, i.e. hair, clothes and make-up, but can also include clients who may be conservative in their appearance yet like to make a bold statement with their nails whether it be their colour, decoration or extreme length. This client may choose nail art but will certainly like the more unusual colours from the range!

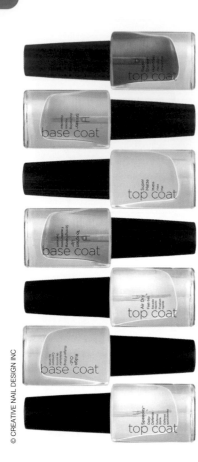

When helping your client to choose the colour they would like, pay attention to your initial consultation and any conversation during the treatment for clues to the three categories of *grooming*, *fashion* or *statement*.

This will give you a starting point to suggest some colours or effects.

Skilful painting, like all other skills, needs plenty of practice. An excellent manicure can so often be let down by bad painting and the client takes away the proof of that lack of skill to look at many times a day.

The results of good painting are:

- colour that stays on for more than 5 days; it should stay on for 7 or more (this can depend on the condition of the natural nail as it is difficult to stop paint chipping from a peeling nail, for example) and good homecare advice can extend the life of the paint

- a smooth and even surface

- a neat, even edge that neither touches surrounding tissue nor shows any unpainted nail

- a layer that is not so thick that it takes an unreasonable time to dry.

Nail varnish is actually quite a difficult medium to work with. It dries too quickly to give the user time to paint neatly and repair mistakes but it dries too slowly to allow the hands to be used for quite some time after. It is affected by air so if you leave bottles open the varnish will get thicker over time and can become unusable long before it is used up.

Several coats of varnish actually take over 2 days to totally harden. The surface will dry quickly, but deeper varnish will stay soft for a long time, hence the dented surface when thick polish has been touched many hours later. As a rule, thicker varnish will take longer as will those with a denser pigment. Therefore a thin, sheer varnish will dry much faster than a thick dark red. The reason for this is the ease with which the solvents contained in the varnish can evaporate. Dense pigments prevent solvents at the lower levels from escaping easily.

The fast dryers available on the market will certainly dry the surface very quickly to make the varnish dry to the touch but not to any pressure. Some paint-on fast dryers will form a hard layer very quickly to help prevent damage from pressure but few, if any, can harden a thick layer of pigmented varnish so it cannot be damaged easily in a short space of time.

Therefore avoid thickened varnish. Even very deep colours will dry quickly if two (or more) thin coats are applied as the solvent evaporates from each layer before the next is applied. It is not necessary – and it is impractical in a salon environment – to wait for each coat to dry before applying the next. A thin coat will have dried sufficiently after painting 10 nails and the next application with its solvents will wet it again anyway.

Most nail polishes are **thixotropic**. If they thicken due to exposure to air or if they have been sitting for a long period, a good shake will thin them out enough to make painting easier.

TOP TIP

Some general tips about varnish:

- Make sure lids are tight.
- Wipe the neck of the bottle before replacing the lid if any varnish has spilled down the outside.
- Keep out of sunlight and away from heat (bottles can explode!).
- Throw away any bottle where the varnish has become thick due to being half (or less) full; it is not worth the effort of trying to use it.
- If you find a bottle that has a perfect brush, when the varnish is finished, clean the brush and keep it; sometimes you will come across a very poor brush that makes painting very difficult and you can substitute the clean one.
- It is permissible to mix varnishes. If you have a bottle where the level of varnish is too low for the brush and it is still thin in consistency, mix it with another either to make a new colour or to consolidate several opened bottles of the same colour. Make sure the bottle is shaken well to mix the varnish.

There are no magic tips about painting. There are no foolproof steps to follow to produce a perfect result. Each varnish will be different to use depending on the brand, the colour, the brush and the temperature. There are, however, some guidelines that may help, but practice is what really counts – and then more practice.

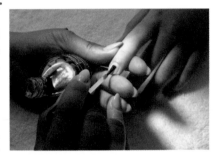

Apply base

Holding the polish bottle General guidelines:

- Practise holding the bottle in the palm of the hand that is holding the client's finger. This is also safer than using the bottle on the desk top where it can get knocked over by your brush. It is quicker to reload the brush and it is useful to be able to do this comfortably as sometimes there are situations when you will not be working on or near a desk.

- Hold the client's finger either side of the nail pulling back the skin to expose the side of the nail plate. This will make painting much easier.

- When removing the brush from the bottle, lift it out in a spiral motion, wiping the shaft of the brush on the neck of the bottle. This will prevent varnish on the shaft running down and flooding the brush or dripping off.

- Wipe the brush away from you on the neck of the bottle. This will leave the brush with sufficient varnish loaded on the side you are going to place onto the nail.

- Try to load the brush with sufficient varnish to cover the nail and so avoid the need to go back in the bottle for more. Varnish is drying while you are painting, so you want a good coverage quickly. Remember to be aware of the size of the nail being painted, i.e. a small nail will need much less varnish than a long nail or the thumb.

- A good brush will fan out when slight pressure is applied to it on the nail. This will greatly assist a neat and even edge at the cuticle area. The way to do this is to load the brush and place it in the centre of the nail plate first. This will avoid flooding the cuticle area with too much varnish. Then ease the brush towards the cuticle putting a slight pressure on it by holding it fairly upright (see picture) and allowing the straight edge of the fanned brush to create the edge of the varnish, then pull the brush down the length of the nail to the free edge. For a wide nail, repeat this either side of the first paint stroke. Otherwise, sweep the brush around each side and make sure that the sides of the nail are painted and have a neat edge also.

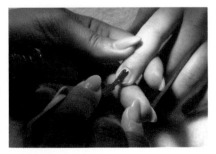

Apply colour

- Avoid overworking the varnish on the nail. Use the minimum number of strokes, as overworking will start to drag the varnish off and make it bumpy.

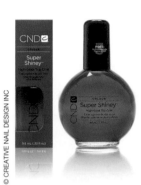

- Whatever the colour, don't worry if the coverage is uneven after the first coat. Keep the layers thin and, if necessary, apply a third coat of the colour to get a good, even coverage.

- This is the final stage of the manicure and it is essential that there is no trace of any oil or moisture on the surface of the nail plate, as it would cause the varnish to peel off the nail very quickly. Thoroughly wipe the nail with varnish remover from the free edge towards the cuticle (this direction will avoid any moisture from the skin being wiped onto the nail plate) to ensure it is clean and dry. Some removers have oily conditioners in them and these can leave a film on the nail plate and cause a problem with the varnish. It could peel off very quickly or sometimes bubble. This is when small imperfections in the surface of a newly painted nail can appear.

- Always use a base coat. These products are formulated differently from coloured varnish. They are developed to create a stronger bond with the natural nail than coloured varnish and help to form a barrier between the nail and the varnish. Deep pigments can stain the natural nail but pale colours can also have this effect, especially when worn in sunlight or on a sunbed. The barrier of the base coat may not prevent this, but it will certainly minimize it.

- Special base coats are also available and can be used if appropriate. Ridge fillers can be useful, but remember that the thicker the layers, the longer the varnish will take to dry. Ridge fillers work by being slightly thicker and smoothing the ridges. This should not be a problem with a thin varnish, but it will create a very thick layer with a thick, densely pigmented varnish. There are also many base coats that are an important part of a branded manicure system and are developed to help improve various nail conditions. These should be used as the manufacturer's instructions suggest.

- A top coat should also be used. Like the base coats they have a different formulation as their job is to create a good shine and be hard wearing. In addition they are often quick drying. After painting the nail plate, run the side of the brush around the edge of the nail. This will seal the nail plate and also the layer of varnish to help protect the nail and avoid chipping. It is very good homecare advice to recommend that the client reapply a top coat every other day and reseal the edge. This will refresh the varnish, help to avoid chipping and protect the edge of the nail.

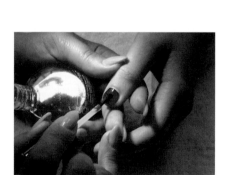

Apply top coat

- Painting is the last stage of the manicure treatment and the client will need to wait for a while before collecting their belongings, putting their coat on, etc. Without offending, it is good practice to suggest that the client may like to settle her bill and book her next appointment before this stage. This will help to avoid damaging the wet varnish by diving into handbags and purses. Some clients even like to put their coat on and get their car keys out so they are ready to leave as soon as practicable.

- There are many quick drying top coats available. Some of them use heat or UV light. It is worth trying a selection of them to decide which is best.

- If the varnish does not look good or if you make a mistake, it is far better to remove the varnish and reapply (even if the next client is waiting). The client must leave with proof of a first class manicure that took a little longer rather than a second rate one that was rushed.

- It is a good practice to apply a small drop of oil after painting to the cuticle area with the nail angled down to allow it to run over the surface of the nail. This will ensure maximum hydration of the skin, and the coat of oil on the surface will stop the varnish being tacky and attracting fluff or hairs, etc.

Procedure for painting

1 Wipe over the nail with polish remover to remove any trace of moisture. Remember to include the edges of the nail down inside the nail walls.

2 Apply a thin layer of base coat or appropriate treatment base.

3 Apply two thin coats of the chosen colour.

4 Assess the coverage of the varnish and apply a third coat if necessary.

5 Apply a top coat and seal the edge.

6 Apply a drop of oil to the cuticle and let it run down the nail.

7 If appropriate, escort your client to an area where she can wait for a while until her nails are dry enough to leave. Carry her belongings for her to avoid damage to the wet varnish and make sure she is comfortable.

French manicure

This is a term used to describe varnish effect that is close to nail art, but is a very popular service for clients. Once again, it needs plenty of practice and only perfect results are acceptable.

A French manicure is the use of two colours of varnish to create an effect that:

a. makes the nail look natural, clean and healthy, or

b. has a stronger looking effect but with similar colours.

Sometimes the term French manicure is used to describe the method but performed using different or unusual colour combinations. It always applies to the effect where the free edge of the nail is painted a different colour from the rest of the nail.

In a traditional French manicure, the free edge, or tip, is a variation of white while the rest of the nail is a sheer neutral colour. However, there are many variations of this in addition to the most well-known version of a white tip with a sheer pink top coat.

1 The natural versions use many variations of white on the tip. The range can be from an opaque off-white or cream to a semi-opaque white or even one with a shimmer. The top coats can be sheer pinks of various shades, sheer beiges or slightly more milky versions. The 'smile line' (the boundary between the free edge and the nail bed either genuine or created by varnish) has a more indistinct and therefore more natural appearance. When deciding which of the many combinations is right for the client there are a number of things to take into account:

   – Client preference i.e. what type of effect she likes.

   – Her skin tone, i.e. does it suit a pink or beige and does she want it to tone with her skin or not?

   – Does the free edge need to be made to look longer than it is by painting a deeper tip? This will require the more opaque white.

   – Is a cream or white-based tip colour most suitable for the top coat?

   – Are there any imperfections on the nail plate that need disguising? If there are, then a milky top coat will be more effective than a sheer one.

   – What will the colour of the nail bed do to the colour of the top coat? It is worth trying it out on one nail to see the effect.

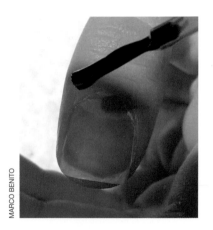

A short and unattractive nail

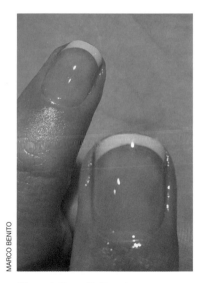

After painting with French

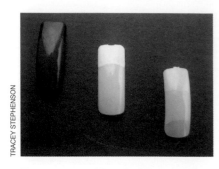

TRACEY STEPHENSON

Three versions of French: different, bold, natural

TOP TIP

White varnish needs to be a thin consistency. Thick varnish is difficult to paint and chips very quickly. Discard a bottle if varnish is thick.

2 The stronger looking French manicure uses a very opaque bright white or cream that produces a very sharp edge at the 'smile line'. The top coat can be sheer, so the nail bed can be seen clearly or a milky version so the nail bed is less obvious but the white tip is still strong.

3 The more unusual variations involve any combinations of colour, e.g. black tip with white nail, silver tip with red nail.

Variations 2 and 3 are the most difficult to paint perfectly, so should be practised the most. It is also worth practising the various combinations of tip and top colour to discover the effects.

General guidelines:

● As with all painting use a base coat.

● Decide if the nail colour is being painted under or over the tip colour. The effect is different for each method.

● Do not paint the tip colour straight across. This looks ugly and is not what this effect should be.

● When painting the tip colour, create an even curve around the 'smile line' taking great care to take the colour to the sides of the nail in a sharp point and not a rounded finish. (This shape is sometimes called 'dog ears' and they should be pointed not rounded!)

● Try to paint the tip from one side of the nail to the other in one brush stroke and, if the nail is long, blend the varnish up over the whole free edge. This can be tricky but it is worth practising until it is perfect. Opaque white is very thick and too many brush strokes make it lumpy and uneven.

● Have a clean, small brush available. This can be dipped in remover to make the smile line sharp and remove any mistakes if necessary.

● Don't worry about getting the polish on the skin at the sides of the nail. This is often necessary to achieve a good 'smile'. It can be cleaned off with remover very quickly.

● Don't paint the white too thickly, as it will chip off very quickly.

● When painting the nail colour over the white tip, use a few light strokes as the still-wet white can get picked up by the brush and streaked over the nail plate.

● Even when using a sheer pale colour, pay attention to a neat edge in the cuticle area and side walls.

● Always finish with a top coat.

Some people refer to an 'American manicure'. This usually means an opaque cream tip and a deep but totally sheer pink/red.

Paraffin wax treatment

This is an additional treatment that is offered in many salons either as part of a luxury manicure or as a specific treatment for conditions such as dry or rough skin. It can be very soothing for arthritis sufferers. It has many benefits:

● it is very relaxing and soothing

● it will soften dry, rough or calloused skin

- it temporarily gives the skin a younger-looking appearance
- it improves blood circulation during the treatment
- it softens cuticles ready for removal
- it soothes aching joints and tired muscles.

It is not advisable to paint the nails after a paraffin wax treatment as the nail will have absorbed oils and the paint will probably peel off very quickly.

Although this treatment is called paraffin wax, as well as paraffin wax obtained from the petrochemical industry, beeswax from beehives can also be used. Some salons and clients are unhappy using petrochemical derivatives, so this should be taken into account when choosing the wax.

There are many waxes available on the market and some have other beneficial additives, for example tea tree oil, which is soothing, slightly **antiseptic** and with certain healing properties. Some have aromatherapy oils added for a range of additional benefits. All wax is solid at room temperature and is supplied in either a solid block, smaller bricks or pellets.

This is a relatively inexpensive treatment from the salon's point of view. Set-up costs consist primarily of a heater for the wax, but the wax itself is a reasonable price and the only other necessity is a disposable method of wrapping the hands after application.

The specialized heaters available for this treatment heat the wax to approximately 53°C (but the manicurist must always check the temperature before using on a client) and can be used for immersing both hands and feet.

A less expensive version of these heaters can be used if cost is an issue or, due to their smaller size, by a mobile manicurist. These heaters are not big enough to immerse a hand or foot, but the melted wax can be painted on with a wide brush. *All* used wax must be discarded and not returned to the heater.

Procedure for a paraffin wax treatment.

1   Make sure the heater is on for sufficient time before it is needed.

2   Have a disposable wrap ready (this could be plastic gloves, cling film or foil) together with clean towels. (This treatment can be used with heated mitts, in which case have them ready to use with relevant accessories.)

3   Make sure client's hands are clean by wiping them over with a damp disposable towel (this will prevent the wax from being contaminated).

4   Check the temperature of the wax.

5   Hold the client's arm just above the wrist and dip the hand in the wax and remove, keeping the hand over the heater. Repeat this several times until a thick coat of wax is covering the hand.

6   Wrap the hand in the prepared disposable wrap and then a towel or place in the heated mitts.

7   Repeat with the other hand.

8   Leave wax in place for approximately 10 minutes.

9   Remove one hand from wraps and peel away wax. Discard used wax and disposable wrap. Repeat with other hand.

10 Continue with manicure treatment.

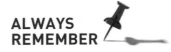

ALWAYS REMEMBER

Paraffin wax treatments should not be used if the hand has any infected areas or open wounds of any kind.

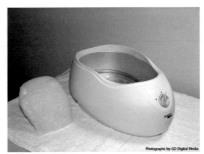

A hand and foot wax paraffin bath

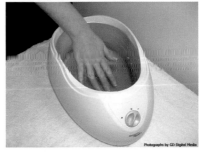

Dipping a hand in the bath

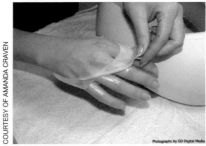

Peeling after the wax hand bath

Masks

In luxury and treatment manicures it is now usual to treat the hands just like the face and a beneficial treatment is to apply a mask to the hands. This is not necessarily used in addition to the other treatment possibilities but it can be an alternative to paraffin wax and heat treatment masks are useful when used in conjunction with an exfoliation treatment.

There are many brands of hand masks on the market each having different effects. Choosing the right one will depend on the condition of your client's skin. There are deeply moisturising masks for dry or calloused skin, collagen masks to help plump up the skin and make it look more youthful, stimulating masks to help skin tone by increasing the circulation, toning masks to refine the surface of the skin and many others.

As with all products, the manufacturer's instructions must be followed. Some masks need to be kept moist and, therefore, after application the hand should be wrapped in film and a towel; others need to dry out so the hand must be left exposed.

Warm oil treatment

While a paraffin wax treatment is beneficial for the hands, a warm oil treatment concentrates just on the nails and cuticles. It is a quick, effective treatment for dry and brittle nails that have a tendency to snap off in a clean break (as opposed to split). It will also help to improve the condition of dry skin around the nail and an overgrown nail fold. In the same way as with paraffin wax, the nail plate will absorb the oil and may make painting less effective, with a tendency to peel off.

Soaking the nail in oil is more effective if the oil is warm as it encourages better penetration into the nail plate and skin. There are several ways of achieving this, both in the salon and as a mobile manicurist:

1   Place the oil in a small bowl that is big enough to accommodate all the fingers and place this in a larger bowl containing hot (not scalding) water.

2   Soak cotton wool pads in the oil, wrap these around the fingers, and then wrap in foil and a towel. The heat from the fingers will be trapped and will aid the penetration of the oil. A desk lamp that gives off heat can be placed above the hands to increase the warmth.

3   Small electric heaters are available that heat the oil to the correct temperature. The oil is placed in a small disposable bowl and then in the heater. After the treatment oil and bowl are discarded.

4   Heated mitts can be used in place of the foil and towel as above.

This treatment will soften the cuticles very effectively so should be carried out before this stage in the manicure, but after the hands and nails are cleaned and the nails have been shaped.

There are some proprietary oils available for this treatment but an inexpensive alternative is to mix wheatgerm oil with almond oil (slightly more wheatgerm oil).

Thermal mitts

These are a convenient way of using heat to increase the benefits of the application of moisturising creams and oils. It is also soothing and relaxing for the client. The heat opens the pores of the skin and softens the cellular membranes allowing nourishing ingredients in the creams to penetrate to a deeper level and so benefit the lower layers of the skin. Only ingredients of a small molecular size can penetrate deeper and manufacturers create formulations that take this into account. Products like paraffin have large molecules of hydrocarbons so cannot penetrate to any depth.

Thermal mitts are readily available and although they may represent a substantial outlay initially, they will last a long time if looked after. As with all electrical equipment in the salon, they must be regularly checked by an electrician to ensure their safety.

General guidelines:

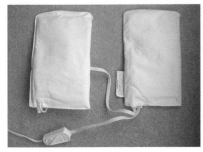

Heated mitts

- Make sure they are ready for use before the manicure.

- When heating, it is inadvisable to put one on top of the other as they may overheat. Place them side by side.

- Most mitts have three heat settings: low, medium and high. If the high setting is chosen for a speedy heating time, check that they are not too hot before placing the client's hands in them and do not leave them on this setting while in use. Medium or low is usually sufficient.

Procedure for a heat treatment

1 When hands and nails are cleaned and the nails have been shaped, lightly apply the appropriate cream to the hands and oil or cream to the cuticles. Do not massage in.

2 Wrap hands in disposable gloves or cling film and place them into the protective plastic bag that is supplied with the mitts.

3 Check that the mitts' temperature is right and place the wrapped hands into the mitts.

4 Make sure the client is comfortable and leave the mitts on for 10 minutes.

5 Remove and unwrap one hand and massage with the cream remaining on the hand. Discard disposable wrapping.

6 Repeat with the other hand.

Exfoliation

Exfoliation is a treatment that has long been associated with facial treatments but, as the skin on the hands is the same as the skin on the face, it is an obvious step to include this in some luxury manicure sequences.

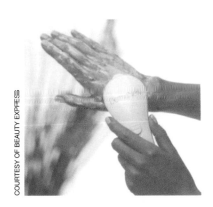

Helping with exfoliation

The uppermost layer of the skin is composed of keratinized skin cells that form a protective layer. They are held together with natural fats or lipids. As more are produced by the epidermis, older cells become detached and are continually being shed (desquamation). Sometimes it is worth removing this layer of older cells (exfoliation) to speed up the cell renewal process and create clean, brighter looking skin.

This treatment also helps to unblock the pores and soften and dry areas on the skin. The skin on the hands is not prone to the problem of dead skin cells in the same way as, for example, the face or the feet because hands are always being washed and exposed to detergents and other harsh chemicals. However, the treatment will improve the texture of the skin and help to treat dry areas.

Another benefit of exfoliation is that as well as removing dead skin cells, it removes other debris from the surface, leaving the skin exceptionally clean and able to absorb moisturisers. This means that the treatment that follows will be more efficient.

Exfoliants are usually creams containing a stimulating ingredient such as menthol and small particles that feel quite rough. The stimulant helps to increase blood circulation to the area, which aids cell renewal and also increases the efficiency of absorption. The particles will physically remove the dead skin cells on the surface as the cream is massaged into the hands.

General guidelines:

- When removing the cream from the container, always use a spatula that can be disposed of or sanitized. Never use your fingers as this will contaminate the product.

- Massage the cream into the hands, but do not over-massage as the skin could become sore.

- Avoid using an exfoliant on delicate or sensitive skin as it could cause an irritation.

- When removing the exfoliant, make sure to remove all the grit. Dipping the hands into a bowl of water will do this or use a wet disposable towel to clean the hands, including in between the fingers. If this is not done effectively little particles of grit will interfere with the massage sequence.

- If your manicure product brand does not have an exfoliant, then you can use a soft facial brush in small circular movements to remove the dead skin and aid desquamation.

Procedure for exfoliation treatment

- Remove a small amount of product from the tub or tube, using a spatula as necessary.

- Place the cream onto the back of one of the client's hands.

- Supporting your client's wrist with one of your hands, gently spread the cream over the hand with the pads of your fingers, using small circular movements.

- Turn the hand over and repeat on the palm, paying extra attention to any hard skin areas.

- When all areas of the hand have been exfoliated, remove excess cream with a disposable towel and either wash the client's hand in a bowl of warm water or use a wet towel to remove all the grit.

- Repeat with the other hand.

Manicure treatment alternatives

The sequence of the manicure treatment depends on two main factors, the practice of the salon and the manicure brand being used. There are many alternatives that suit different situations, and this section includes a list of sequences that are logical progressions for various types of treatment. They are offered as guidelines, and you should be careful to follow the sequences supplied by the manufacturers of the products you use.

General guidelines (i.e. for all treatments):

- The work area must be prepared before the client arrives with all relevant tools and equipment clean and ready for use.

- A consultation with the client must be carried out, even if a specific type of treatment has been booked. An alteration to this booking is acceptable following the consultation.

- It is also acceptable that, following the consultation, additional equipment is collected and prepared for use.

- Make sure the client is comfortable and has clean hands before starting the treatment. The client can either be asked to wash their hands or to use a sanitizing hand cleaner.

- The client's jewellery should be removed and placed close to her where it can be seen.

- Sleeves should be rolled up and protected if this is appropriate.

- Your hands should be clean and you should be sitting comfortably and safely.

- Any existing varnish should be removed before the consultation so the condition of the nails can be seen.

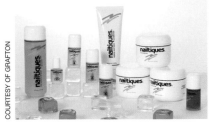

Manicure system products

Reshape and varnish

Timing: 15 minutes.

1 Shape nails on all ten fingers.

2 Clean under the free edge with a disposable orange stick.

3 Apply base coat, coloured varnish and top coat.

4 Apply oil.

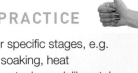

BEST PRACTICE

Timings for specific stages, e.g. massage, soaking, heat treatments, etc. have deliberately not been given. This is because these are stages that can take more or less time as required. Some clients want minimal shaping or cuticle work; others will need more. The manicurist must learn to keep an eye on the timing and make up time if necessary.

EQUIPMENT LIST

hand sanitizer   base and top coats

varnish remover   coloured varnish

nail wipes   nail oil

orange sticks   file

Mini manicure

Timing: 20 minutes.

1 Apply a cuticle softener to all ten fingers.

2 Shape nails on all ten fingers.

3 Remove the cuticle on each finger and tidy the nail fold.

4 Wipe nails to remove cuticle softener.

5 Apply hand cream to both hands.

6 Clean under the free edge with a disposable orange stick.

7 Wipe nails with remover.

8 Either apply varnish or buff nails.

EQUIPMENT LIST

hand sanitizer	hoof stick
varnish remover	hand cream
nail wipes	orange sticks
cuticle softener	three-way buffer
file	base and top coats
cuticle knife	coloured varnish
cuticlc nippers	nail oil

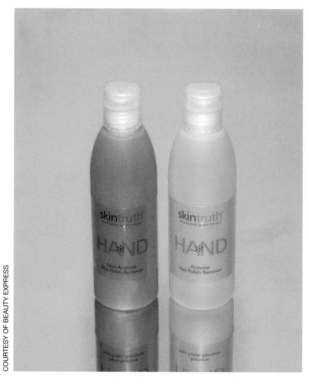

COURTESY OF BEAUTY EXPRESS

Varnish removers for natural and artificial nails

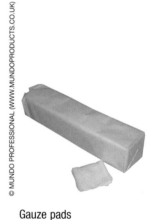

© MUNDO PROFESSIONAL (WWW.MUNDOPRODUCTS.CO.UK)

Gauze pads

EQUIPMENT LIST

hand sanitizer	hoof stick
varnish remover	hand cream
nail wipes	towels
file	orange sticks
cuticle softener	three-way buffer
bowl of warm water with softener	base and top coats
cuticle knife	coloured varnish
cuticle nippers	

Step-by-step: Manicure 1

Timing: 30 minutes.

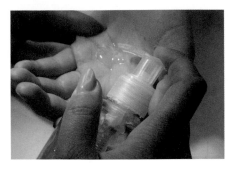

1 After washing the hands with soap and water, sanitize both the client's and your own hands.

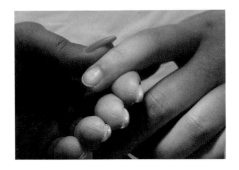

2 Examine the hands and nails in order to diagnose their condition and to look for any contra-indications.

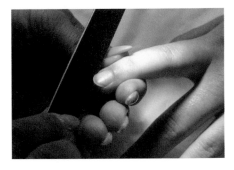

3 Shape the nails on one hand with a 240 grit (or higher) file after discussing with the client as to what shape they prefer. Keep the file angled slightly under the free edge.

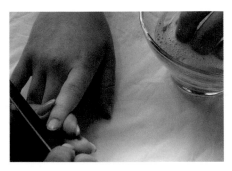

4 Place the fingers in a bowl of warm water to which a skin softener has been added. In the meantime, shape the nails of the other hand.

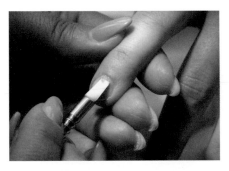

5 Remove the first hand from the bowl and dry. Apply cuticle remover and remove the cuticle with a disinfected cuticle knife

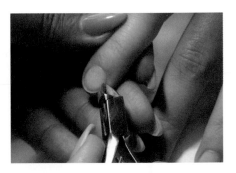

6 Using clean nippers, remove any hangnails. Remember to squeeze the nippers and release. DO NOT pull the skin.

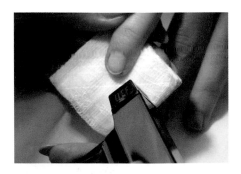

7 Clean the nails to remove any trace of cuticle remover.

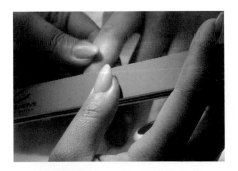

8 Using a three-sided buffer or a glosser, buff each nail to a high shine. Repeat steps 5 to 8 to the second hand.

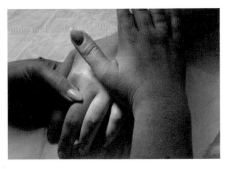

9 Using a massage oil or cream, spread it over first hand and lower arm with effleurage movements ready for a massage.

Manicure 2

Timing: 40 minutes

This is similar to manicure 1, but involves a full hand and arm massage (please refer to the massage step-by-step on page 109) and, if time, the nails can be buffed and varnished.

Treatment manicure 1

Timing: 45 minutes:

1 Shape nails of both hands

2 Apply appropriate cream and oil to both hands

3 Wrap hands and place in heated mitts

4 Remove one hand

5 Remove cuticles and tidy nail fold

6 Remove second hand and repeat

7 Provide hand and arm massage to both hands

8 Clean under nails and wipe them with remover

9 Apply varnish or buff

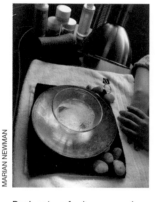
Desk set up for luxury manicure

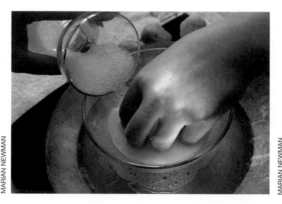
Luxury soak

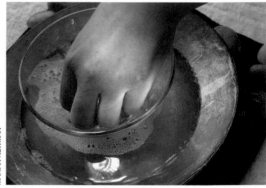

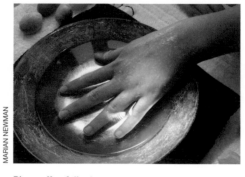
Rinse off exfoliant

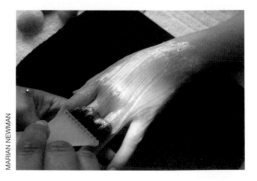
Spread mask

EQUIPMENT LIST

hand sanitizer	cuticle knife
varnish remover	cuticle nippers
nail wipes	hoof stick
file	towels
cuticle softener	orange sticks
hand cream	three-way buffer
disposable wrap/gloves	base and top coats
heated mitts	coloured varnish

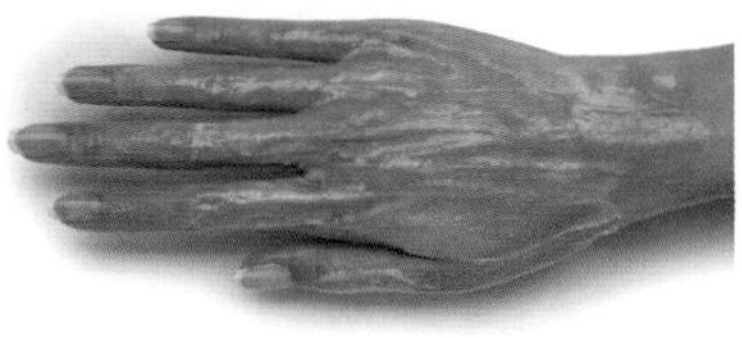

Step 3

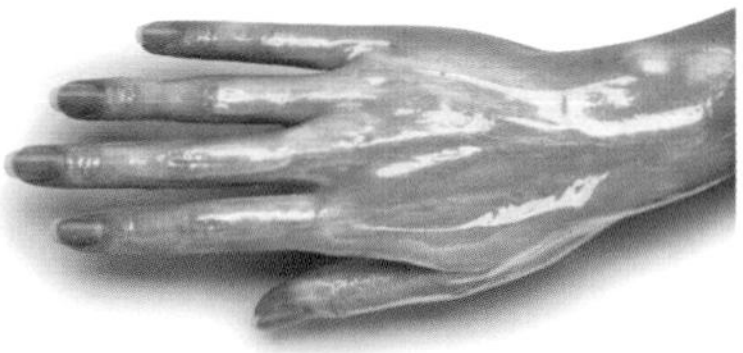

Step 4

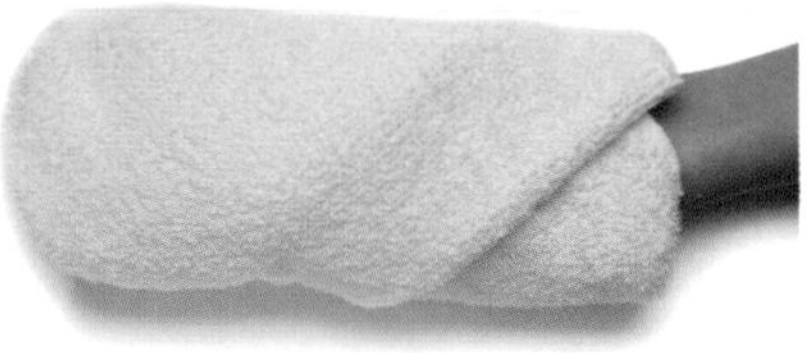

COURTESY OF CND AND SWEET SQUARED

Step 5

Treatment manicure 2

Timing: 60 minutes:

1. Apply cuticle softener to cuticles
2. Shape nails of both hands
3. Apply exfoliation treatment
4. Apply appropriate mask
5. Wrap in disposable material and then a towel to keep warm
6. Remove all traces of mask with wet disposable towel
7. Provide massage to hand and arms with appropriate cream
8. Buff nails
9. Tidy nail fold and clean under edge of nail
10. Apply varnish

EQUIPMENT LIST

hand sanitizer	wet towels
varnish remover	cuticle knife
nail wipes	cuticle nippers
file	hoof stick
cuticle softener	towels
exfoliating cream	orange sticks
mask	three-way buffer
disposable wrap	base and top coats

Male manicure

Timing: 15 minutes:

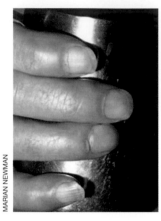

Men's hands also need some care and attention!

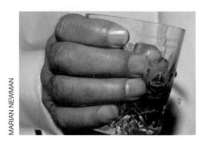

A good manicure can completely change the appearance of a man's hands. Just by shaping the nails, removing the cuticles and tidying up the skin will help towards overall grooming.

1 Shape nails of one hand. Follow shape of the end of the finger and leave a very short, even free edge (unless otherwise requested).

2 Put the fingers in a bowl of warm water to soak, with or without the application of cuticle softener.

3 Shape nails of second hand.

4 Remove first hand and place in towel.

5 Put fingers of second hand to soak.

6 Thoroughly dry first hand.

7 Remove cuticles of first hand. Avoid nipping the skin as it will just get harder.

8 Repeat sequence with second hand.

9 Apply hand cream with a short hand massage to both hands.

10 Buff nails but check with the client if he wants a shine. Some men like shiny nails while others prefer them just smoothed.

11 Clean under the free edge.

EQUIPMENT LIST

hand sanitizer	cuticle nippers
varnish remover	hoof stick
nail wipes	hand cream
file	towels
cuticle softener	orange sticks
bowl of warm water with softener	three-way buffer
cuticle knife	

Male treatment manicure

Any of the treatments are appropriate for a man's hands. Men often have very tough skin that can benefit from the softening effect of, for example, paraffin wax or heat treatment.

Manicure treatments for common nail and skin conditions

Conditions that restrict the manicure

Minor nail separation There are several things that cause the nail to separate from the nail bed (see Chapter 4). If the separation is very slight and there is no evidence of an infection under the nail, the manicure may continue. However, if separation is present, the seal at the edge of the nail bed (hyponychium) has been broken and this can allow bacteria under the nail that could cause an infection.

To prevent passing or spreading bacteria during treatment, make sure every piece of equipment is disinfected and do not, under any circumstances, put any tool under the free edge of the affected nail. Advise the client that they must do the same and keep the nail clean. The use of tea tree oil can sometimes help this condition as it has mild antiseptic properties.

Minor eczema and psoriasis If there is some eczema present and the skin is not broken or sore the treatment can continue. Avoid the use of perfumed products and proceed as if you were dealing with sensitive skin. Be very gentle over the affected area and avoid heat treatments. These conditions benefit more from moisturisers.

Damaged nails As it is impossible to list all the possible forms of damage to nails, it is easier to list some general guidelines:

- do not treat where there is broken skin
- do not treat where there is any evidence of infection
- do not treat if there is any pain
- be very gentle in the area in case the problem can be made worse.

Bitten nails A manicure can often help a nail biter to give up the habit. Obviously, there is nothing that can be done to the shape of the nails, but a biter usually also has cuticles in very bad condition. Spending extra time on making the cuticles and the skin around the nail look better is sometimes all the encouragement the client needs.

If the cuticle area is particularly bad, the extra skin that is lifted could be nipped off, but the client must be made to understand the implications and what aftercare treatment will be required.

Even though there may be little or no nail to shape, the nail plate will benefit from buffing to stimulate growth and improve its appearance.

Sometimes, even on a tiny nail, it is worth painting. The paint must be very neat and a colour that the client particularly likes, but it is another incentive not to bite and the taste of the varnish will remind the client when biting is done without thinking. A series of manicures will result in a vast improvement in the appearance of the hands and nails and, eventually, even the worst set of bitten nails will look natural.

Broken bones

If a client has broken bones in the hand or arm, it can make a manicure very difficult, but a client wearing a cast may want the nails to look good almost as compensation for the inconvenience of the break. It is possible to very gently deal with the cuticles and nails without causing any movement. Painting the nails in a bright colour can cheer up the client.

Conditions that can benefit from a manicure

Weak nails

A client may have thin and weak nails in the same way as they can have thin weak hair—either as a natural characteristic or as a result of a systemic condition. Weak nails can also be due to external effects, for example damage from artificial nails, the effect of chemicals, bitten but growing nails, etc.

Whatever the cause, the treatment is the same. The nails must be treated gently and buffing should be avoided other than with the final side of a three-sided buffer as a stimulation. Filing should also be kept to a minimum.

Weak nails benefit from wearing varnish, whether coloured or clear. This will offer some measure of protection by providing an extra thickness to the nail and also by sealing the edge to help prevent peeling. Several layers can be applied to the nail and reapplied every 2 days. If the nails are bending, the polish may peel away but can easily be reapplied. Applying nail oil and massaging it into the skin and nail is also essential to help nourish the nail and replace any oils lost.

If a base coat for weak nails is used, care must be taken that this is not used for too long as it can cause the nails to become brittle and snap. Alternating its use with a different base coat and using nail oil will help prevent this.

Brittle nails

Like weak nails, brittle nails may be a characteristic or caused by external influences. A manicure can proceed as usual for this condition, which would obviously benefit from the treatments that use plenty of creams and oils, for example warm oil or heat treatments.

Basic base coats can be used for this condition and, of course, those for brittle nails. The most useful treatment would be the application of a nail oil every day and hand cream several times a day. If the nails are very brittle then it is best to keep them quite short to avoid painful breaks.

Ridged nails

There are different types of ridged nails. Those that are found on thick, usually brittle, nails and those found on thin nails. It is important that you know which type you are dealing with. If the nail has thickened into ridges and minimizing the appearance of them by buffing will not result in the overall thickness of the nail plate becoming too thin, they can be treated. However, if the nail plate is the same thickness throughout and the ridges are folds created by the nail bed or matrix, they should not be buffed as the ridges will become splits.

Aftercare advice

During all manicure treatments, you should explain to the client exactly what you are doing, why, how this benefits them and how any improvements can be maintained following the treatment.

At the end of the manicure, the specific recommendations you are making that are relevant to the client's nail and skin condition should be repeated and reinforced. These should be supported by suggestions of retail products that will help and suggestions of other or further treatments. Treatment manicures should definitely be followed by further treatments as the improvement in condition is a relatively slow process. As improvements become visible, the treatment may need to be varied slightly. Remember to note your aftercare and retail recommendations on the client's record card.

If your client's nails are very slow to grow and she wants quicker results, you could recommend that she has a set of artificial nails for a short time while work continues to improve the condition of the skin. The natural nails will grow with the artificial set and they can then be removed.

General tips:

- Apply hand cream several times a day, especially last thing at night.
- Massage nail oil into the nails and surrounding skin.
- Reapply a top coat every few days to refresh the varnish.
- Wear gloves when using cleaning materials.
- Wear a barrier hand cream if gloves are impractical.
- Do not use nails as tools to open things.
- Do not pick or bite the skin or nails.
- Use a hand cream that has some sun protection, even in the winter.

Possible retail recommendations:

- hand cream
- nail oil
- top coat
- nail treatment base coat
- varnish remover
- gentle nail file
- varnish colour.

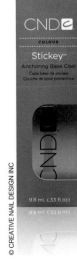
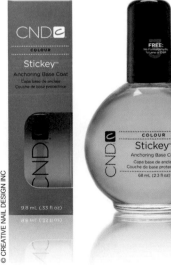

Summary

This chapter has provided the information on all manicure techniques, products used, alternative treatments and homecare advice.

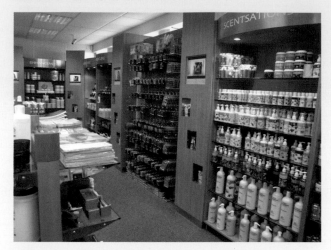

Well stocked professional wholesalers

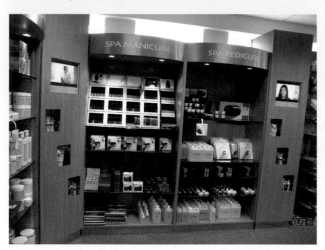

wholesalers

ASSESSMENT OF KNOWLEDGE AND UNDERSTANDING

1 What are the correct methods of filing natural nails?

2 Describe the nail plate with regard to the layers.

3 Why should the nail plate layers be kept sealed and how can this be achieved?

4 What is the cuticle and why should it be removed?

5 Name three ways of softening the cuticle.

6 What are the benefits and effects of massage?

7 What is a paraffin wax treatment and what are the benefits?

8 What would be your recommendations to a nail biter?

9 How would you treat:
  • weak nails?
  • brittle nails?
  • peeling nails?

10 Why is aftercare advice important to the client?

6

Providing a pedicure treatment

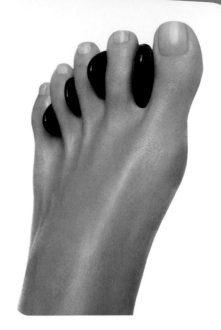

Learning objectives

In this chapter you will learn about:

- **what a pedicure is**

- **all the techniques used in a treatment and their purposes**

- **the purposes of the products being used**

- **additional treatments, their procedure and purpose**

- **various treatment alternatives and their timings**

- **aftercare advice.**

Introduction

There are many treatments that can improve the condition of the feet and toenails. This chapter explains in detail the various techniques that may be used during these treatments, their purpose and value, and gives procedural steps for a variety of treatments.

Why a pedicure?

Our feet are obviously a very important part of our body and should be kept in good condition: not only to make them look attractive (as they are not usually the prettiest part of the anatomy) but also to keep them in good condition for our comfort. Appearance is important to most people and good looking feet and nails are a part of good grooming; and paint on the toenails is very much part of today's fashion culture. It is a fact that those who are not comfortable wearing coloured varnish on their fingernails often wear colours on their toes, or perhaps a much brighter or bolder colour on their toes. This is probably more to do with the distance away from their face and painted toes do, usually, look more attractive.

A **pedicure** is still often thought of as a real luxury, but those who regularly receive one consider it to be an essential; not only for the sake of grooming but it is also a perfect form of relaxation with a result that improves comfort.

Pedicures have many similarities to a manicure: treatment of skin, nails, cuticles, massage, painting, buffing, etc. However, there are a different set of conditions.

The hands suffer greatly from external influences, for example detergents, sun damage, accidental damage to nails. The feet have different problems: in summer they need to look attractive, in winter they need to be maintained for comfort and at all times they need treatment and protection from some very common foot conditions such as fungal infections (easily picked up from others, by wearing the wrong shoes and as a result of ineffective hygiene) or hard skin (due to the nature of their job). The feet do not often suffer from dry nails and cuticles (although this is possible) and dry skin is usually found on the soles rather than on the hairy skin on top of the foot (conversely the hands are usually dry on their backs). Other conditions such as ingrown toenails and excessive sweating are also common.

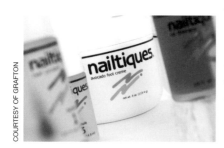

Pedicure products

Foot and toenail treatments

There are several levels of treatment that are relevant to the feet and toenails. The manicurist can carry some out, but others will need qualified medical advice.

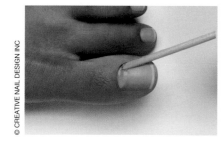

- The simplest treatment (other than good homecare) is a short pedicure that temporarily improves the appearance of the foot and/or nails. This would be appropriate for a client whose feet and toenails are in excellent condition and wants this to be maintained plus perhaps having the nails painted. Alternatively, it would suit for a client who has time or financial restrictions and needs a fast or inexpensive treatment maybe in the form of an application of moisturiser or a reshape of the nails and some paint.

- The next level would be a pedicure that was part of a treatment plan that improved the condition of the skin and nails suffering from common conditions such as dry, rough skin or long nails. The condition of the feet and toenails cannot be dramatically improved immediately, so this type of treatment would form part of a plan for the client that was working towards permanently improving these skin conditions. It could also be a one-off treat for a client who wanted a bit of pampering.

- A manicurist is not qualified to diagnose or treat anything more than simple nail or skin conditions. A recommendation to see a chiropodist should be given to the client. A pharmacist can treat some conditions, such as minor fungal or bacterial infections.

- If a condition is difficult to diagnose or treat by a chiropodist then the client will be referred to a dermatologist who may recognize the condition or conduct various tests in order to accurately diagnose and treat the condition.

Pedicure or chiropodist?

As a general description, a pedicure will improve the appearance of the foot and the toenails. It will also treat very minor nail and skin conditions. A **chiropodist** is a foot specialist and is able to medically treat a number of foot and toenail problems, having studied a 3-year degree course. They do not, however, work towards improving the appearance of the feet! In fact, they often want to cut the nails down to a length that is unacceptable for fashion. A chiropodist or **podiatrist** (there is no difference) carries out a variety of treatments and it is important to understand their role so that recommendations can be made.

Chiropodists treat people of all ages and from all walks of life. For example:

- children sometimes have pains in their legs or feet as they grow or have problems walking

- diabetics may have problems with the circulation or sensation in their feet

- sports men and women often suffer from injuries to the legs and feet

- dancers who spend long hours rehearsing and performing put stress on their feet and legs that can cause injuries

- people needing minor surgery such as nail surgery or laser treatment

- some people do not need treatment but just want advice about footwear or foot health.

Chiropodists will:

- assess and treat ailments that may, range from problems such as verrucas to deformity

- analyse a person's walk or run and correct misaligned anatomical relationships between the different segments of the foot; orthotics – custom-made soles – are often prescribed to achieve this

- monitor and manage foot problems and deformities caused by diseases such as rheumatoid arthritis

- advise and treat patients at high risk of foot problems and amputation such as those who suffer from diabetes

- carry out nail surgery using a local anaesthetic.

The following section looks at each stage of a pedicure treatment, explains its purpose and benefits and describes how the procedure is carried out. Although the stages are in a logical order they do not necessarily relate to a complete treatment.

Pedicure techniques

Foot preparation

As with hands, feet must always be clean before you touch them. There are various methods of cleaning feet and this is something the manicurist must do (unlike with hands, where a wash with soap and water or sanitizing hand gel is carried out by the client).

The method will depend on the products used in the salon. The feet could be dipped into warm water with an antiseptic additive and then dried or sprayed with a foot cleanser or wiped over with an antiseptic wet wipe. Whichever method is used, it should be done first

ALWAYS REMEMBER

A manicurist must never diagnose a skin or nail condition that has a medical or systemic basis. Simple environmental damage, such as minor hard skin, are part of the manicurist's remit, together with individual characteristics that result in similar, common conditions such as weak, thin nails or delicate skin. The manicurist will come across many different conditions on many different clients and must be able to recognize all the more common ones and know when a pedicure can continue and improve the condition, when a pedicure can continue but with certain restrictions (e.g. when bruising or minor eczema are present) or when a pedicure treatment cannot be carried out and a client should be referred to a pharmacist or GP (e.g. for ingrown toenail, fungal or bacterial infections).

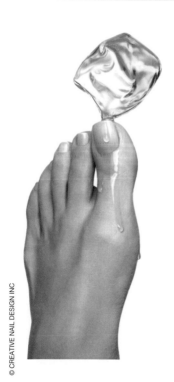

© CREATIVE NAIL DESIGN INC

before the feet are touched. During this cleansing process, the feet can be inspected for any conditions that may prevent treatment such as fungal infections or viral infections.

When the feet are clean, any varnish should be removed and the nails inspected for any problems.

Filing

It is easier to file a nail into a good shape when it is at its hardest (that is before it is soaked in water or soaked with oils). This is because an over-hydrated nail will have a tendency to bend and it will be difficult to achieve a smooth and even edge. Also, the moisture may disturb the natural bonds between the nail plate layers and filing could cause the layers to separate.

For all natural nails, a very fine file or emery board must be used. Causing trauma to the layers easily damages the edge of the nail and a harsh abrasive will splinter the layers and cause them to part.

Remember the comparison of nails to plywood in Chapter 5 (p. 102). The toenails are constructed in the same way as fingernails but they do have some minor differences. The big toenail is usually much bigger and often thicker than any other nail. It protects a very important part of the foot: the big toe is essential for balance. Remember the discussion of the arches of the foot in Chapter 2 (p. 36): it is a shaped like a tripod. That is, there are three main points of contact with the ground. The big toe is a crucial part of this shape and it is also important in gripping. Without a strong toenail the big toe would not be so efficient.

The nails on the next three toes are usually quite small and thinner. Their role is protection and they do not suffer the wear and tear of fingernails or the big toenail. The little toenail differs because it often suffers from pressure from tight shoes. It may have a misshapen, thickened nail or sometimes a nail that can barely be seen. This toe frequently suffers corns, again from rubbing against tight shoes.

If nails need to be shortened, cutting with a sharp pair of scissors or clippers followed by filing with a fine emery board is safe. When using clippers on the big toenail do not cut the whole width of the nail in one cut as this could cause the nail to split and also puts pressure on the sides of the nail.

Make small cuts all along the nail from one side to the other. For minor length reduction, a file is all that is needed.

Toenails do not suffer from the same abuse as fingernails. They are not continually plunged into water and detergents, etc., but they can suffer from being enclosed for long periods.

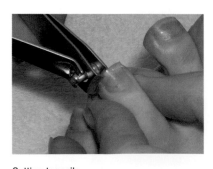

Cutting toenails

The shape of the filed nail should be to the preference of the client who may follow the current fashion or have a personal preference. If the client has real preference and leaves the decision to the manicurist, the nail shape can be straight or slightly curved. The important point to remember is not to file down the side of the nail. Let the sides of the nail reach the top of the toe before you shape the free edge. Taking the sides of the nail away may cause a problem when the foot is in a shoe that will squash it. The nail can then grow into the skin and result in an ingrown toenail. If the sides of the nail are already below the top of the toe, shape the corners of the nail so there is not a sharp point that can dig into the skin.

During the winter months, the toenails should be no longer than the toes. Closed-in shoes can press on the nails, particularly the big toenail or the longest toe. Continual pressure on the nail in this way can cause it to start to separate from the nail bed and infection under the nail can result.

In summer, when open-toed shoes are predominantly worn, the nails can be kept slightly longer if the client wishes. However, if the client wears closed shoes or trainers, the nails must be kept short.

Hard skin removal

This is an essential part of a pedicure treatment and is the main difference between this treatment and a manicure. Nearly all feet have some areas of hard skin to varying degrees. It is most common on the heel and the ball of the foot; on the pressure areas of the feet, in fact. It can also occur on the sides of the heel and either side of the foot near the toes.

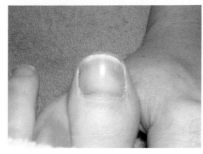

Rounded toenail

The hairless skin on the soles of the feet and palms of the hands has the structural ability to become very hard and tough. Those who use their hands for hard manual work develop thick, hard skin that can withstand a great deal of abuse. People who walk barefoot have a very thick layer of hard skin on their feet to protect against rough ground. This is an example of the body's natural protection systems working.

However, clients requiring a pedicure are unlikely to be the 'barefoot' type of person as they want their feet to look and feel attractive. Hard skin on the feet tends to look very dry and can even start to 'crack' on the heels.

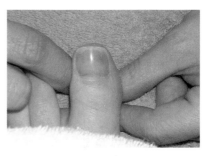

Square toenail

Although many people associate pedicures with summer and wearing sandals, it is important that the feet are also looked after in the winter as enclosed shoes and man-made fibres cause the feet to sweat. The dry, dead skin should be removed regularly to prevent a build-up resulting in thick patches of hard skin.

A manicurist can only deal with superficial hard skin. If the areas are very thick, it is worth recommending that the client visits a chiropodist who can remove hard skin to a deeper level using scalpel blades. The alternative to this is for the client to have more regular pedicure treatments and maintain the hard skin prevention treatment at home.

Manicurists should only use an abrasive and exfoliator during a treatment. An open blade should *never* be used to remove hard skin. Most insurance policies and local authority licensing does not allow for instruments of this kind at this level of treatment. There are many excellent abrasives available on the market designed for this use, plus many pedicure brands that have very efficient hard skin removal products. These produce excellent results without the need for cutting skin away.

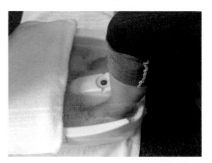

Place feet in bowl of warm water and foot soak

Hard skin can be removed when the skin has been softened but take care not to remove too much. Or on cleaned feet before the soak. The usual method is a soak in warm water containing a small amount of liquid soap, for cleansing and softening, and an antiseptic solution. (Many inexpensive foot soaking solutions are readily available.) Feet can be soaked in a clean plastic bowl but, ideally, a specific piece of equipment with a thermostat to control and maintain the temperature of the water is preferable for the comfort of the client. Those with disposable inner bowls are perfect for hygiene purposes.

After the toenails have been filed and shaped and cuticle remover (if used) has been applied to the toes, the feet are placed in the water for around 5 minutes. This is very relaxing for the client, especially if the bowl has a massaging facility. Five minutes should give sufficient time for the hard skin to soften, especially if a suitable solution has been added.

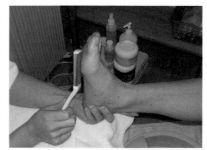

Removal of hard skin

Remove one foot from the bowl and place it onto a clean towel. Feel with your fingers for the areas of hard skin and, using the rough side of the abrasive, buff off the skin until the area feels smooth and soft to your fingers. Feel all around the foot taking care not to miss any areas.

After all the areas of hard skin have been removed with the harsh abrasive it is important to smooth the skin. As with using a three-way buffer on the nails, the abrasive leaves the surface feeling rough and, when the skin dries out, this will be unpleasant. Most foot files have a hard and soft side, so buff over all areas with the softer side to smooth and 'polish' the skin.

If an exfoliator is used, manufacturer's instructions should be followed.

When all the hard skin has been removed and the skin feels smooth, return the foot to the bowl so any debris can be washed away. This will also serve to keep the foot warm while the process is repeated on the other foot.

If a heated bowl is not being used, the water will get too cold for the foot to be returned. In this case, after the hard skin removal, continue to the cuticle removal then wrap the foot in a towel to keep it warm while the second foot is treated.

It is advisable to remove the bowl of water at the end of this stage.

Cuticle removal

As for manicure, it is important to understand this area of the nail unit. The structure on the toes is the same as on the fingers.

The cuticle (as its name implies: a thin layer on the surface) is a layer of epidermal skin that grows from under the nail fold and sticks to the nail plate. It is this that can be removed, but not as far back as the seal of the eponychium.

As in a manicure, this skin should be removed and it is usually very easy to do so. On toes, the nail fold is not always so evident, but there is plenty of cuticle waiting to be removed.

When the cuticle is softened with water, oil or proprietary removers, it is very easy to remove it from the surface of the nail. Usually, the correct use of a good cuticle knife will make an efficient job of this with the very occasional use of a pair of clean, sharp cuticle nippers. Often there is so much cuticle that the use of nippers is desirable after the skin has been lifted from the nail plate.

This is an important part of the treatment. It will make the toes look better, neater and well looked after. It will also make painting easier and more effective.

Cuticle should only be removed when it has been softened. During a pedicure this is almost always after the feet have been soaked.

The methods used during any kind of pedicure will depend on salon procedure or the brand of pedicure products being used. It is always advisable to closely follow manufacturer's instructions.

Buffing

This is a useful procedure for several reasons:

- the stimulation to the nail plate increases blood circulation in the area
- it can remove superficial staining caused by polish
- it produces a very healthy looking shine that will last several weeks
- it will minimize ridges
- it helps to make the nail plate less porous
- polish bonds better and is therefore less prone to chipping
- when used on the free edge, it will help to seal the layers and make the edge smooth and rounded.

A three-way buffer is a tool that has progressively finer abrasives on its three surfaces. Usually it is coloured for the first and most abrasive side, then white for a finer abrasive and finally grey for a smooth surface.

Care must be taken not to over-buff as this can thin the nail, particularly over ridges. The full three-side buffing should only be done about once a month as any more could thin the nail. The last two sides can be done more often to bring up the shine.

Sometimes the big toenail has excessive ridges. If the nail itself is quite thick these ridges can reduced before the use of a three-way buffer. This can be done with a clean white block buffer or a 240 grit file. Be careful not to buff too much and thin the nail. Never do this to a nail that is thin and delicate.

The end of this stage is a good time to clean under the nails. Buffing dust has probably collected there and the nail bed on the toes sheds dead skin cells. Use a clean orange stick and have a tissue or cotton wool disc in your hand to wipe the orange stick after cleaning under each nail. Take care not to break the seal of the hyponychium.

TOP TIP

Buffing the toenails makes varnish stay on much longer.

Massage

Clients often say that the massage is the best part of the pedicure as it so relaxing. It is also definitely the only stage that they cannot carry out effectively at home and it can turn a pedicure into a real treat and luxury treatment.

Apart from keeping the client happy, there are many reasons why a massage of the foot or, time allowing, foot and lower leg is beneficial. The hands and feet are the extremities of the body and often the first to feel the cold or suffer from sluggish or poor circulation. The benefits of massage include the following:

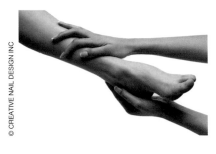

© CREATIVE NAIL DESIGN INC

- blood circulation is stimulated and, therefore, during the period of the increase, becomes more efficient at delivering nutrients and oxygen to the cells of the area and removing cellular waste

- the improved circulation will also help with muscle tone, skin tone and colour

- lymphatic drainage is improved by the manual friction, so waste from the tissues is removed and the body's mechanism for dealing with infection has a period of increased efficiency

- absorption of the nourishing cream used during the massage is improved so its nutrients reach deeper tissues

- a good massage can relieve tension in the muscles and joints

- it is relaxing and soothing for the client.

There are situations and conditions when massage must be avoided or restricted. Avoid massage:

- over open cuts or wounds, as cross-infection could occur or bacteria could be introduced to the open skin

- over recent scars as they could be stretched

- in inflamed or infected areas

- over areas of bruising.

Restrict massage:

- over painful, inflamed joints, for example in clients with arthritis whose joints should be avoided during the massage

- at any joint that is painful.

Movements See Chapter 5 (p. 108) for the main movements.

A massage routine

- Make sure you have sufficient massage medium in your hands for the complete massage of one hand and arm. Knowing how much to use will only come from experience with the specific product and your client's skin.

- Depending on your working conditions, the massage may be carried out with your client's foot on your lap or resting on a foot stool. Make sure your lap or the stool are covered with a clean towel.

- Once you have started the massage, do not take both hands away from the area at the same time. This can be disconcerting for the client. One hand may be removed to move position but never both.

- When the massage is coming to an end, slow the movements down and finish by placing the client's foot down on the floor. Make the final stroke down the foot and off at the toes.

- Encourage the client to keep her feet very relaxed and remind her if the foot or leg starts to tense.

Step-by-step: Massage

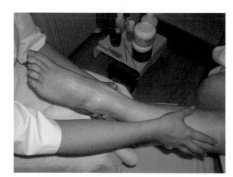 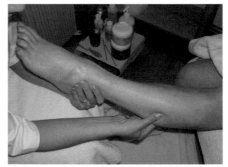 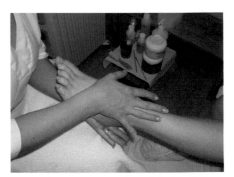

1 With the chosen massage medium on both hands, take your client's foot with one of yours to support the foot and leg and, with the other, spread the massage medium up the leg to just below the knee. Repeat with the other hand so the area to be massaged has been spread with sufficient medium for the treatment. Repeat these actions two or three times as a relaxing start to the massage.

2 Support the foot and leg on your lap or stool with one hand and, using the fingers and thumb of the other, gently squeeze and release the calf muscle near the ankle on one side and repeat this up the leg to just below the knee (petrissage). Slide your hand back down to the ankle. Repeat this once or twice more then repeat with the other side of the leg.

3 Holding the client's foot in both your hands, apply effleurage movements over the top of the foot in a rhythmic movement. Apply more pressure on the stroke towards the ankle.

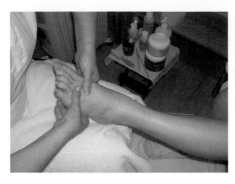

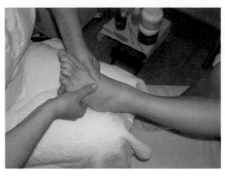

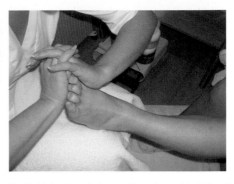

4 Supporting the foot, use your thumb to apply small friction movements between each meta-tarsal on the top of the foot from the toes to the ankle.

5 Repeat, but use a deep sliding movement with firm pressure on the upward stroke. This is a lymph drainage movement.

6 Hold the toes between the palms of both hands (using the heel of the hand, that is the part of the palm nearer to the wrist) and 'grind' the toes. This is very relaxing.

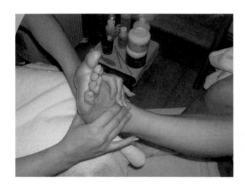

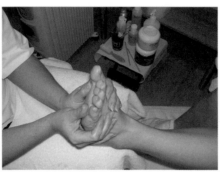

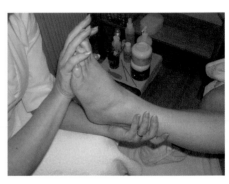

7 Supporting the heel of the foot, flex the foot up and use your thumbs to apply deep friction movements all over the sole of the foot. With the side of your forefinger and thumb, squeeze the outside edge of the foot.

8 With both your hands, place your fingers on the top of the foot and with your thumbs on the sole just below the toes, spread the foot while applying small friction movements with your thumbs.

9 Grasp the client's ankle and rotate the foot from the ankle a few times in each direction.

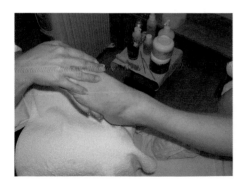

10 Apply a few gentle effleurage movements to the foot and leg becoming slower, and finish off with the last down stroke coming off at the toes as you place your client's foot down on the towel.

Wrap your client's foot in the towel to keep warm. Repeat for the other foot and leg.

Painting

Not every client will want painted nails, but those who do should be delighted with the result and the colour or effect achieved. A beautiful, professionally painted set of nails should be better than most clients can do for themselves. The paint should last longer and the finish should be perfect.

Clients will often choose a colour that is bolder than one they would wear on their fingers. If they are unsure, follow the general rules given for a manicure to help them decide.

Skilful painting, like all other skills, needs plenty of practice. An excellent pedicure can so often be let down by bad painting and the client takes away the proof of that lack of skill to be seen several times a day.

The results of good painting are:

- colour that stays on for more than 5 days; it should stay on for 7 or more (Paint on toes usually lasts longer than fingers as it is not immersed in water several times a day.)

- a smooth and even surface

- a neat, even edge that neither touches surrounding tissue nor shows any unpainted nail

- a layer that is not so thick that it takes an unreasonable time to dry.

There are no magic tips about painting. There are no foolproof steps to follow to produce a perfect result. Each varnish will be different to use depending on the brand, the colour, the brush and the temperature. There are, however, some guidelines that may help, but practice is what really counts – and then more practice.

General guidelines for painting toenails:

- Toes need to be kept apart while painting and drying. Use a clean pair of toe separators for each foot or roll a tissue up and wind it around the toes (the tissue can be discarded once the varnish is dry).

- Make sure you and your client are in a comfortable position and that the foot is at an angle that allows you to see the toenails properly.

- Practise holding the bottle in the palm of the hand that is holding the client's toe. This is safer than using the bottle on the desk top where it can get knocked over by your brush. It is also quicker to reload the brush and it is useful to be able to do this comfortably as sometimes there are situations when you will not be working on or near a desk.

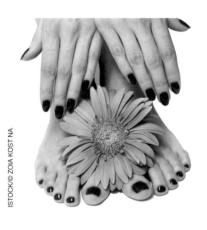

- When removing the brush from the bottle, lift it out in a spiral motion wiping the shaft of the brush on the neck of the bottle. This will prevent varnish on the shaft running down and flooding the brush or dripping off.

- Wipe the brush away from you on the neck of the bottle. This will leave the brush with sufficient varnish loaded on the side you are going to place onto the nail.

- Try to load the brush with sufficient varnish to cover the nail and so avoid the need to go back in the bottle for more. Varnish is drying while you are painting so you want a good coverage quickly. Remember to be aware of the size of the nail being painted, i.e. a small toenail will need much less varnish than the big toe.

- Avoid overworking the varnish on the nail. Use the minimum number of strokes, as overworking will start to drag the varnish off and make it bumpy.

- Whatever the colour, don't worry if the coverage is uneven after the first coat. Keep the layers thin and, if necessary, apply a third coat of the colour to get a good, even coverage.

- Always use a base coat. These products are formulated differently from coloured varnish. They are developed to create a stronger bond with the natural nail than coloured varnish and help to form a barrier between the nail and the varnish. Deep pigments can stain the natural nail but pale colours can also have this effect, especially when worn in sunlight or on a sunbed. The barrier of the base coat may not prevent this, but it will certainly minimize it.

- Special base coats are also available and can be used if appropriate. Ridge fillers can be useful, but remember that the thicker the layers, the longer the varnish will take to dry. Ridge fillers work by being slightly thicker and smoothing the ridges. This should not be a problem with a thin varnish, but it will create a very thick layer with a thick, densely pigmented varnish.

- A top coat should also be used. Like the base coats they have a different formulation as their job is to create a good shine and be hard wearing. In addition they are often quick drying. After painting the nail plate, run the side of the brush around the edge of the nail. This will seal the nail plate and also the layer of varnish to help protect the nail and avoid chipping.

- Painting is the last stage of the pedicure treatment and the client will need to wait for a while before collecting their belongings, putting their coat on, etc. It is a good idea if a client brings sandals with her for a pedicure treatment. This means that she does not need to wait until the nails are dry before leaving. As varnish takes a long time to dry, putting on shoes will almost always leave dents in the varnish, even if the surface is dry.

- This is the final stage of the pedicure and it is essential that there is no trace of any oil or moisture on the surface of the nail plate, as it would cause the varnish to peel off the nail very quickly. Thoroughly wipe the nail with varnish remover from the free edge towards the cuticle (this direction will avoid any moisture from the skin being wiped onto the nail plate) to ensure it is clean and dry. Some removers have oily conditioners in them and these can leave a film on the nail plate and cause a problem with the varnish. It could peel off very quickly or sometimes bubble. This is when small imperfections in the surface of a newly painted nail can appear.

- If the varnish does not look good or if you make a mistake, it is far better to remove the varnish and reapply (even if the next client is waiting). The client must leave with proof of a first class pedicure that took a little longer rather than a second-rate one that was rushed.

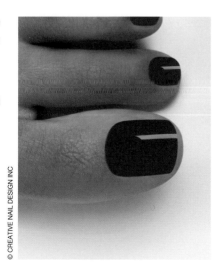

© CREATIVE NAIL DESIGN INC

- It is a good practice to apply a small drop of oil after painting to the cuticle area with the nail angled down to allow it to run over the surface of the nail. This will ensure maximum hydration of the skin, and the coat of oil on the surface will stop the varnish being tacky and attracting fluff or hairs, etc.

Procedure for painting

1   Wipe over the nail to remove any trace of moisture.

2   Apply a thin layer of base coat or appropriate treatment base.

3   Apply two thin coats of the chosen colour.

4   Assess the coverage of the varnish and apply a third coat if necessary.

5   Apply a top coat and seal the edge.

6   Apply a drop of oil to the cuticle and let it run down the nail.

7   If appropriate, escort your client to an area where she can wait for a while until her nails are dry enough to leave.

French pedicure

See Chapter 5 (p. 115) for details on French manicure, which can be applied to the feet.

Paraffin wax treatment

This is an additional treatment that is offered in many salons either as part of a luxury pedicure or as a specific treatment for conditions such as dry or rough skin. It can be very soothing for arthritis sufferers.

This treatment in a pedicure has all the same benefits as in a manicure:

- it is very relaxing and soothing
- it will soften dry, rough or calloused skin
- it temporarily gives the skin a younger-looking appearance
- it improves blood circulation during the treatment
- it softens cuticles ready for removal
- it soothes aching joints and tired muscles.

It is not always advisable to paint the nails after a paraffin wax treatment as the nail will have absorbed oils and the paint will probably peel off very quickly.

See Chapter 5 (p. 116) for details on types of wax and heaters.

Procedure for a paraffin wax treatment

1 Make sure the heater is on for sufficient time before it is needed.

2 Have a disposable wrap ready (this could be plastic bags, cling film or foil) together with clean towels. (This treatment can be used with heated bootees, in which case have them ready to use with relevant accessories.)

3 The feet need to be soaked to make sure they are very clean. After this, it is usually advisable to remove hard skin with an abrasive. This will allow the wax to have a better softening effect on the skin.

4 Check the temperature of the wax.

5 If the heater is big enough, hold the client's ankle and dip the foot in the wax and remove, keeping the foot over the heater. Repeat this several times until a thick coat of wax is covering the foot. If the heater is too small for this, place the foot on the disposable covering that is being used (e.g. foil or cling film) and paint several layers of wax onto the foot using a clean small paint brush.

6 Wrap the foot in the prepared disposable wrap and then either in a towel or place it in the heated bootee.

7 Repeat with the other foot.

8 Leave wax in place for approximately 10 minutes.

9 Remove one foot from wraps and peel away wax. Discard used wax and disposable wrap. Repeat with other foot.

10 Continue with the pedicure treatment.

ALWAYS REMEMBER

Paraffin wax treatments should not be used if the foot has any infected areas or open wounds of any kind.

Masks and exfoliators

As with manicures, there are many brands that have a full range of pedicure products that loosely follow the treatments of a facial (after all, it is all skin).

It is important that manufacturer's instructions are followed for the sequence of these treatments and their recommended usage.

See Chapter 5 (p. 118) for general observations about masks.

Warm oil treatment

On the feet, as on the hand, hard, brittle and dry nails and dry cuticles benefit from an oil treatment. It is not possible to dip just the toes into a heater and it is not very practical to fill a whole foot bath with oil especially as it should be discarded after use! Fortunately, there is an easy method for providing an oil treatment:

1 Soak cotton wool pads in the oil. Apply a generous amount of a moisturising foot cream to the foot. Wrap the oil-soaked cotton wool around the toes, then wrap the foot in foil and a towel. The heat from the foot will be trapped and aid the penetration of the oil. Meanwhile the benefit of the foot cream can be enjoyed.

2 Heated bootees can be used in place of the foil and towel, as above.

As with paraffin wax, oil will be absorbed by the nail plate and may make painting less effective, with a tendency to peel off.

Thermal bootees

See the details on thermal mitts in Chapter 5 (p. 118).

Procedure for a heat treatment

1 When the nails have been shaped, the feet have been soaked and most of the hard skin removed, lightly apply the appropriate cream to the feet and oil or cream to the cuticles. Do not massage in.

2 Wrap the feet in disposable plastic bags or cling film and place them into the protective plastic bag that is supplied with the bootees.

3 Check that the bootees' temperature is right and place the wrapped feet into the bootees.

4 Make sure the client is comfortable and leave the bootees on for 10 minutes.

5 Remove and unwrap one foot and massage with the cream remaining on the foot. Discard disposable wrapping.

6 Wrap the foot in a towel to keep it warm.

7 Repeat with the other foot.

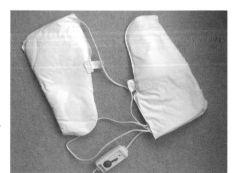

Heated bootees

Pedicure treatment alternatives

The sequence of the pedicure treatment depends on two main factors, the practice of the salon and the pedicure brand being used. There are many alternatives that suit different situations, and this section includes a list of sequences that are logical progressions for various types of treatment. They are offered as guidelines, and you should be careful to follow the sequences supplied by the manufacturers of the products you use.

BEST PRACTICE

Timings for specific stages. e.g. massage, soaking, heat treatments, etc., have deliberately not been given. This is because these are stages that can take more or less time as required. Some clients want minimal shaping or cuticle work; others will need more. The manicurist must learn to keep an eye on the timing and make up tlme if necessary.

General (i.e. for all treatments):

- The work area must be prepared before the client arrives with all relevant tools and equipment clean and ready for use.

- A consultation with the client must be carried out, even if a specific type of treatment has been booked. An alteration to this booking is acceptable following the consultation.

- It is also acceptable that, following the consultation, additional equipment is collected and prepared for use.

- Make sure the client is comfortable before starting the treatment and has removed all footwear.

- Trouser legs should be rolled up and protected if this is appropriate.

- Your hands should be clean and you should be sitting comfortably and safely.

Reshape and varnish

Timing: 20 minutes:

1 Thoroughly clean feet with an antiseptic wipe or spray.

2 Shape nails on all ten toes.

3 Clean under the free edge with a disposable orange stick.

4 Apply base coat, coloured varnish and top coat.

5 Apply oil.

EQUIPMENT LIST

antiseptic wipe/spray	orange sticks
varnish remover	base and top coats
nail wipes	coloured varnish
file	nail oil
hoof stick	

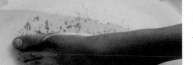

Mini pedicure

Timing: 30 minutes:

1 Thoroughly clean feet with an antiseptic wipe or spray.

2 Apply a cuticle softener to all ten toes.

3 Shape nails on all ten toes.

4 Remove the cuticle on each toe and tidy the nail fold.

5   Wipe nails to remove cuticle softener.

6   Apply foot cream to both feet.

7   Clean under the free edge with a disposable orange stick.

8   Wipe nails with remover.

9   Either apply varnish or buff nails.

EQUIPMENT LIST

antiseptic wipe/spray	hoof stick
varnish remover	foot cream
nail wipes	orange sticks
cuticle softener	three-way buffer
file	base and top coats
cuticle knife	coloured varnish
cuticle nippers	nail oil

Step-by-step: Pedicure

Timing: 45 minutes

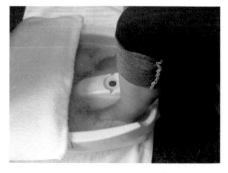

1   Place feet in bowl of warm water and foot soak.

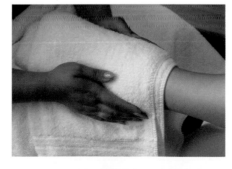

2   Remove one foot, dry, remove any polish and inspect foot for skin and nail condition and any contra-indications or other conditions that may affect the service.

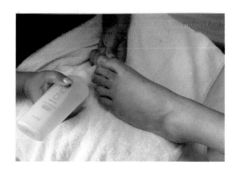

3   Apply cuticle remover.

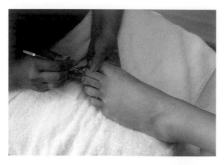

4   Remove cuticle with cuticle knife. (Note the cotton pad under the foot to wipe the cuticle knife on.)

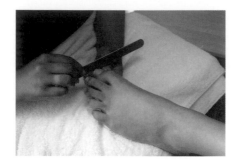

5   File nails. Return foot to bowl and repeat steps 1-5 to other foot.

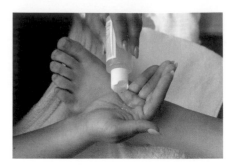

6   Remove first foot from bowl, remove hard skin with foot file, prepare for massage.

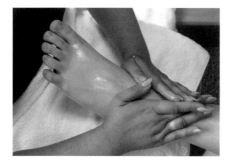

7   Using long effleurage movements, spread the massage oil over foot and up the lower leg to just below the knee.

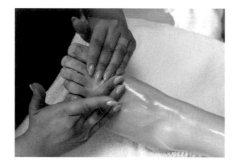

8   Using circular petrissage movements, massage the top of the foot, up the front of the leg and down the back of the leg.

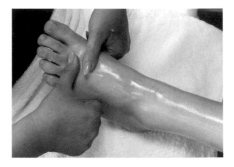

9   Using circular frictions, firmly massage the top of the foot, up the front of the leg and down the back of the leg.

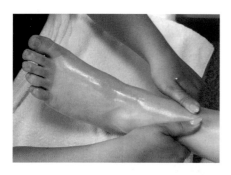

10   With more petrissage movements pick up the skin in small firm movements up the sides of the leg and down the back of the leg.

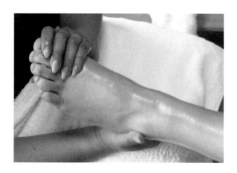

11   Supporting the foot with one hand under the heel, rotate the foot to the extreme of its movement but without forcing it.

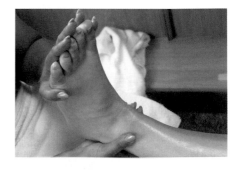

12   Using a similar movement, push the foot towards the leg to release tension at the back of the leg.

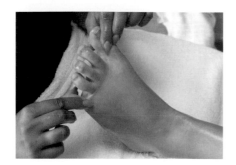

13   Gently rotate each toe in both clockwise and anti-clockwise directions.

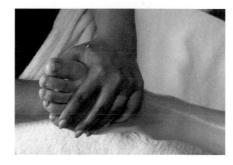

14   With one hand on the top of the foot, use the knuckles to very firmly massage under the foot. Wrap the foot in a towel to keep warm and repeat with the other foot.

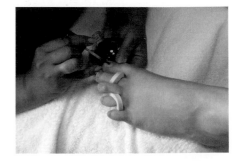

15   With the first foot, place toe ropes or a rolled-up tissue between the toes. Wipe the nails with polish remover to clean away any oils and apply a base coat. Repeat with other foot.

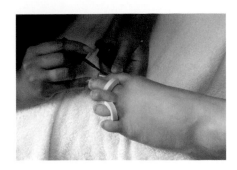

16 Apply the chosen nail varnish to the toes of first one foot then the other.

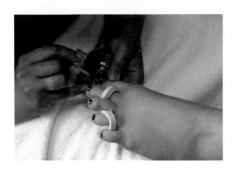

17 Apply a top coat to toes of both feet and clean away any mistakes.

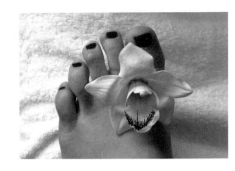

18 Finished foot! Bright colours look great even on short toenails.

EQUIPMENT LIST

antiseptic wipe/spray	cuticle nippers
varnish remover	hoof stick
nail wipes	foot cream
foot spa	orange sticks
towels	three-way buffer
cuticle softener	base and top coats
file	coloured varnish
cuticle knife	nail oil

Step-by-step: Luxury pedicure

After all the work on the toes but before the massage, a luxury pedicure provides exfoliation to the skin and a moisturising mask.

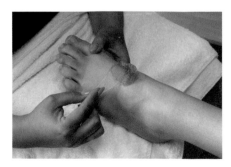

1 Apply the exfoliation product.

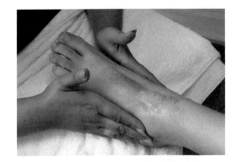

2 Massage the product all over the foot working on the harder skin areas. Place the foot back in the bowl and repeat to the other foot.

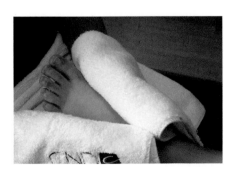

3 Make sure the product has been washed off the foot, remove it from bowl and dry.

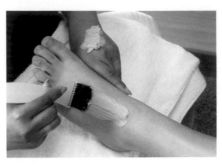
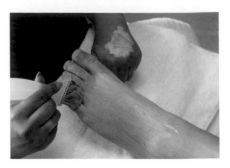

4   Apply mask and spread over the foot. Wrap the foot in a towel to keep warm and repeat with the other foot. Then, depending on the product used, the foot can either be massaged with the mask or it is removed and a massage oil used.

Treatment pedicure (thermal bootees)

Timing: 60 minutes:

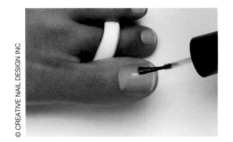

1   Ask client to place her feet in the prepared bowl for 2 to 3 minutes. Remove one foot and roughly dry while inspecting the condition of the skin. Wrap in the towel, leaving the toes exposed.

2   Remove any varnish and inspect the condition of the nails. Clip, file and shape the nails.

3   Return foot to the bowl and repeat with the other foot.

4   Remove the first foot from the bowl, pat dry and remove the hard skin. Wrap foot in towel to keep warm.

5   Remove second foot, pat dry and remove hard skin. Apply foot cream and cuticle treatment and wrap the foot in the disposable covering.

6   Apply foot cream and cuticle treatment to first foot and wrap in disposable covering.

EQUIPMENT LIST

antiseptic wipe/spray	cuticle knife
varnish remover	cuticle nippers
nail wipes	hoof stick
foot spa	towels
file	orange sticks
cuticle softener	three-way buffer
hand cream	base and top coats
disposable wrap/gloves	coloured varnish
heated bootees	

7   Place both feet in thermal bootees for 10 minutes.

8   Remove first foot from bootee and briefly massage in any remaining cream.

9   Remove cuticles and buff nails. Wrap foot to keep warm. Repeat with second foot.

10 Massage foot and lower leg of second foot. Massage foot and lower leg of first foot.

11 Clean under nails of the first foot with orange stick. Wipe nails with remover.

12 Apply varnish if required. Repeat cleaning and polishing on second foot.

Treatment pedicure using a mask

Timing 60 minutes:

You should follow the manufacturer's recommended procedure for a pedicure using a mask.

Pedicure treatments for common nail and skin conditions

Chapter 5 (p. 127) discussed conditions that restrict manicure treatments, and these are all – with the exception of bitten nails! – applicable to pedicure treatments. Similarly, conditions that can be improved by manicure can also be helped by pedicure.

Aftercare advice

Following a pedicure treatment, it is pleasant for the client to apply a product suitable for the condition of the feet. This may be a refreshing foot spray in the summer or a foot powder in the winter to help keep the feet dry in shoes.

During all pedicure treatments, you should explain to the client exactly what you are doing, why, how this benefits them and how any improvements can be maintained following the treatment.

At the end of the pedicure, the specific recommendations you are making that are relevant to the client's nail and skin condition should be repeated and reinforced. These should be supported by suggestions of retail products that will help and suggestions of other or further treatments. Treatment pedicures should always be followed by further treatments as progress is relatively slow. Remember to note your aftercare and retail recommendations on the client's record card.

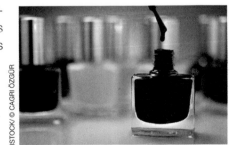

ISTOCK/ © CAGRI ÖZGÜR

General tips:

● Apply moisturising foot cream last thing at night, paying attention to the areas of hard or dry skin, such as the heels.

● Massage nail oil into the nails and surrounding skin.

● Reapply a top coat every few days to refresh the varnish.

● Do not pick the skin or nails.

● Wear well-fitting shoes.

● Visit a chiropodist if there is any sign of corns or bunions, infections or ingrown toenails.

Possible retail recommendations:

- moisturising foot cream
- refreshing foot spray
- nail oil
- top coat
- foot file for use in the bath at home
- varnish colour
- varnish remover.

Summary

This chapter has provided the information on all pedicure techniques, products used, alternative treatments and homecare advice.

ASSESSMENT OF KNOWLEDGE AND UNDERSTANDING

1 Explain a pedicure treatment and what it can achieve.

2 What treatments can a chiropodist provide?

3 What skin and nail conditions prevent treatment?

4 What skin and nail conditions restrict treatment?

5 Explain the four main massage movements.

6 Describe the benefits of heat treatments.

7 What after care advice is appropriate following a pedicure?

8 Why are feet more prone to fungal and bacterial infections?

7
Essential chemistry of artificial nails

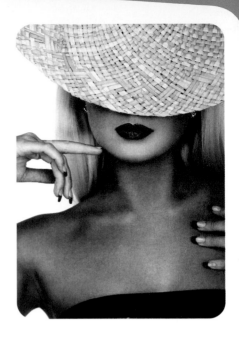

Learning objectives

In this chapter you will learn about:

● the artificial nail 'systems' used in the professional nail industry

● the critical differences between the 'systems'

● ways to choose the right one for you

● the basic chemical processes in all artificial nail products

● how to find the cause of a problem and put it right.

Introduction

Every person who considers themselves to be a professional should strive to be a master of their craft. A nail technician should be skilful at applying nails to all types of nails; they should also be knowledgeable about the products and tools they use. This chapter provides the nail technician with a basic understanding of the chemicals, chemical processes and generic products that underpin all aspects of artificial nails.

In the nail industry, the information available about the products in use tends to be provided by manufacturers of brands and this information is usually tied up with marketing exercises. A technician needs to have a basic knowledge of the chemistry involved and then add specific product knowledge to this, almost as 'postgraduate' learning. You may use the same products every time, but the client, their nails, the circumstances and the environment will differ every time. By understanding how the chemistry of the products works and what can influence the chemical reactions and performance, the professional technician will be equipped to use all products to their best potential and solve any problems that may arise.

'Systems' in the nail industry

Although all types of artificial nails result in either longer or stronger nails that, hopefully, look natural, there are several different ways of achieving these results using different sets of products. These different methods are called **'systems'** in the nail industry. The name 'system' has evolved as a group of specific products working together to produce artificial nails: there is a system of using them together and a chemical system that makes them work.

The three main systems in use

There are three main 'systems' that the industry is familiar with—**acrylic**, **UV gel** and **fibreglass** – but the names that are now in common usage are inaccurate and can be misleading. The inaccuracy of the names of the systems is unimportant as they are widely accepted and understood, but an understanding of the underlying chemistry will show the discrepancies. The three main systems have several derivatives that confuse the situation even more, but the different systems refer more to application methods than the system components and chemistry. We can briefly look at each of them.

- *Acrylic* – This system uses a liquid monomer and a powder polymer that, when mixed together, form a solid. This should more accurately be called liquid and powder (L&P).

- *UV gel* – This system uses a gel that is supplied as a 'pre-mixed' product and forms a solid when exposed to UV light.

- *Fibreglass* – This system utilizes the additional strength of a **fibre** mesh – that can be man-made fibreglass or natural silk or cotton – together with a resin that hardens.

The way in which each of these systems works from a chemistry point of view is actually very similar. The application and type of product differs enormously.

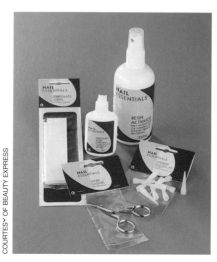

COURTESY OF BEAUTY EXPRESS

A fibre system

TOP TIP

Concentrate on one system first, understand how it works on a wide variety of clients before moving on to another.

When a nail technician starts their career, or is thinking of starting, one of the most confusing and difficult decisions is which system to learn. It is important, in spite of any advice to the contrary, to concentrate on one system at the beginning. The application of artificial nails is a practical skill that needs lots and lots of practice. Experience can be achieved only by working with different clients, as experience cannot be taught. A deep understanding will provide the knowledge of how to deal with every situation. While these skills and understanding are being gained it is better to avoid the complication of trying to understand system differences and characteristics. Once the skills have been achieved and the technician has plenty of experience of different situations and problems, it will be a very easy matter to 'add on' another system. In this way the intricacies of the system can be concentrated on.

Choosing a system

When choosing which system to learn, there are five main things to take into account:

- **Which one you enjoy**. This is the most important. When learning anything new, an enjoyment of the subject or skill will aid learning enormously. There will be one system that an individual will enjoy or find easier than another. The best way of making this decision from an informed point of view is to look at every system, watch their application by an experienced nail technician and, if possible, have a go yourself. A

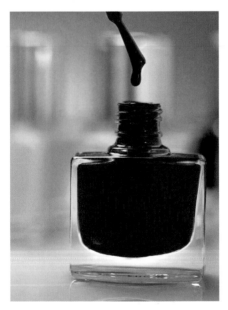

good technician will make every system look incredibly easy, but a few minutes of trying it out will show you that none of them is as easy as it looks.

- **Your existing confidence and knowledge**. It may be that you have been a client of a technician and have been impressed with the system that has been used. You will also have an amount of knowledge as you have been watching the process. Perhaps you work in a salon where a specific system is used very successfully. These are good reasons for choosing a system but remember that every system is only as good as the technician: every system will work in the correct hands.

- **The financial cost**. Starting any new career or skill can be very expensive. It may be that the cost of a student or starter kit influences this decision. This need not be a problem as the basics are the same for all, and the basic knowledge will provide a good foundation for any system. It is also worth knowing the cost in terms of products for a full set of artificial nails, as this will influence what you can charge your clients for your services.

- **Availability.** Nail products, like hair and beauty products, are available in several ways. There will be one way that suits you better or a combination of several. There are many items that are required for nails, not just the system products, such as cotton wool or nail wipes, disposable towels, terry towels, tools and much more (see Chapter 3). Products are available from direct sales companies that supply them via mail order. Some of these outlets will only sell their products to those who have taken training courses with them or can prove that they are already trained. Others will supply products to anyone. When buying via mail order, you will need to find out: what charges are made for postage and packing; whether there is a minimum order level; how long deliveries take; and how payment is made. You will also need to be available to accept delivery of packages. Direct sales companies do not always sell basic items, such as cotton wool, so you will need to go to a wholesaler for these items. If you prefer to see products before you buy, you will need to go to trade shows. However not all the direct sales companies attend these shows, so you will need to rely on their catalogues.

Another way of buying products is via a local wholesaler. There are hundreds of these all over the country and, as they are professional wholesalers, most of them require proof that you are in the trade.

Many wholesalers operate a delivery service and always sell the additional items needed for 'nails'.

What is convenient for you may affect what system you choose. Some direct sales companies only sell one system of a specific brand, others sell more than one system of specific brands. You may choose the brand rather than the purchase method, but take into account what is the most convenient for your situation and how much extra you are prepared to pay (and wait) for delivery or how much time (and petrol) you are prepared to pay for visits to wholesalers.

- **Company advice**. Most product companies are more than willing to give you lots of advice on what to buy. One word of caution here: the company may advise you that a specific system is the only one for you. This may be the case but if the system is the only one that the company sells there may be another reason why they are promoting it.

As a general piece of advice, do not rush into anything when choosing a system. Do your research, gather information, talk to others, attend trade shows, buy trade magazines. When you have lots of information you can decide for yourself from an informed position rather than being persuaded by others.

TOP TIP

Understanding how systems work will allow you to 'troubleshoot' when things go wrong.

TOP TIP

Never underestimate the value of product company training provided for technicians. They are not always the right people to provide training for beginners, but technicians should always attend a session for product knowledge and application techniques. Update these sessions regularly and never stop learning.

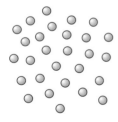

Fig 1 Water (H_2O)

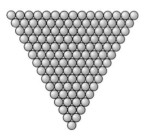

Fig 2 Molecules of water forming a pyramid of ice (solid)

Fig 3 Molecules of water forming a liquid

The chemistry of nail products

The chemistry of nail products for all brands is similar. In the same way as beauty therapists who learn how moisturisers work on the skin and how various electrical currents affect tissues, as hairdressers learn how perming solutions curl or straighten hair and hair colours work on the hair, nail technicians need to know how nail products work together and on the nail. Once this is understood, the specific product knowledge provided by manufacturers and distributors will enhance your skills and understanding and make you a better and more professional technician – especially if you have the essential attitude that a technician never stops learning.

When the word '**chemicals**' is mentioned, many people immediately think of danger! This is not so. Everything in the world is made of chemicals, including us! The only exceptions are heat, light and electricity, which are energies that affect chemicals.

Atoms and atomic structures The smallest state in which a chemical can recognizably exist is an **atom**. This is a microscopic piece of matter that is organized in a way that is specific to the simplest chemicals in existence, that is **elements**. Examples of elements are oxygen, carbon, hydrogen and calcium; there are over 100 different elements, each with its own kind of atom.

The atomic structure is specific to the different elements but each atom can have a negative or positive charge. As we all know from playing with magnets, a negative charge will attract a positive charge and vice versa. When a negative charge is joined to a positive charge a **chemical bond** is created. It is the joining together of these elements in various combinations and configurations that creates all the millions of chemicals that make our world.

Molecules When an atom joins other atoms it forms a molecule. An example of a molecule is H_2O (Fig 1). The letter H is the symbol for the element hydrogen, the letter O is the symbol for the element oxygen; H_2O means 2 atoms of hydrogen joined to 1 atom of oxygen – which makes 1 molecule of water.

This specific molecule is the smallest form in which the chemical known as water can exist. How many molecules there are in a space or how they are joined together determines the form that the water is taking:

- lots of molecules tightly packed together will be water but in the form of ice (Fig 2)

- fewer molecules loosely packed together will be flowing water (Fig 3)

- very few molecules with only some packed together will be steam (or vapour gas) (Fig 4).

Water has the chemical symbol of H_2O but, if only one more element is added, for example carbon, and the number of hydrogen, oxygen and carbon elements varied, the chemicals that are formed are vastly different from simple water: alcohols (such as the one found in alcoholic drinks: ethanol C_2H_5OH), fatty acids (such as acetic acid in vinegar: CH_3COOH) and even solvents (such as acetone, widely used in the nail industry).

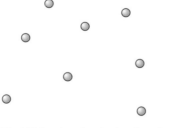

Fig 4 Molecules of water forming steam vapour

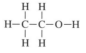

Ethanol C_2H_5OH

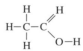

Acetic acid CH_3COOH

We are very familiar with each of these chemicals in their liquid form but should already be aware of possible dangers. Water is quite safe to drink, but too much of it in the wrong circumstances is dangerous; we can drown in it. The ethanol in our favourite alcoholic drink is good in small quantities, but a little too much has very unpleasant effects and considerably too much causes alcoholic poisoning and death. There is no one who would wish to consume too much vinegar and no one who would want acetone in their stomach, but we are quite happy to use it to remove nail varnish. Chemicals used correctly and in suitable quantities are neither dangerous nor harmful.

Vapours, fumes and odours Molecules of chemicals can escape into the air and become **vapours**. Water does not smell, but is present in the air all the time. Some chemicals can escape into the air much more easily than others. For example, water under normal conditions does not escape too readily, but if left long enough will evaporate. Other types of liquid chemicals, such as solvents, that can escape very easily are known as 'volatile' and this property is useful for fast drying. Molecules of the actual chemical are in the air when this happens but they cannot necessarily be detected by smell. These molecules are called vapours and the liquid is said to be vaporizing. Volatile liquids vaporize very easily so should be kept in closed containers that prevent this.

The smell of these liquids are often called **fumes**. This is very inaccurate. We refer to car exhaust fumes and this is accurate. Fumes are burned particles in gasses, e.g. from chimneys. What is often found in the context of nails is vapour – that is, the volatile chemicals escaping into the air. There are NO fumes in a salon.

Smell or **odour** is different again. We can detect some chemicals via our noses, others we cannot detect, but that does not mean they are not there. A strong smell of nail products suggests that the chemicals have escaped into the air as vapours and are now being breathed in. (The effects of this were discussed in Chapter 3.)

Bonding

A basic understanding of how molecules bond together to create something different will be useful in understanding the chemistry of nail systems. It is also important to understand that some molecules will bond together naturally owing to their positive and negative attractions; others need help. The help required could come in the form of heat, light or another chemical to speed up the process. This process is a crucial part in the understanding of nail systems, as the methods used and the speed of reaction affects the results and the application.

Acrylics, polymerization and monomers Almost every product used in the various nail systems belongs to a vast family of chemicals called 'acrylics'. An acrylic is a man-made type of plastic and those that are used in the nail industry use the same chemical process to form a solid from a liquid or from a semi-liquid: this process is called '**polymerization**'.

- Polymerization is a process that joins single but complex molecules called monomers together to form a solid even more complex structure called a polymer. The term 'monomer' is made up of 'mono': single + 'mer': unit; 'polymer', similarly, is 'poly': many + 'mer': unit. If we think back to the water molecules discussed earlier, single molecules can flow around as a liquid; when their temperature is drastically lowered, they join together to form a solid that is ice. It is the lowering of the temperature that has made this happen. (This reaction is not strictly the same as polymerization, but thinking of it in this way makes it easier to understand.)

- Monomers are present in some form in all nail system products. As explained, the single units or molecules are monomers; there is also a slightly different arrangement where a few units are formed together. These are called '**oligomers**'. As a general rule, monomers are the products that are liquid in form and oligomers are in a semi-liquid form, such as a gel or **resin**.

Monomer (liquid)

Oligomer (semi-solid)

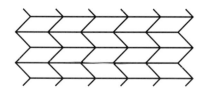

Polymer (solid)

Thinking back to how proteins are formed, you may remember that amino acids join together in long chains and these chains are linked together by amino acid bonds. These too can be described as polymers as they are single units (the amino acids) joined together to form long chains. Nails are made up of keratin so therefore nails are also polymers.

- The cells that are formed in the matrix on the nail unit have in the nucleus (or 'brain') of the cell the instructions to create the keratin. The nucleus initiates the process by collecting the relevant amino acids and causing them to link together in a specific format that will make the protein, keratin. This is a process of polymerization, but notice that an instruction from the nucleus was needed to make it happen. To relate this to nail products is now a simple exercise. Monomers (or oligomers) are present in a nail product. When the polymerization process is initiated, the single units join together to create long chains with bonds linking them together and a solid is formed. This solid is what becomes the artificial nail. The precise way in which this happens is different for each of the systems.

The initiator and the catalyst: these are chemicals that start or promote a chemical reaction. Polymerization needs an **initiator** to start the process but the initiator needs to be told when to do this and how fast the chemical reaction will take. This is where the **catalyst** comes in.

An example of this in a UV-cured gel system is that the initiator is already in the gel but it will not start the polymerization process until a catalyst is present that starts it off and determines the speed of the reaction. In this case the catalyst is the **UV light**.

The pairing of the initiator and catalyst in all systems is carefully balanced chemistry! If polymerization is too fast the resulting nail overlay will be brittle and the chemical reaction could burn the nail bed. Too slow and the overlay will take far too long to harden or cure.

The chemistry of systems

The liquid and powder system (L&P)

This system is the most popular in the UK and the US, holding probably about 50 per cent of the nail market. It is also popular in Europe, but other systems hold the largest market share in some countries, such as Germany, where a UV gel system is favoured. The acrylic system was the first to be used commercially, and came, as we saw in Chapter 1, directly from the dental industry. This is why it became to be known as 'acrylic nails'. Now this system is referred to as L&P. Even the colours that are used came from dentists, as they used pink for dental plates and various shades of white for dentures. (Pink and white is often used to create a natural-looking nail with a white free edge.)

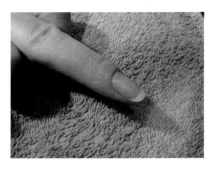

Finished nail

The L&P system is a two-component system using a liquid monomer and a powder. As already explained, the monomer (liquid) needs to polymerize and become a solid, and it needs an instruction to do this. If a liquid monomer is left exposed to light at room temperature, it would start to polymerize of its own accord, but this reaction would occur very slowly and the resulting polymer would be very soft and jelly-like. L&P comes from the methacrylate family.

Two conditions are needed for the process to be successful for the nail industry. An initiator is needed to start the process off and a catalyst is needed to determine the speed of the process. Two different chemicals, when they come together, create these two conditions. They start the process by giving the monomers a 'blast' of energy. This comes from the **chemical reaction** that occurs when the two come together – a release of energy that 'kicks' the monomers into linking together.

The two chemicals are both essential. The amount of each is also an important factor, and a balance that was created for a different application (such as making dentures) could produce problems. The blast of energy that is produced needs to be controlled, as too much would speed up the process too quickly, not enough would result in a very slow polymerization.

The catalyst and initiator process: When these two react together they create the 'instruction' for the monomers to join together. A similar reaction is used in permanent or semi-permanent hair dyes. Hydrogen peroxide and **amines** are used to create the necessary reaction to allow the pigments in the hair dye to enter the hair shaft. Every acrylic system needs an initiator and catalyst to create the acrylic polymer used for artificial nails.

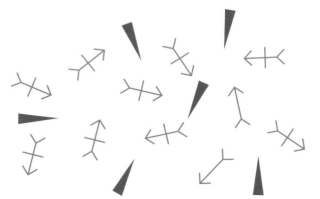

+ Acrylic monomer with initiator to 'kick-start' the polymerisation process

ALWAYS REMEMBER

Never mix systems. Use products and UV lamps that are designed to work together.

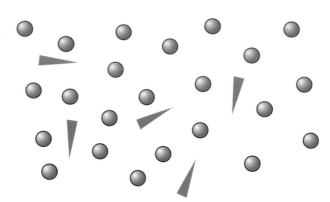

= Acrylic polymer powder with catalyst to regulate the speed of the process

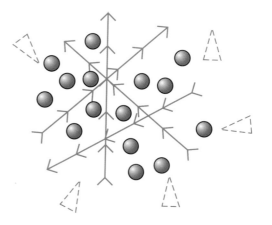

Solid acrylic with polymer chains and polymer beads. Catalyst and initiator used up

The polymer beads: The polymer beads have several roles, including the delivery of the 'instruction' to polymerize. The polymer beads remain as beads during the process and after polymerization is complete. They stay in among the long polymer chains that are being formed and give support and strength to the final structure. The monomer alone would produce a soft and flexible structure but, with the polymer beads, the structure remains flexible but also has the strength of the supporting spheres.

The liquid and the powder: The amount of the liquid and powder that is mixed together, that is the 'ratio', is important to the finished solid. Too much powder can make a very hard solid that may be brittle. Too much liquid can result in a soft and weak solid. The correct ratio plays an important role in the performance of the system and needs practice, together with some guidance from the manufacturer.

Another role of the powder is to carry coloured pigment. Technicians and their clients like to have the choice of a natural nail or a permanent 'French manicure' (with a very white free edge that is often created by nail varnish). This can be achieved on artificial nails by using a pink or peach toned powder over the nail bed and a white powder on the tip.

There are also opaque powders is a variety of skin tones that can be used to great effect to enhance the appearance of the artificial nail. For example, a nail biter can have an artificial nail that hides the unsightly, bitten nail to create an aesthetically pleasing nail. A client with a short nail bed can have this extended with opaque powder matched to their own skin tone to create a more elegant enhanced nail.

There are powders that have strong colour pigments and are designed to take the place of coloured varnish or can be used in nail art or to colour the free edge of the nail to create a vast variety of effects. (If these are used over the whole, the overlay should be removed every few weeks to make sure that there is no problem with the natural nail, as this will not be seen through the opaque overlay.)

Methacrylates – EMA and MMA: The chemicals used in this system commonly belong to the methacrylate family. The two most common are **ethyl methacrylate (or EMA)** and **methyl methacrylate (or MMA)**. Both of these were used at one time as monomers, as they were in the dental industry. However, it was discovered that MMA caused a great many allergic reactions and was too aggressive for skin. As a liquid monomer, it is now banned in the US although the very low-cost acrylic systems available there are sometimes MMA. MMA is a stronger polymer but, as a monomer, produced very hard and brittle overlays. The method of bonding MMA to the nail plate is to use deep scratches to allow the overlay to penetrate these scratches and hold on. Accidental damage to the nail could mean that the natural nail is ripped from its bed rather than the overlay ripped from the nail plate. This physical etching of the nail plate, often done with electric filés, severely damages the nail and leaves it thin and weak when the overlay is removed and prone to nail separation and infection.

EMA is most commonly used for monomers. Like all products it can cause allergic reactions but by working correctly this should not cause a problem. Monomers are a highly reactive substance in that they have a great deal of energy, with the molecules rushing about all over the place. They want to polymerize and, as stated earlier, will do so given enough time. This is one of the reasons why they can cause allergic reactions if they touch the skin too often. When they are polymerized, their energy has gone and it is then less likely that clients will react to them.

Use of EMA in a L&P system does not require etching of the nail plate, just gentle removal of the shine. The resulting overlay is thin and flexible but is structured for strength. Although the bond with the nail plate is strong it is not as strong to the bond between the nail plate and the nail bed so in the event of an accident the overlay will break before the nail plate is ripped away from the bed.

Powders in acrylic nail systems: Powders in this nail system are usually made from the same chemicals, as members from the same family tree will have very similar characteristics. Powders are already polymers and they can be a 'homopolymer' – that is, it is made from one polymer, either MMA or EMA, or, more usually from two or more polymers, MMA plus EMA, which is called a **copolymer**.

EMA will form a softer, more flexible polymer so, when used as a monomer, it needs the strength of a good polymer powder to support it. However, a homopolymer reacts faster with a monomer that is the same. Therefore, an EMA liquid monomer will react faster with an EMA powder polymer, but will produce a relatively soft overlay. An EMA monomer reacts slower with a MMA powder polymer, but can produce a stronger overlay. A regularly used mixture is an EMA monomer with a copolymer of EMA and MMA. This will result in a reasonably fast reaction with a good combination of flexibility and strength.

When a liquid monomer and a powder polymer are mixed together, the resulting product goes through several stages, which are 'stage managed' by the catalyst system. Timings are infinitely variable and are brand specific:

- The first stage is when the monomer meets the powder and the additives to the powder, or beads, are released, which can be called 'swelling'. This is when the reaction really gets going and it happens quite quickly. It can be seen as the product starts to melt.

- The next stage is when the polymerization starts and the mixture stops melting. It begins to have more of a gel consistency. At this **gel stage**, the product can be moved around the nail. The length of this stage varies for different brands.

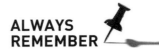

ALWAYS REMEMBER

There are many cut price salons that use MMA for their liquid and powder nails. The product is not banned for use in the UK. It is easily recognizable. The overlay is usually thick and milky looking. When filing it there is a slightly fishy smell to the dust. Any client who has these overlays should be advised to have them removed after explaining what damage is being done to their nails. Removal is by soaking in acetone for about 1 hour.

- The next stage is when the product leaves the 'gel' stage and goes into the beginning of the final 'cure' or setting stage. The product cannot be moved around easily now without leaving dips or bumps. Once this stage has been reached, the final cure will not be far away. This whole process can take anything from 3 minutes to over 10 minutes and finishes when the product is hard enough to file (or produces a clicking noise when tapped with a brush handle). However, do not be fooled! The overlay may be hard enough to file but the polymerization process will continue within it for many hours. Harsh abrasives or hard knocks to the overlay can interfere with this process and create weak areas in the artificial nail.

Temperature and polymerization: There are external factors that can influence the process, the most obvious of which is temperature. Higher temperatures will speed up the process.

Fast polymerization can create a heat sensation on the nail. The process itself produces a small amount of heat as it is an '**exothermic**' reaction (one that gives off heat), but this is too small to be felt by a healthy nail plate under normal circumstances. Fast polymerization can also create a brittle overlay with weak areas. Normal room temperature is ideal, and this is one reason why technicians are advised not to work under desk lamps that get hot.

A low temperature will slow down polymerization. The result of this can be seen when the liquid monomer is cold or the client's hands are cold. When the overlay is applied, crystals or frosting can be seen in the area near the cuticle. This occurs because the process is slow to start and the **volatile** monomer evaporates leaving some of the powder on the nail. Using the monomer at room temperature and keeping your client's hands warm can prevent this.

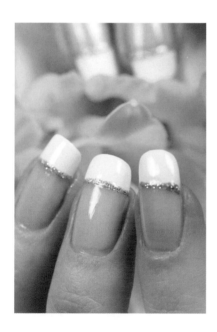

When the chemical engineering is unbalanced: The acrylic nail system, as can be seen, is a delicately balanced piece of chemical engineering. Several things can affect this balance. The addition of extra chemicals, for example, can have disastrous results – the most common chemical is brush cleaner, which can contaminate the mix.

The traditional acrylic system is prone to discoloration, or yellowing, caused by UV light from either the sun or sunbeds. Some brands of the system have an additive (called a **UV absorber**) that prevents this type of discoloration by working in a way that is similar to sunscreens for the skin. Some have a blue or violet colour added to the liquid. This is present as an **optical brightener**, to make the white look whiter and the pink look pinker, but it will also cover any slight yellowing.

Some brands of the system require the application of a **UV block**, in the form of a varnish, over the finished nail. The block needs to be reapplied regularly. However, all brands are prone to discoloration owing to **contamination**, which is dealt with in Chapter 9.

The chemical balance in this system is crucial to its performance. You are strongly advised not to mix brands – that is, a liquid monomer of one type with a powder from another. The catalyst system may not be compatible and other additives may not work together. Always use products that are designed to be used together.

As with anything, good quality costs more. The chemical engineering needed for a L&P system that is efficient and easy to use costs more than a standard version. Many of the cheaper brands are manufactured in the same factory and packaged by specific brands. This is often why technicians try mixing brands and don't believe they have any specific problems in doing so. There is no guarantee this is the case! *Do not mix brands.*

The choice of brand is personal. As a beginner or newly qualified technician it is worth trying out a few different brands. It is sometimes false economy to just buy the cheapest as it can lead to problems that cost more in the long term.

Removal of L&P nails is done by soaking them in acetone. Acetone breaks down the links between the polymers and allow it to, in effect, be scraped off. It DOES NOT melt the overlay, just breaks it down.

An L&P overlay is relatively porous. That is to say, there are spaces between the polymer chains that will allow molecules that are small enough to pass into the spaces. This means the removal can be quick depending on the thickness of the overlay. This characteristic is also useful as regular application of nail oil will penetrate the structure and help to keep it flexible.

HEALTH & SAFETY

Always follow the Manufacturer's instructions.

The UV gel system

This system is sometimes called a 'pre-mixed' system, as it does not need another product or chemical for it to work. What it does need, however, is UV light to make it cure, or set. Like the acrylic system, it has, for the most part, been derived from the dental industry where light-cured materials are used to seal teeth.

This system is in the **acrylate** family but there are some newer and more advanced products that utilize the methacrylates like the L&P system

The initiator and the catalyst: Like the L&P system, the semi-liquid gel that is applied to the nails needs to polymerize or cure. The acrylic system uses a catalyst system that initiates the process with a blast of energy. The initiator that gets its 'instruction' from the energy from the catalyst is in the gel and it is a 'photoinitiator' in that is responds to light energy. The energy needed to start the polymerization process in this system is UV light. Light, as we saw earlier, is a form of energy. You may remember learning about light from your school days. Light energy either comes from the sun, or from electrical energy converted into light. We see the visible light spectrum – that is, light from red to violet, as in a rainbow. At either end of this spectrum, but just outside of the visible range, there is UV at one end and infrared at the other. Also outside the visible spectrum are microwaves, X-rays and radio waves.

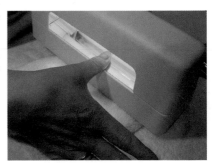

Cure for recommended time

UV light: There has been some concern about using UV light in a nail system, as it is perceived to be harmful. UV light can be very harmful, but in the case of nail systems this is not the case. There are three different 'strengths' or wavelengths of UV light: UVA, UVB and UVC. All of these are emitted from the sun in various amounts. When getting a tanned skin from the sun or a sunbed, the skin produces a pigment called melanin that protects the underlying tissues from the harmful effects of the dangerous wavelengths of UV light. This process needs relatively large quantities of UVA, which is safe, and smaller quantities of UVB, which can be harmful. 'Fast-tan' sunbeds sometimes have a higher percentage of UVB to speed up the process. It is possible to burn the skin under sunbeds when overexposed. The size of these tubes are usually 100 watts and an average sunbed has about 24 such tubes: a blast of 2400 watts of UV light!

The story is different for nail systems. The tubes in most nail lamps emit only UVA, it is not necessary to have UVB. Tubes are usually six or nine watts and lamps can have from one to five tubes, depending on the design. The maximum 'blast' is therefore only 45 watts of UVA.

As with all L&P systems, it is important to use the lamp designed for use with the gel. Wattage of the tubes does not relate to the emission of UV light energy. Depending on the type of tube more UV energy can be produced than one of a higher wattage. A lamp designed for a specific gel will have many factors taken into account:

- the energy emission of the tubes
- the number of tubes
- the configuration of the tubes in the lamp
- the distance of the fingers (or toes) from the tubes
- the design of the internal cavity and reflectors.

ALWAYS REMEMBER

Use the lamp recommended by the manufacturers for the best and safest results!

It is worth remembering these brief facts in case your client asks, 'Will my fingers get a tan?' or 'Is the UV light harmful?'.

As with L&P systems, many of the more inexpensive UV gels will be of a similar formulation and will work with a generic lamp but not without problems!

UV gel, oligomers and polymerization: So now we understand a bit about UV energy, how does it affect the UV gel? All the nail systems need some type of energy to make them form a solid structure on the nail. An acrylic system needs the energy generated from a chemical reaction. UV gel needs UV energy to turn it from a semi-liquid into a solid. The process of forming a solid, as with all other systems, is called polymerization.

- The gel used in this system varies between the brands, but many are from the acrylate branch acrylic family. Some advanced ranges are from the methacrylate branch. The liquid in the L&P system has single units of monomer, hence the liquid form. Gels have short chains of units, called oligomers, that are not long enough to be called a polymer. This gives the gel its consistency and makes the creation of polymers from light energy easier as they are partially formed already.

- When a UV gel is subjected to the energy of UV light, the polymerization process starts and continues in much the same way as with acrylics. As with acrylics, the process is exothermic – that is, the chemical reaction gives off heat. This is relatively easy to control with acrylics as it is the carefully balanced chemistry that does most of the controlling. This is not always the case with UV gels as there are many variables that can cause a much stronger exothermic reaction.

TOP TIP

The extreme heat is often called 'heat spike'. Modern systems should not have this problem unless the layer is too thick. If it does happen, remove the fingers and wait for the heat to go which it will quite quickly. Then replace the fingers. It should not happen the second time. If this is a common occurrence, place the fingers on the desk just in front of the lamp but in its glow for about 10 seconds. Then place them in the lamp. This sometimes works as the exposure to the UV light is minimal so the 'blast of energy' is lessened. Once the process has started there should not be any heat.

- When a blast of energy is applied to the oligomers, they literally rush around at great speed, linking up with each other. All this rushing about creates a heat that is similar to the friction caused by rubbing two things together: the faster the rubbing, the greater the heat. This happens in the gel if the energy blast is too high, if the output of the UV lamp is too high for the specific gel. It can also happen if the layer of gel is very thick. This is because there are more oligomers rushing around in a greater space and creating the friction effect. (To put this picture into perspective: if the nail was the size of the UK, the oligomer would be about the size of an ant!)

- This excess heat is a problem, for two reasons. First, the heat can be so great that it is felt by the nerve endings in the nail bed and the pain can be very severe and very frightening. This is obviously unpleasant for the client and it can damage the nail bed. Some clients are more prone to feeling this heat sensation than others and the nail bed will be particularly sensitive if it is damaged or thinned owing to excess buffing. Second, such a fast polymerization will create a very brittle polymer that could easily crack or shatter. This can be avoided by using the correct UV lamp and avoiding thick layers of a gel. Always follow the manufacturer's instructions.

- Modern gel systems have a much better polymerization control system in place. When using the correct lamp with a gel there should not be any excessive heat.

UV gel and oxygen: Polymerization does not like oxygen! The presence of oxygen slows down, or inhibits, the process. This is also the case with polymerization in the acrylic system, but the method is not so sensitive to it. Gel, however, is sensitive to oxygen. There are many gels available on the market that, when cured under the UV lamp, still have a sticky surface. There have been stories that this happens because the gel cures from the bottom up and liquid is pushed to the surface. The truth is due to the role that oxygen plays in its hindrance of the process. Oxygen is all around us; the surface of the gel is exposed to oxygen and therefore does not polymerize as the oxygen inhibits the process.

This sticky layer is not a problem if it is removed correctly and thoroughly. It is the oligomers that are not polymerized and, like the liquid monomer in the acrylic system, are likely to cause allergic reactions if the skin is touched. This sticky layer, known as the 'inhibition layer' must be removed with an alcohol based solvent. Ideally, start with the smallest finger and work up to the largest and wipe from the cuticle to the free edge so as to avoid the unreacted monomer touching the skin.

Viscosities of gels: The chemical formula of the gels is very complicated and the different types of gel that are available all have variations in both their characteristics and their make-up. One of the first things that can be seen about the gels is the thickness of each of them. This thickness is called '**viscosity**'. A thick liquid is described as viscous; water or any liquid that is free-flowing has a very low viscosity.

Gels, depending on their nature and on the manufacturer, are available in various viscosities. The low-viscosity gels are used for painting thin layers onto nails and building up a sufficient coating to strengthen a natural or artificial nail. They are also used, depending on their characteristics, as a finishing layer that has a very high gloss shine.

Thicker, or more viscous, gels are applied in fewer layers and, again, depending on their characteristics, can be applied to create a specific structure to provide maximum strength to the nail. Some gels do not hold their shape for long before curing and care must be taken to avoid the gel running into the sides of the nail and onto the skin. Other types of thicker gels do hold their shape and stay where they are placed. These, however, have a consistency that is similar to that of petroleum jelly and can be difficult to apply without plenty of practice.

The simplest UV gel systems consist of one type of gel that is painted on in thin layers. This creates a flat layer without any structure.

More advanced UV gel systems have a variety of gels;

- Bonder gel: a thin gel that creates a strong bond between it and the nail plate.

- Builder gel: a thicker gel that is used to create a structure and shape that will provide strength and aesthetic appeal. These are often available in skin tones that are either clear or opaque.

- White gel: these can be very thin to apply over the builder gel or thicker to use for sculpted nails.

- Coloured gels: opaque or semi-opaque gels that are used instead of polish for application on either an enhanced nail or natural nails.

- Gloss top coat: usually a thin, clear gel that is the last to be applied and provides a long-lasting gloss. (This is sometimes used over the top of L&P if the client prefers the appearance of a UV gel gloss.)

In addition to the types of gels used in a system there are:

1 Buff off gels.

As the description suggests, these need to be removed by buffing. The polymer structure is such that it doesn't allow acetone to penetrate it to break down the links. This makes it a strong system that is resistant to all solvents so keeps its glossy appearance. These are usually acrylate gels.

2 Soak off gels.

Usually in the methacrylate branch of the acrylic family, these allow removal with acetone. They are not usually quite as strong as the buff-off version and are very flexible. Although they can be used for artificial nails their slightly lesser strength make them suitable for natural nail overlays for semi-permanent colour.

Shrinkage of UV gel: Polymerization of any kind is prone to some shrinkage as the chains form. Gel is particularly prone to this and, if the shrinkage is severe, the overlay will lift from the nail plate or the client may feel a tightness that can make the fingertip throb. If shrinkage is severe the nail could be lifted from the nail bed. A good-quality gel should not shrink too much, but thicker layers will shrink more that thinner ones. Therefore several thin layers are much better than one thick layer. Even the builder gels do not need to be thick. If they are formulated well the artificial nail can be structured and the overlay will be strong without any bulk.

UV gel 'hybrids'   Although not strictly a hybrid, there is a system available on the market that is a UV gel but also uses an acrylic powder. The powder is similar to that in an L&P system a catalyst/initiator system as this is unnecessary.

Before the gel is cured under the UV lamp, powder is sprinkled onto the overlay. The buff-off gels are strong if applied correctly but the addition of the powder will help towards preventing too much shrinkage. As with an L&P system, the polymer beads will remain untouched but will support the network of polymer chains created by the gel when it has been polymerized (cured).

The fibreglass system

Rather than from the dental industry, this system has been developed from the beauty industry! Before artificial nails and all the accompanying products, manicurists developed a way of repairing split nails that involved using tissue paper and clear varnish. A split in the nail was sealed by painting the nail with a clear varnish then applying a small piece of tissue paper to hold the split together and then painting several layers of clear varnish over the top to give it strength and a smooth finish. This method could work, but was not always satisfactory as it was not very strong, could peel off and came off with nail varnish remover. If the split was close to the end of the nail, however, it could be saved temporarily in this way until it could be filed away.

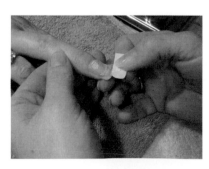

Applying fibre

Stick-on nails were introduced into both the retail market and professional market where a whole plastic nail was attached with strong adhesive over the natural nail. These adhesives were useful to repair natural nails and also to stick on the paper used to hold the edges together.

Again, this system is in the acrylic family but this time it's in the cyanoacrylate branch.

The three-component system: This is called a three-component system because there are three products necessary within the system–fabric mesh, resin and a resin activator.

- **Fabric mesh**: fabric is used to provide a cross-linked structure and to give the overlay strength (a bit like the polymer beads in the acrylic system). Any thin fabric will work, but those in common use and produced specifically for the job are a fibreglass mesh and a natural silk. These are both supplied as a fine mesh with a sticky back and are used to reinforce the overlay. The one you use is a matter of personal preference.

  - *Fibreglass* is, as the name suggests, fibres with a high glass content. Of the two, this is slightly stronger as the glass remains untouched by the resin as a linked structure, but it is more difficult to 'wet' than silk.

  - *China silk* is a very fine mesh of natural silk fibres. It does reinforce the structure, but the resin soaks into the fibres and the silk becomes an integral part of the resin. It is easier to 'wet' than fibreglass.

  The mesh is supplied either as strips that are cut, using special scissors, to the width of the nail or in pre-cut 'fingers'.

- **Resin**: The second component of this system is a 'resin'. This, again, belongs to the acrylic family of chemicals and is a **cyanoacrylate** of a specific chemical structure and viscosity. Cyanoacrylates are used as the adhesive to apply tips to nails. It is excellent at bonding with the nail plate so it is ideal for the nail industry. It is used to 'wet' the fibre, so that it cannot be seen, and then built up to an overlay. Cyanoacrylate is a monomer, but it has a different chemical structure to the ones used in other systems. It is sensitive to air and moisture and will cure (polymerize) when exposed to either.

  - Cyanoacrylates are used in a great many industries as an adhesive, in the motor industry, plumbing, woodworking and many others including the medical industry where it can be used as a skin or bone adhesive.

  - There are different kinds of this adhesive and different grades or qualities. The type most suitable for nails is an **ethyl cyanoacrylate**. The viscosity is infinitely variable, as is the speed at which it cures. A high-grade cyanoacrylate is preferable. This chemical is used as an adhesive for nail tips but a specific viscosity and chemical make-up is called a resin and is used in the fibreglass nail system.

    Although not impossible, cyanoacrylates rarely cause allergic reactions. It does eventually break down in water. Its chemical structure makes the overlay very porous so it is quick to remove (in acetone) but is also subject to staining. When using, it is advisable to use a base coat before any polish or a top coat if leaving 'natural'.

  - It is the least strongest of all the systems but is ideal for shorter nails, clients who are not heavy on their nails or have, perhaps, developed a sensitivity to the other systems. It is also a quick and easy overlay, minus the fibre, for 'weekend nails' which, as their name suggests are only needed for a few days.

- **Resin activator**: The resin will set, or cure, in time, on its own as it uses moisture from the air to set. As this takes at least 15 minutes and results in a very pliable coating that can peel off easily, it is not practical for the technician. To speed up the process and produce a strong overlay, an activator (or accelerator) is used. This is either in a spray or a brush-on format.

  - Spray: care MUST be taken when using a spray as large quantities of the chemical will be put in the atmosphere. (See chapter 3 on ventilation). Only a tiny amount of the product is needed to cure the resin. Controlling the cure is difficult with this method as too much accelerator will cure it too fast and create a painful exothermic reaction (heat spike) and result in a very brittle or damaged overlay. A very short spray from about 30 cm is all that is needed and a second layer of resin will usually cure immediately due to the accelerator being present on the nail.

— Brush-on: this will produce a slower cure with less chance of heat. The brush can be used to spread the resin while the accelerator mixes with it. There is not so much danger of overexposure from breathing in the vapours by using this method.

Polymerization: As with other nail systems, this system is based on acrylic polymers. When the resin is polymerized, it forms long chains but does not have any cross-links and needs the added strength of a fibre mesh. Owing to the lack of cross-links, it needs special care when removing nail varnish or using household cleaners.

The process of polymerization, as we know, gives off energy in the form of heat. When the process is properly controlled at the right speed, this heat cannot be felt. If the process occurs too quickly, then excessive heat is produced, which can be very uncomfortable for the client and produce a weak overlay.

By applying the resin and spraying it with **activator**, the polymerization process is started as the reaction is given the blast of energy required. To control the speed of the process, a very small amount of activator should be sprayed from a distance of about 30 cm. If the client feels any heat at all, the spray is too close. A fast cure is not only uncomfortable but also produces a brittle and cloudy overlay that has thousands of tiny cracks.

Fibre mesh: When introducing the fibre mesh into this system, it is important that the mesh is not visible through the overlay. To make it invisible it needs to be '**wetted**'. This is the term used to describe the application of resin to the fibre to make sure it penetrates the mesh and makes it invisible. It is essential that this is done with care as an artificial nail with the fibre showing through does not look natural. The mesh must be soaked with the resin before any further layers are applied. (This method is described in Chapter 6.)

Fibre system 'hybrid' As with the UV gel system, there is a version that uses acrylic powder to give the overlay extra strength. When the resin has been applied but before curing, the nail is dipped in the powder. If the nail is dipped, the remaining powder should be discarded in case of contamination. Sprinkling the powder may be a better option.

Other important chemical reactions in nail systems

Tip adhesives

The chemical reaction that takes place within tip adhesives is closely associated with the fibreglass system as it involves cyanoacrylates. Tip adhesives are always an ethyl cyanoacrylate that is sensitive to moisture and the cure of which is inhibited by oxygen. The viscosities can vary from a water-like liquid to a thick gel. As a general rule, the thicker the adhesive, the slower the cure and variations will apply to personal preference and to the job in hand.

- Tip adhesives, as the name implies, are used to stick a plastic tip to the natural nail. As the adhesive is sandwiched between the tip and the nail, the oxygen is expelled (therefore no inhibition to the cure) and there is sufficient moisture in the nail to encourage polymerization. Thin adhesives cure very quickly, in a couple of seconds, the thicker ones take a little longer.

- Personal preference relates to how quickly the technician wants the tip to stick firmly. Beginners tend to prefer to have a bit longer to position the tip before it is too late, experienced technicians like to work as fast as possible. However, speed is not always the main consideration. A thin adhesive can produce only a thin layer of adhesive between the tip and the nail, which is fine if the tip fits the nail exactly and the nail plate does not have any irregularities. If this is not the case, air pockets are created that not only look bad but can also create problems later. A thicker adhesive can form a thicker layer and fill up any irregularities. The gel-like adhesives are an invaluable help when dealing with a severe nail-biter or a nail shape that tilts upwards, as the surfaces can be safely filled with adhesive (see Chapter 6).

● Cyanoacrylate adhesives can, over time, break down in water, so, in the artificial nail you should not put too much confidence in the strength of the bond between the tip and the nail. The strength needs to be between the overlay and the nail.

Primers

Function of a primer There are some brands that do not require any help for the overlay to bond to the natural nail; they may just need a very clean, oil-free surface that has had the shine removed. Some systems have a built-in method of bonding a man-made plastic to a natural surface of keratin. Many need some help to create this bond and the product is generally known as a '**primer**'. Primers are seen in many areas: metal, wood and ceramic tiles all need a primer before they can be painted; natural nails should have a base coat before varnishing; even teeth need a primer before a veneer can be applied. A primer is necessary in these cases as whatever is being applied to the surface must bond with it, otherwise it will peel or fall off. A primer prepares the surface to accept a substance that does not naturally bond with it. Shiny surfaces do not bond together and a roughened surface will accept another substance more readily. Nails, when shiny, almost have a seal on the surface that prevents too much penetration by substances. When the shine is removed, the surface bonds more readily with adhesive or overlays and allows a small amount to penetrate and create a stronger bond.

Methacrylic acid Some nail systems require extra help in the form of a separate primer. A common primer in use is a chemical called **methacrylic acid**. As can be seen from the name, this chemical belongs to the acrylic family and therefore will have an affinity to the overlay. The acid part of it, although mild, will gently etch the surface of the nail and encourage it to accept the overlay. It forms both a chemical and a mechanical bond by holding the overlay onto the nail plate.

Methacrylic acid is a strong irritant and is corrosive. Care must be taken when using it not to allow it to touch any soft tissue. Bottles must be kept with the lid on and spillages dealt with carefully.

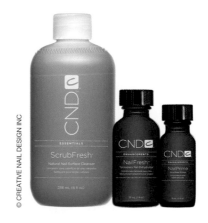

Acid-free primers There are other primers available, which are generally called 'acid-free'. They will work in such a way as to hold on to both the natural nail and the overlay. They 'interface', or soak into, the nail plate and, as a type of monomer, will polymerize with the overlay to create a complete structure.

The best primer to use is the one that is recommended by the manufacturer of your system, as they will have developed the primer to give the best results with its own system. As with all nail systems, information on how to use products efficiently and safely must come from the manufacturer. A technician should spend some time learning, in depth, all there is to know about the products and a reputable company will provide this information. There may also be some application techniques that are best to use with specific brands and that make an application quicker or more effective. Do not consider that such training is a waste of time or money – it is the complete opposite, every product that is on the market will work properly in the right hands; in the wrong hands, where there is insufficient knowledge, most products will not work.

Artificial nail removal

A final explanation of the chemistry of artificial nails is their removal. The most commonly used method of removal is to soak the nails in acetone or some other solvent. The solvent does not dissolve the overlay but breaks down the bonds between polymer chains. The stronger the bonds, the more difficult it is to break them down.

Using a solvent

In the various systems, the cyanoacrylate resin in the fibreglass system has the weakest bonds as there are no cross-links in the structure. UV gel is usually the most difficult to remove, as the bonds are exceptionally strong and cannot be penetrated. There are many gels that cannot be removed with solvents and the only way is to buff them off.

When the nails are soaked in the solvent, the bonds break down and the structure becomes soft. While in the solvent, the overlay can be scraped off quite easily. If the nails are removed from the solvent before this is done, the softened acrylic immediately becomes hard again.

In order to imagine what happens to the acrylic in the solvent, imagine putting paper in water (those with children may have had to fish out a roll of toilet paper from the lavatory in the past!). The paper becomes very soft and liable to break up, it is still, however, paper and does not dissolve in the water. When the paper is removed from the water and dries out, it may feel a little harder and the separate sheets may have moulded together, but it is still paper. This is very similar to the effect that acetone has on acrylic.

The use of acetone

There have been some worries about using acetone to remove acrylic nails. All solvents are classed as hazardous chemicals and all chemicals, even water, are hazardous if care is not taken in their use and storage. Overuse of any hazardous chemical is a danger but sensible use should not be a problem. Continually soaking skin in acetone, or any other solvent, could cause problems, but this would need daily soaking. Usually, the only reasons to remove artificial nails are if a problem with the natural nail or skin is suspected or if clients decided that they no longer want or need them. Correctly maintained artificial nails do not need to be removed. Occasional removal by soaking in acetone or similar solvent is not a problem, as long as the correct procedures are followed and the used solvents are disposed of carefully.

Nail Polish

Millions of bottles of nail polish are sold every day throughout the world. It is such a commonly used cosmetic product but I wonder how many technicians understand what it is?

There are many formulations of nail polish some of which are very specific to a brand with a 'secret' formulation, others are general and used for many brands. Essentially, all formulations are similar in that they all have:

- Nitrocellulose: a polymer that produces a hard and shiny layer.

- A resin: that combines well with the nitrocellulose to make a good bond with the nail plate. This could be TSF (toluene sulfonamide formaldehyde resin) or TAF (tosylamide formaldehyde resin). This is NOT formaldehyde (see below). Or it could be an epoxy resin.

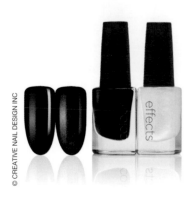

- Plasticizers: that give the polish flexibility.

- Solvents: these could be butyl acetate, ethyl acetate, ethyl alcohol, toluene. It is the evaporation of these that make the polish dry.

- Suspension agents; these make the polish easier to use. Nail polish is thixotropic. This means that when a bottle is shaken the polish becomes thinner.

- Pigments: a vast variety of coloured cosmetic pigments and effects are used to create the colour.

- Stabilizers; to prevent colours from fading or changing. These can include a UV blocker to prevent discoloration from the sun.

TOP TIP

If a polish becomes thick while you are using it, don't struggle on and end up with very thick layers. Put the top back on and give it a good shake. It will become thinner.

The drying of polish all depends on its formulation and lots of other external influences. A thinner polish will be quicker to dry as the solvents can escape easily. A sheer or semi sheer polish will be fast for the same reasons. An opaque colour will take a bit longer as the solvents need to make their way through the pigments. The same for a thick layer.

There is no need to wait for each layer to dry. This is an unnecessary waste of time. As soon as the next layer is applied the solvents in it will wet the previous layer. The few minutes it takes to complete ten fingers and return to the beginning is sufficient time for the previous layer to be on the way to drying.

The solvents evaporate in air. If a top is left off a bottle it will evaporate quickly making the polish thick and unusable. The bottle needs an airtight seal so the neck of the bottle should be kept clean.

When a bottle is used there will be an airspace where the solvents will evaporate into. Shaking the bottle before every use is necessary to mix the pigments (that is why ball bearings are put in every bottle) but it will also help to mix in the solvents too.

If bottles are kept in sunlight or somewhere too warm and they are close to full, the evaporation of the solvents due to the heat can make the bottles shatter!

There are many 'quick dry' formulations marketed today. These have higher levels of solvents to encourage this speed but this results in a brittle coating that is prone to chipping. As is often the case, it is compromises that need to be decided upon: fast dry with shorter longevity or a slower dry for longer-lasting results.

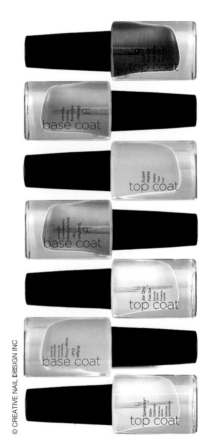

© CREATIVE NAIL DESIGN INC

Base and top coats

As you will see all the ingredients in nail polish have a part to play. Base and top coats are very similar but have a greater percentage of the relevant ingredient. Resin improves nail plate **adhesion** so there will be more of that in a base coat and less nitrocellulose. Top coats need to be more resistant and shiny and go over polish. They do not need so much adhesion but need more nitrocellulose for shine and durability.

Neither have coloured pigments as a general rule.

What is 3 free?

This refers to polishes that do not have formaldehyde, toluene or DBT (dibutyl phthalate). As professionals, we should know and understand what the implications of this are.

Formaldehyde This is a gas. It becomes a liquid when combined with water to create formalin. This has been used in nail hardeners for many years. Problems can arise as it can cause allergic reactions and when used for too long will make the nail very brittle and therefore prone to snapping. Its use in polishes was highlighted a few years ago in the US and lobbyists called for its removal due to potential sensitivities. There is no real evidence to suggest this is the case. In fact it has only been present in nail polishes in the form of a resin (TAF resin), not formaldehyde (or formalin). The potential danger it poses is negligible. It is still the best resin to use for this purpose and its replacement in many polishes has resulted in a less efficient polish.

Toluene   A solvent that has been used in polishes since the 1930s and it helps the application and results. The concern (in the US) was its evaporation into the atmosphere. Studies showed that there was no potential danger but its use was banned from retail polishes but not professional polishes.

DBT (dibutyl phthalate)   This has been used as a plasticizer in polishes for years. The EU decided that there is a risk with these ingredients. There have been studies into the use of phthalates in cosmetics. Although there has been no evidence to prove that there is any genuine health implication to their uses, the authorities have remained suspicious.

In conclusion, there are many suspicions about these ingredients and there is no doubt that some people will be sensitive to one or more of them. To allay any fears many polish brands have developed a '3 free' approach. This has resulted in an inferior polish but formulations are being worked on all the time to try to make them as effective as they were with the removed ingredients.

Polish removers and solvents

Polish removers are solvents. The fastest solvent for this is, without a doubt, acetone. However, this is so fast that it is also used to remove artificial nails (except for buff-off UV gels). Acetone is a very safe solvent but, like any other must be used correctly and safely. There are no known health risks with proper use although clients should be discouraged from removing their polish every day as this could lead to overexposure.

Acetone will also act as a solvent for natural oils. This makes it drying to the nails and skin. Acetone mixed with one part water to ten parts acetone will help to reduce this and there is no reason for it to be used so often that the oils cannot be replaced immediately.

The 'acetone-free' removers usually use ethyl acetate or methyl ethyl ketone. These do exactly the same job but slower! It is almost a perception that they are kinder to the nails and skin as a remover but they take longer to remove polish. They are certainly too slow to remove artificial nails and this is why they are recommended to remove polish from artificial nails.

Warmer solvents will act faster. Care must be taken when doing this (see Chapter 11 on removal procedures).

There are retail versions of polish removers that have conditioners in them. These just give the impression that the solvent is not drying out the skin but they can often leave a film on the nails that can cause polish to lift.

Care must be taken when using any solvents. They must be handled and stored correctly and used liquid and cotton pads disposed of correctly (see Chapter 3).

Quick dry products   Polish will only be dry when all the solvents have evaporated and this, realistically can take many hours depending on the polish and other conditions. There are many sprays, some of which will speed up the process. As before, care must be taken with sprays and the environment.

Drops are another format of a 'quick dry' product. These often contain dimethicone, a silicone oil, that encourages evaporation while protecting the sticky surface.

Those that have an oil base are most useful as they will help to condition the skin and keep the polish flexible.

Beware of some quick dryers as they will dull the surface of the polish.

Some electrical polish dryers may help as the heat will help speed up evaporation but a fan speed that is too high may effect the surface of the polish.

Service breakdown All the systems are designed to work perfectly together. If they are not used exactly how they are meant to be there will be 'service breakdown'. Each system has its own characteristics and situations that adversely affect it. Most of these will be covered in the relevant chapter but an understanding of the chemistry will usually provide the skilled technician with the information to work out what is causing the problem.

Organic products There are some nail products on the market that use marketing stories based on 'organic' hype. This marketing suggests that the products are 'natural' and 'safe' etc. However, there are two meanings of 'organic' in this context.

1 Occurring naturally; without the use of synthetic ingredients or products; examples of this could be organic food grown or reared under strict conditions without synthetic additives.

2 A branch of chemistry that involves chemicals or compounds that have the carbon atom in their molecular structure. Plastics and acrylics fit very firmly into this category and most nail products, including polishes, involve this chemistry.

Summary

This chapter has explored the chemical reactions that underpin the three main 'systems'– acrylic, UV gel and fibreglass – used in artificial nail technology and what the choice of system entails for both the technician and the client.

TOP TIP

Nail Structure and Product Chemistry, Douglas D Schoon.

ASSESSMENT OF KNOWLEDGE AND UNDERSTANDING

1 What are the three main artificial nail systems available?

2 Explain: (a) vapours, (b) fumes, (c) odours.

3 Ventilation is essential for the safe removal of (a), (b) or (c) in Question 2?

4 What is the name of the chemical process that changes an artificial nail overlay into a solid?

5 How can room temperature affect artificial nail products?

6 What is the purpose of an initiator in any artificial nail system?

7 What are the initiators in each of the three main systems?

8 Name some problems that could occur as a result of contamination of artificial nail products.

9 What is polymerization?

10 What is the sticky layer on a cured UV gel and why should it be removed?

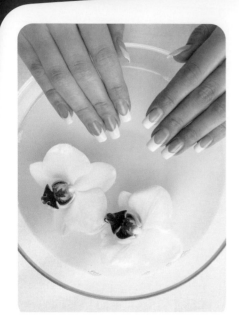

8

Applying tips to the nails

Learning objectives

In this chapter you will learn about:

● how to prepare the natural nail plate for artificial nail products

● about the different types of tip and their uses

● how to apply and blend a tip

● how to apply a tip to various nail shapes in a way that improves their appearance

● how to apply tips to bitten nails

● the use and application of tip varieties.

Introduction

There are two methods of lengthening nails: one is by applying a plastic tip to provide the length and then an overlay over the top; the other is by 'sculpting' the overlay onto the nail to provide the length (see Chapter 10). This chapter deals with the application of plastic tips and is relevant to all the different nail systems, as it forms the basis of this method of applying artificial nails.

Preparing the natural nail

Before any artificial product is applied to nails, they must be carefully prepared. If steps in this stage are missed or done inefficiently a problem with the artificial nail will result, for example lifting of the overlay. This procedure must be carried out before any artificial product is applied and precedes tip application.

As a beginner to the nail technicians craft, there are many problems and situations to learn about and overcome. One of the most frustrating is when a carefully applied overlay lifts from the nail plate. Almost always the cause of this will be something missed in the preparation stage.

It is worth spending more time on this stage and making sure the prep is carried out with complete accuracy. In the long term, results will be worth the extra effort.

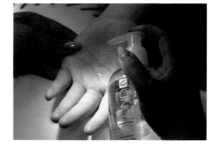
Sanitize hands

Stage 1: Sanitize the hands and the nail plate

The nail plate must be perfectly clean before any work is carried out. There are many specific products available for this purpose and every system brand usually has one. In effect, the nail plate is cleaned of surface debris and oils using a solvent. It is possible to use a varnish remover as long as it does not have conditioners, as these can remain on the nail plate.

A cotton wool disc or a disposable nail wipe is used and the nail should be wiped from the edge to the cuticle. In this way oils from the skin will not be drawn onto the nail plate.

Stage 2: Removing the cuticle

The cuticle is a thin, clear layer of dead skin cells that are attached to the nail plate. It is shed continually from under the nail fold and there is always some to be removed. It is possible, if a client has not had a manicure or any nail treatment for some time, that the cuticle could be covering the lower part of the nail. As it is so thin and transparent it is difficult to see. Removal of this is essential as any overlay products will not bond to this skin, they will bond only to a clean nail plate. A little area of missed cuticle will cause lifting of the overlay that, in turn, can result in other problems. The nail fold at the base of the nail must never be pushed or forced, especially when it is not softened. It is important to follow the manufacturer's instructions as to the correct product to use at this stage. If the nail fold is unsightly, the technician should recommend that the client has a few manicures first to minimize the skin.

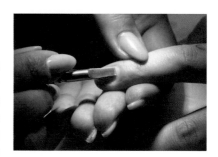
Remove cuticle

Before applying artificial nails, the most efficient method of removing the cuticle is with a clean cuticle knife on softened cuticle. Some can have a very sharp blade, but every metal tool needs to be used carefully as they can cause severe damage to the nail plate.

This stage must never be missed and the whole nail must be checked for cuticle. With practice, it is often easier to feel the cuticle rather than see it. With so many different cuticle tools available, it is advisable to get advice from the distributor on their correct use.

As a general guide, hold the cuticle knife reasonably flat on the nail plate and, starting around the centre of the nail, gently scrape down towards the nail fold. Any cuticle on the nail plate will be easily removed if the knife is held at the correct angle and the nail will not be affected. If the knife is held upright it is possible to dig into the nail. Once the whole nail has been checked for cuticle, special attention needs to be paid to the sides of the nail. The skin can be pulled back by a finger and thumb and the cuticle knife can check for cuticle down the side walls.

The nail fold at the base of the nail should be gently lifted, never forced. An efficient cuticle knife in the correct hands should accomplish this without any problems. The knife should then be used to clean away any debris from around the edges and nail fold.

Some technicians like to use a cuticle softener at this stage. However, remember how porous the nail plate is and unless the product is removed thoroughly, including under the lifted skin of the nail fold, there could be a problem with lifting later.

A wooden orange stick is not suitable for removing the cuticle. It is good for gently lifting and shaping the nail fold during a manicure, but is not able to remove cuticle as efficiently as a good cuticle knife.

Any product that has been used at this step must be carefully removed. A water spray with a cotton pad will work efficiently but care must be taken in drying the nail plate thoroughly.

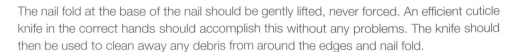

TOP TIP

If the client has a nail fold that has grown too far down the nail, it may be necessary to suggest a manicure first.

Stage 3: Removing the shine

A nail plate is naturally smooth and fairly shiny. Two shiny surfaces do not bond together well with an adhesive as there is not enough 'grip'. (This could be likened to a shiny leather sole on a new shoe and a smooth pavement. There is no grip, but if the sole is scored to make it rough, it will grip much better.) The adhesive or overlay has more surface to hold onto if the shine of the nail has been removed.

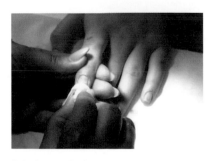

Remove shine

The nail plate, like the skin all over the body, has bacteria living on the surface. Some of these bacteria are harmless and sometimes useful. Other bacteria may not be so friendly so, when applying artificial nails, it is safer to try to remove all the bacteria. Using a gentle abrasive to remove the shine on the nail will also help to remove some of these unwanted 'visitors'.

The natural nail should never have an abrasive used on it that has less than a grit of 240 as it would cause too much damage. The end of a file of 240 grit or less is ideal to remove the shine. The end shape can get very close to the nail fold without causing damage to the soft tissue, and the sides of the file are perfect for getting down inside the side wall and ensuring there is no area of nail missed. The file should be used in the direction of nail growth, that is from the cuticle area towards the free edge. Keeping to this one direction only will minimize any trauma to the nail plate and help to avoid any more of the surface being removed than is necessary. It is literally only the shine that needs to be removed and **not** a layer of nail or any amount of nail that will make the nail plate thinner.

The process can be likened to using the first side of a three-way buffer as it should not leave any scratches on the surface of the nail.

Shape free edge to fit stop point on tip When the entire surface of the nail has been gently filed the free edge, if there is any present, can be tidied up and shaped to fit into the stop point of the tip. (See features of a tip on p. 176) At this stage the nail plate should look dull all over.

Stage 4: Dehydrating the nail plate

It is essential that the nail plate does not have any trace of oil or moisture on the surface immediately before application of the overlay. Oil or moisture could be carrying bacteria or fungal spores that could cause problems, and any overlay or adhesive will not bond to the nail if there is any oil or moisture present.

Obviously, the nail bed is excreting natural oils and moisture that keep the nail healthy and flexible and this will continue. This moisture will not affect the overlay once it is bonded to the nail, but the bond must occur while the nail plate is moisture-free.

Dehydrate nail plate

As the nail plate has a surface that is slightly more porous than usual, owing to the removal of the shine, any dehydrator used on it will penetrate the upper layer very slightly and remove excess moisture that is present. Dehydrators used on the nail plate not only remove excess moisture, but they also act as sanitizers. Most bacteria and fungi require moisture to live, and by removing this essential moisture any organisms that are present will not be able to survive. The mild products used for this purpose will not necessarily kill the organisms, as the products must be mild enough to be used on the skin, but they will stop or inhibit their growth.

As before, the product designed for this job should be applied following the manufacturer's instructions. Alternatively, the dehydrator can be wiped over the nail on a cotton wool disc or nail wipe towards the finger. This will remove the dust that has been generated by filing.

The nail is now perfectly clean and prepared and ready for the application of artificial products. It is at this stage that the client must be prevented from using the prepared hand and the best way to avoid this happening is to ask the client to keep their hand flat on the towel. It is likely that the client will touch her face or head then all the preparation of the nail will be spoilt as oil, moisture or make-up may have been transferred to the nail plate.

If the nail system being used does not involve a UV lamp for curing, it is best for each hand to be prepared and all artificial nails applied before the next hand is started. In this way, the client has one hand free and there is no chance of contaminating the prepared nails.

If a UV system is being used, both hands must be prepared, as one hand is worked on while the other is under the lamp. The technician must ensure that the nails are kept away from any contamination.

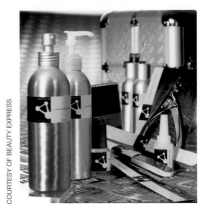

COURTESY OF BEAUTY EXPRESS

System nail preparation products

Adhesives

Tips are applied to the nail with an adhesive (glue is an incorrect term as this describes a product made from natural materials). The adhesives used in the nail industry are cyanoacrylates, specifically ethyl cyanoacrylates. It is widely used in artificial nails, as it is used for applying tips and is also the basis of the resin in the fibre system.

Adhesive is manufactured in several viscosities (thicknesses) and speeds of cure. It also has several grades. The highest grade is used in surgical procedures. That used for nails should be high grade, while its viscosity and speed are another area for personal preference.

As a general rule, thin adhesives cure very quickly and thicker versions more slowly. For the purposes of tip application, a thin adhesive will bond quickly but is prone to air bubbles and will not fill up any irregularities in the nail surface; a thick adhesive will take longer to bond and will cushion the nail and fill irregularities (this type is ideal for a bad nail biter).

Adhesives are broken down with solvents, the most efficient being acetone. If any skin is bonded together during its use, cotton wool on an orange stick soaked in acetone will quickly solve the problem.

Applying a plastic tip

Plastic tips come in many shapes and sizes, colours and lengths. Some of them are amazing to behold and all of them, to the beginner, look impossible!

Applying the tip is a skill in its own right and one that is often hurried during training in an effort to get on with overlay application. The application of the tip must be perfect and, on completing this stage, the nails must look like they actually grew on the finger and are not a

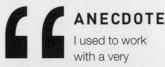

ANECDOTE

I used to work with a very good technician, but one who was prone to accidents, large and small. A common occurrence for her was to get adhesive on skin, usually her own but sometimes the client. When adhesive dries on skin it can be easily peeled off without any damage although, ideally, it should be soaked off with acetone. On one memorable occasion, I heard noises coming from my colleague that were obviously designed to attract my attention and sounded a bit panicky. When I looked, her finger was in her mouth. I quickly understood what had happened. She had got some adhesive on her finger and had tried to peel it off with her teeth (not recommended on any occasion). The adhesive was still wet and promptly stuck her finger to her teeth! The bond was not strong and her finger came away but not before the moment of panic!

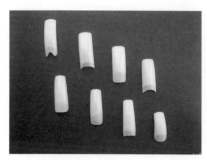

Various tip shapes

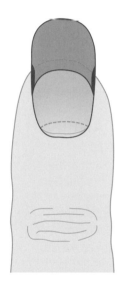

Nail with area of tip highlighted to demonstrate reinforcement of vulnerable area

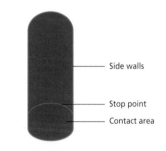

Side walls

Stop point

Contact area

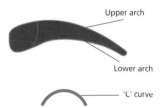

Upper arch

Lower arch

'C' curve

Features of tip (a) the front (b) the side (c) the end

piece of plastic stuck to the end. If the tips are not a perfect fit, they cannot be corrected by the overlay. The shape of the overlay has its own rules and requirements, and must not be concerned with correcting a badly applied tip.

The tip plays only a small part in the strength of the finished nail. The most important area of strength is provided by the overlay. The tip alone is only as strong as the bond between it and the natural nail and this is not a good bond. If the real strength is not provided by the overlay, the tip will snap off. A well-applied tip does provide some strength in one area and that is the side wall near to the free edge. This area of nail, either real or artificial is very vulnerable, and is the most usual place for a nail to break. A tip will add some strength here.

ABS plastic or acetate tips

A good-quality tip is made from 'virgin' ABS plastic. **ABS** is a plastic within the acrylic family; it is relatively strong and can be made in many different colours. Most tips today are made from ABS plastic, but occasionally a tip may be made from another type of plastic called acetate. These tips have a translucent quality and are usually more transparent than traditional tips. They tend to be cheaper and were originally made for the false nails that were sold for retail use to be stuck over the whole nail. These are not suitable for artificial nail systems as they are difficult to blend into the natural nail and have a higher oil content that may affect the overlay.

Making the tip

Tips are manufactured by pouring liquid ABS plastic into a mould that is shaped rather like a tree with a central 'stalk' and the tips coming out of the side-like branches. The little rough bits on the end of tips show where they were removed from the main 'stalk'. The 'stalks' that are left after the tips have been removed are sometimes melted down by manufacturers and reused to make more tips (rather like remould tyres). This obviously helps manufacturers to keep costs down but, like some remoulded tyres, the tips can have weak spots. 'Virgin' plastic is a plastic that has been freshly made and not mixed with the melted 'stalks'.

Important features Every tip, whatever its shape or size, has a number of features that are relevant to the technician:

1   **Contact area or well**. This is a thinner area and the part that is in contact with the natural nail.

2   **Stop point**. This is the demarcation point of the contact area and the actual tip. The natural nail free edge should fit snugly into this without any gaps to trap dirt and it will protect the edge of the nail and stop it absorbing too much water. When the tip is properly blended, this line will produce a natural-looking smile line.

3   **Side walls**. Tips either have parallel or tapered side walls to suit the natural shape. A well-constructed tip will have a reinforced side to the contact area in order to provide maximum strength in this vulnerable area.

4   **Upper arch**. Like natural nails, tips have differently curved upper arches from flat to very curved. Choose the one that fits the natural nail shape or, if the natural upper arch is flat, it will need some correcting and a tip with a curved upper arch will help. If the nail has a high arch, a curved tip will exaggerate this even more so a flatter tip will help compensate.

5 **Lower arch**. Like nails that have grown naturally, a tip needs to have a lower arch. This is not so obvious if the shape of the finished nail is going to be oval, but the lower arch is still there and is what makes the tip look as if it has grown from the finger and not been stuck on top.

6 **'C' curve**. As with the upper arch, this can vary between types of tip, and the shape of the natural nail should dictate which is most suitable. Unlike the upper arch, it is not advisable to choose a shape that is different from the natural 'C' curve. The tip needs to sit on the nail comfortably without distorting the shape of the tip. If the natural nail is quite flat and a tip is applied that has a deeper curve, the tip will need to be flattened to adhere across the width of the nail. Once applied, the tip will try to return to its shape and this will put undue stress on the nail bed. When this happens, clients will feel a great deal of discomfort, as the nail bed will throb as if it is bruised. It is even possible that, if the nail plate is very thin, nail separation could occur where the tip is pulling at the centre of the nail by the free edge. If the natural nail has a deep curve and a tip is applied that is flatter, the only way to stick it to the nail is to hold the sides of the tip onto the nail and make it follow the natural curve. Again, after application the tip will try to return to its original shape that may not necessarily cause discomfort but may result in lifting down the side walls.

Choosing the correct tip

Some guidelines

- The first thing to look for when choosing the correct tip is the 'C' curve of the natural nail. Match the shape of the natural nail.

- The next area to take into account is the natural upper arch. Again, match the natural shape, or choose a tip to correct an over- or under-exaggerated arch.

The above guidelines will help save some time in trying several tips. However, the best way to choose a tip is to try it on the nail. If it follows the curves it is the right one. It is worth a technician having at least two different types of tip available, and more if finances allow.

Size and width Once the correct tip has been chosen, the right size or width must come next. Most tips come in 10 or 11 different sizes with 0 being the biggest and 10 the smallest. Sizes 4–6 are the most commonly used.

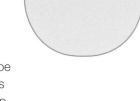
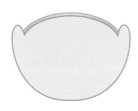
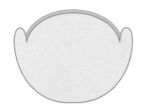

'C' curve of a nail looking from the nail down the length of the finger (a) flat 'C' curve (b) natural 'C' curve (c) deep 'C' curve

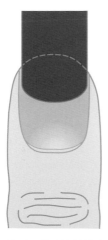

Placing the tip (a) tip too small for nail

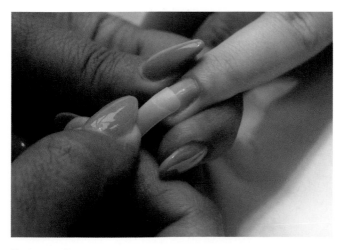

Tip too small

TOP TIP

If you are not sure if the tip is the right size, hold the tip against one side wall and look across at the other side wall. This will show a tip that is too narrow. Sometimes, when looking down onto a nail, the tip will look right but is actually too narrow when this technique is tried (see picture).

TECHNICAL TIP

If a client has a very flat nail and the flattest tip still has the wrong 'C' curve, choose a much wider tip, which will be flatter, and the sides can then be filed until it is the correct width.

TOP TIP

Always **pre-tailor** or shape a tip to fit before application as it cannot be changed when it is on the finger.

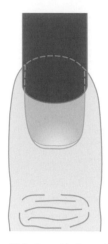

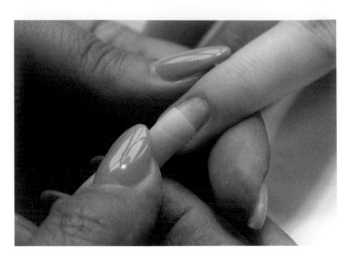

(b) tip too wide for nail

Tip too big

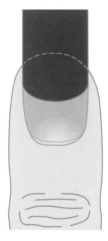

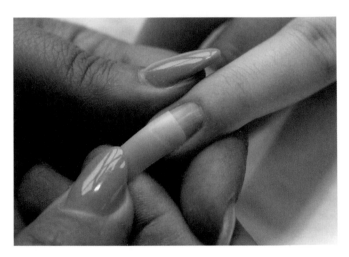

(c) tip of correct size

Correct size

When choosing the correct size, the width of the contact area must be ignored as it is the width at the stop point that is important. This must be exactly the same width as the nail at the smile line (or **onychodermal band**) without any gaps when the skin is pulled back from the sides. It is a very common mistake to fit a tip that is too narrow. It cannot always be seen on a new set but, when the nail grows, there will be a step at the side with some natural nail exposed. Some clients have puffy or thick skin at the sides of their nails and unless this is firmly pulled back, the full width of the nail will not be seen.

If one size is too wide and the next is too narrow, choose the wider one and file away a very small amount from either side until it fits perfectly. If there is any doubt as to the correct size, one side of the tip can be 'tucked down' into one side wall and the other side looked at. Very often this will show that a tip that looked right is actually too narrow.

Full contact area versus reduced contact area   Many tips have a full contact area. These can be applied directly to the nail plate with adhesive or they can be tailored beforehand. There are eight main reasons why it is worth removing most of the contact area before application:

1   When applying a tip with a full contact area it is easy to get bubbles under the tip. If this happens, the tip must be removed. The bubbles are unsightly and are areas where bacteria could grow.

2 The bond between the nail and the tip relies on the adhesive used. This will be a cyanoacrylate and this can eventually break down in water. If the bond covers most of the nail (1) there is a larger area to be broken down.

3 The strongest bond in the artificial nail structure is between the nail and the overlay. If most of the nail plate is left exposed, as in the first diagram, the bond will be more effective.

4 A full contact area needs blending until it is invisible and there is no shadow that can be seen through the overlay. This involves more work and there is a greater risk that the natural nail will be buffed. Blending a small area is very quick.

5 When any tip is applied to a nail with a flat upper arch, the contact area must be completely in contact with the nail. A full contact area will cause the tip to be tilted upwards at a very unnatural angle (2).

6 By having a minimal contact area, the angle of the tip can be placed so that the finished nail looks most natural (3).

7 By placing the tip at the correct angle with a reduced contact area, the line to be blended will be at the top of the upper arch curve and therefore easier to blend without touching the nail plate (4).

8 Sometimes the contact area is almost as long or longer than the client's nail plate and there is very little room left to blend the area without damaging the soft tissue. This is particularly the case with nail biters.

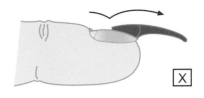

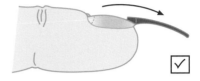

Tip and upper arch (a) tip with complete contact area producing wrong upper arch curve (b) tip with reduced contact area producing correct upper arch

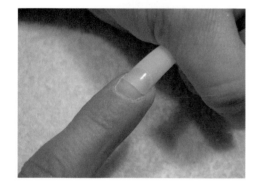

(1) Tip with full contact area on nail

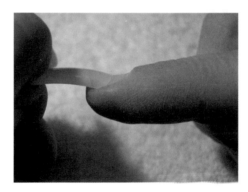

(2) Wrong angle of tip with full contact area

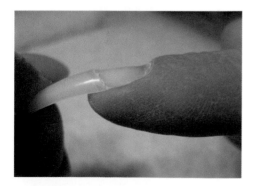

(3) Corrected angle of tip with reduced contact area

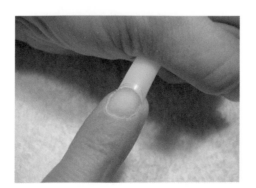

(4) Tip with reduced contact area on nail

Removing the contact area   There is no rule that states that the contact area must be removed or left in place. However, it is a very useful skill and a thorough understanding of the question allows individual technicians to make up their own mind what is right for their client. The most important result is a natural-looking, strong artificial nail that has been applied without damage to the natural nail and under safe and hygienic conditions.

There are two methods of removing the contact area:

1 *Using a file*. By holding the tip and the file at the appropriate angle (see picture), the contact area can be removed very quickly leaving a curved edge. By leaving this shape as opposed to a straight edge, the side walls of the free edge of the natural nail are provided with extra protection and support.

2   *Using scissors or clippers*. Scissors with a curved blade are ideal for snipping around the contact area, following the shape of the stop point. Nail clippers can also be used to cut out a 'V' shape.

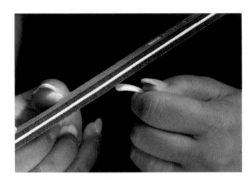
Removal of contact area using a file

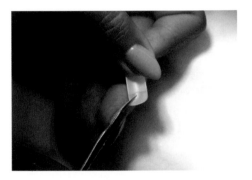
Removal of contact area using scissors

Applying the tip to the nail   Once the tip had been chosen and any necessary tailoring carried out, it must be applied to the nail with adhesive. The choice of adhesive is for the technician unless the client is a severe nail biter or has a damaged nail plate. If this is the case, a thick adhesive or gel should be used that will fill and cushion the irregularities of the nail plate or, in the case of a nail biter, fill the area where the nail has been bitten down below the hyponychium. If this area is left as an air space, there could be problems with bacteria or excess moisture.

A small amount of adhesive should be carefully placed in the contact area of the tip. Placing adhesive here is preferable to it being placed directly on the nail. When placed on the nail, it can easily run down into the side walls or over the edge of the finger. When placed on the tip, it starts affecting the plastic of the tip immediately, softening it ready for accurate placement.

The tip should be brought to the free edge of the nail at an angle of around 45°. This will allow the nail to be placed correctly in relation to the nail plate and then levered down onto the nail, expelling any air bubbles as full contact is made. As soon as the excess adhesive is seen being squeezed out onto the nail plate, the tip should be held in place for a few seconds until the bond is made. At this stage, the finger should be pushed up from underneath by the hand that is holding it rather than the tip pushed down. If the tip is pushed down it is very easy to lift it too high and therefore break the contact at the free edge and pull in air. The lack of oxygen present between the tip and the nail encourages the adhesive, to cure quickly, much quicker that when exposed to the air. However, the thicker the adhesive the longer this curing takes.

This should be repeated for each finger on one hand. When all five tips are applied, they can be cut to slightly longer than the desired finished length. The length should be decided by the client, but with advice from the technician if the requirements are unreasonable, such as too long for the nail bed or lifestyle. At this point, it is worth asking the client what shape is required – oval, square, rounded square or tapered. If the client has no preference, the shape of the base of the nail should be followed to create a good-looking nail.

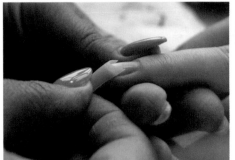

Fit free edge into stop point at 45 degree angle

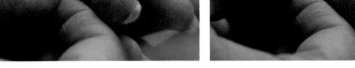

Lever tip onto the nail and hold in place for a few seconds

Angles of one-cut tip cutter

1 = square

2 = rounded square

3 = oval

Cutting techniques

There are several tools on the market designed to make cutting tips easier. They are adaptations of a tool used for clipping animal claws but instead of a round hole that the claw fits through, they have a curved hole for the tip. These clippers are quick and efficient and allow the tip to be shortened with one movement. When using cutters, the metal plate that has the curved hole must be nearer the finger. This will protect the finger from being cut as the blade is on the other side. If the cutter is angled under the client's hand, a slightly curved shape will be cut on the tip. The more upright the cutter is held, the straighter the edge. Care should be taken not to hold the cutter away from the client as this will result in an edge that curves in the wrong direction and, if the cutter is moved during cutting, could result in pulling the tip off.

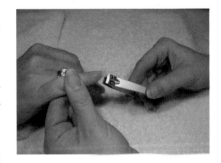

Cutting tips with clippers

Scissors or nail clippers can be used for cutting tips. Plastic tips are easily 'stressed' or bent which results in white areas. When using clippers or scissors, the tip should never be cut across in one action as this will cause the stress lines. Each side should be cut separately (see picture). The angle of the clipper blade will produce an outline of the finished shape – that is, oval, square or tapered. The piece of tip should be discarded as it cannot be used for anything else.

TECHNICAL TIP

During training, this stage often causes damage to the natural nail due to inexperienced blending. To help avoid this as a learner, apply a thin layer of adhesive to the nail plate and allow to cure in the air or activate to protect the nail before applying the tip.

Blending the tip

Once all the tips have been cut to the required length and the unwanted ends discarded, the tips must be blended to the natural nails. The result should be perfectly natural in appearance and look as if the nail grew there. More importantly, there must be no damage to the nail plate.

There are two methods of blending the tip: manually – that is with a file – or chemically with acetone or a branded tip blender.

HEALTH & SAFETY

Only a fine grit of 240 or more should be used on the natural nail. Great care must be taken to avoid buffing the nail plate. This is the stage that causes many problems for beginners and removing the contact area of the tip may help.

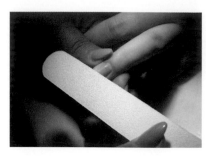

Blending the tips

Manual blending During training, procedures are easily learned if eight easy steps are followed. These steps will help to produce a perfectly blended tip:

1 Holding the file parallel to the finger, 'tuck' it down in the side walls and, with a few strokes, blend the sides of the contact area of the tip so that it is the same width as the nail plate. By keeping the file parallel, the sides of the free edge will remain straight.

2 Shape the free edge to the approximate shape and length required. Look at the tip on the finger as a whole and not just the nail plate to check that it is a suitable length and shape and that it is straight to the finger.

3 Holding the file flat to the tip, gently start buffing the surface, starting at the tip and working backwards towards the contact area. The shine of the tip must be completely removed.

4 Using at least two-thirds of the length of the file, gently buff the contact area. Care must be taken not to buff in the same place for too long. Keep moving the file all over the area but avoiding the nail plate. It is not necessary to press hard with the file as gentle pressure is much more effective. The contact area will become much thinner until it is transparent and cannot be seen. A little nail adhesive often squeezes out onto the nail during the tip application and becomes shiny. This is can be a very useful guide to help know when the tip has been blended and the nail is being avoided. The tip must be completely invisible and there must be no evidence of a 'shadow' where the contact area is.

5 Refine the shape of the free edge until it is perfect and even, and remove any debris that may have collected underneath during filing.

6 Look at the nail from the side to check that the upper arch is correct and even, and that the lower arch is correct.

7 Gently refine the 'smile line' area to produce a neat and natural-looking effect.

8 The tip should now look like a perfect natural nail and is the ideal 'canvas' on which to apply the overlay.

Chemical blending This method works by melting the plastic of the tip as an alternative to blending with a file. Some people, trainees in particular, like to use this method as they feel that damage to the nail plate can be avoided. To a certain extent this is true, but other problems may occur if it is not fully understood. It is not necessarily quicker than manual blending as, once mastered, manual blending is very fast.

Acetone may be used or there are a number of branded products on the market.

1 Once the tips are applied, paint a small amount of the tip blender with either a disposable cotton bud, or a brush used solely for this purpose, over the contact area. Wait a few minutes while the plastic melts. This time can be used to apply the blender to other tips to help speed up the process. Do not apply too much, as any liquid can be absorbed into the nail plate and could cause unnecessary dehydration. Too much liquid will also run into the side walls and cause dehydration.

2 While waiting for the blender to work, the free edge can be shaped to the required length.

3 When the tip starts to look very shiny, use a fine file to file away the melted plastic. The blender can be reapplied if necessary, but too much solvent on the nail plate should be avoided.

4 Follow steps 5 to 8 for manual blending now to ensure a perfect nail.

5 Make sure that there is no melted plastic covering the nail plate, as this could prevent a good bond with the overlay and could result in lifting in the centre of the nail leading to an air pocket.

6 Brush the file as the melted plastic can stick to the abrasive and make it less effective. Discard the file if the plastic cannot be removed.

Although skilful manual blending is usually faster, chemical blending is an excellent standby for the client who has very sensitive nail beds and cannot take any buffing on the surface. It is also useful for a nail biter who has such a tiny nail plate that it is difficult to use a file without damaging the soft tissue.

Removing the dust

Once all the tips are perfect, the dust that has been produced must be removed from the nails. A bristle brush may be used, but thorough hygiene procedures must be followed to keep this very clean. Remove dust inside the nail folds with care, making sure that oil from the skin is not brought onto the surface of the nail. The product being used for preparing the nail plate is often very useful for this job as the moisture will remove the dust and the product will ensure a clean, oil-free nail.

Once the tips are blended and cleaned, they should look like perfect natural nails. If this is not the case and there are shadows on the contact area or the free edge is curving up and not down, they are too wide or too narrow, they cannot be corrected by applying the overlay. No amount of clever overlay application will correct a badly applied tip. It will only make it worse.

Step-by-step: Preparation and tip application

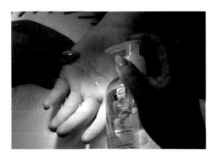

1 Sanitize the hands.

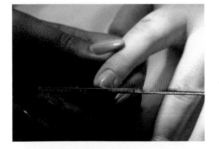

2 Shape the nail to fit the 'stop point' of the tip.

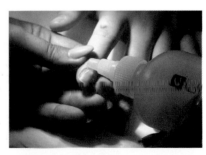

3 Apply cuticle remover.

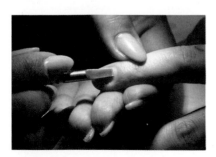

4 Remove ALL traces of cuticle from the nail plate.

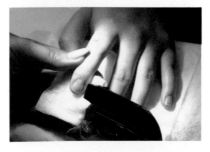

5 Wash the nail to remove cuticle remover.

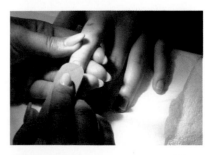

6 Remove the shine from the surface of the nail. ONLY the shine. Use the end of a 240 grit file with gentle strokes from cuticle to free edge. Make sure the file is angled down inside the side walls.

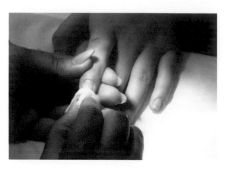

7 **Dehydrate** the nail plate to remove all traces of oil or moisture.

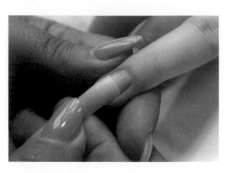

8 Choose the correct tip for the nail and pre-tailor by removing the well. Shape the sides if necessary.

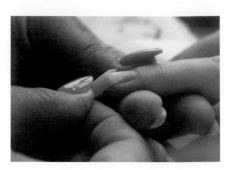

9 Place a small amount of adhesive in the contact area of the tip. Fit the free edge into the stop point at the angle shown (this will avoid air bubbles under the tip).

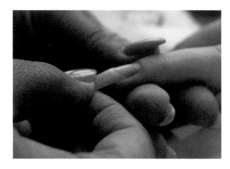

10 Lift the end of the tip so the contact area closes down onto the nail plate pushing out any bubbles that may be under the tip. Make sure the angle of the tip on the nail is correct by looking at the side view. Hold in place for a few seconds.

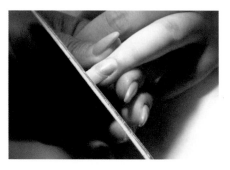

11 Cut the tip to the chosen length and roughly shape the free edge.

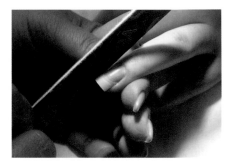

12 Using a thin file, blend the side walls first.

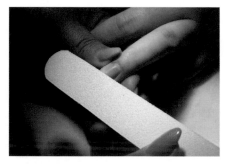

13 Using a 240 grit file blend the tip taking great care to avoid the nail plate. Gently blend until there is no sign or shadow of the tip. Refine the shape.

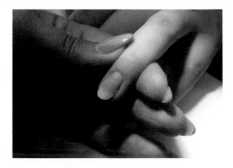

14 The finished nail. The tip should look like it 'grew there'! Perfect fit. Note the side walls are perfectly in line.

Problem nail shapes and how to correct them

Clients come in all different shapes and sizes, and so do their nails. It is a very lucky technician who is presented with lots of nails that have beautiful long nail beds with parallel side walls and neat free edges. Most clients present their technician with all manner of horrors and it is the job (and often challenge) of the technician to make the artificial nail look perfect.

It is not enough to apply nails that follow the natural shape. Many natural shapes are not perfect and are not always very attractive. The technician must correct natural imperfections. Many natural imperfections or problem shapes can start to be corrected with the tip application. This, followed by a planned overlay shape, will result in the desired perfection.

Practice is the only real way to perfect the art and skill of correcting problem shapes, but the following suggestions are a starting point to help that practice along.

Fan-shaped nail

Looking at the nail from the top, the side walls of a good shape should be parallel to each other. A **fan-shaped nail** is very common; this is where the edge of the nail is wider than the base, that is, the side walls 'fan' out. This nail plate is usually quite short and artificial nails can look very wide and clumsy and not at all elegant if the shape is not corrected by the skilful technician.

The correct tip size should be chosen carefully and the width of the nail plate at the free edge is the area which will decide the correct tip size. A tip with a full contact area usually appears much too wide as the contact area will often be wider than the centre of the nail plate. This does not matter as the contact area can be removed. The stop point of the tip must be the exact width of the free edge (a). Once the correct size is chosen, the contact area can be removed. It is likely that most of the area will need to be removed to avoid it being wider than the nail plate. Sometimes it is also necessary to angle the remaining contact area inwards so that it fits the nail.

The tip being tailored should keep being fitted to the nail to make sure the shape is right. This shape of nail is also usually quite flat with little or no upper arch or 'C' curve. A tip that has a flatter shape should be chosen so as to avoid any stress being put on the nail bed by a curved nail. If the flatter tip is still too curved to comfortably fit the nail without pressing it flat, a wider tip should be chosen and the sides filed to the correct width. When this has been achieved and the tip has been applied at the correct angle for a gentle upper arch (remembering that the tip will need to be angled down slightly to help create an upper arch), it can be cut to length. It is inadvisable for the free edge to be any longer than half the length of the nail bed. Anything longer than this will not look attractive and will not be as strong as a shorter nail.

When shaping the free edge, the side walls need to be tapered in to compensate for the wide free edge. An oval is often better for this shape of nail as the base of the nail is usually oval, but a square can be achieved if required that does not look too wide. This is achieved by making the parallel side walls taper slightly towards the tip of the free edge. If done correctly, the sides will still look parallel but more elegant than if left, as this can accentuate the 'fan' shape of the natural nail. The square edge can then be achieved, and the overlay applied.

Hooked or claw nail

A **hooked** or **claw nail** has an exaggerated upper arch and the free edge has a tendency to curve over the end of the finger. Clients with this shape of nail are often unable to grow their nails as the downward curve is unattractive.

The solution for this problem is to remove any free edge on the natural nail, choose a tip that fits (this is often one with quite a deep 'C' curve) and remove a great deal of the contact area. When the tip is applied to the nail, the side view should be checked and the

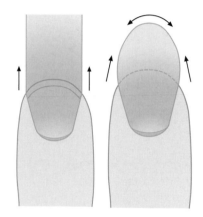

(a) Fan-shaped nail: fit tip to width at free edge (b) Fan-shaped nail with blended tip: tapered sides and oval shape

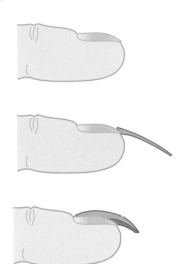

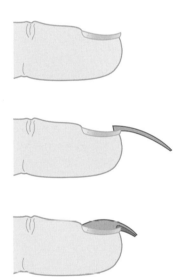

Claw nail (a) claw nail with no free edge (b) tip applied to edge of nail at correct angle (c) tip blended and overlay applied to correct poor upper arch

Ski-jump nail (a) ski-jump nail with no free edge (b) tip applied to give better upper and lower arch (c) tip blended and overlay applied to correct poor upper arch

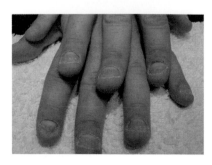

Bitten nails

upper arch corrected. Care must be taken that the underside of the tip does not have a gap between it and the nail plate, as debris could collect and cause problems.

The length should be quite short as, the longer the free edge, the more the curve will appear. Adjustments in the structure of the overlay will further compensate for this shape.

Ski-jump or spoon shaped nail

A relatively common shape, the **ski-jump** is a nail that curves up towards the tip. If a tip was put onto this shape without any correction, the nails would appear to be pointing upwards.

The corrective solution is very similar to that of the claw nail. The free edge should be as short as possible and the contact area of the tip removed. As the strength of the finished artificial nail is in the overlay and not the tip, the contact area can be tiny, if necessary, in order to achieve the correct upper arch. As before, when applying the tip, look at the side view and make sure the tip is curving down, even though the nail bed is curving the other way.

The length should be quite short and the overlay will need to be adjusted to compensate for the unusual shape produced by tip application.

Bitten nails

Bitten nails are probably the biggest challenge for the technician. If a good-looking set of artificial nails can be achieved from a set of severely bitten 'stubs' the technician can do anything! Obviously there are many degrees of nail biting, from the occasional nibbler to the person who bites their nails down past the hyponychium and onto the nail bed. The worst scenario is the experienced biter who not only bites down onto the nail bed, but also chews and picks at the soft tissue around the nail. The technician can do their best with the nails but can do little, other than offer advice, for the surrounding skin.

Obviously, recommending a course of manicures before applying artificial nails is preferable, as the cuticle and nail fold can be improved and some nail growth will help the strength of artificial nails; however, it is unlikely that the client will agree to this or succeed if they do agree. Biters do not usually bite deliberately and often try to stop the habit. They will try quite hard and achieve a little growth but then, while watching a good film, reading a good book or after a stressful day, will unconsciously nibble and spoil all the hard work. When this happens, there is often little point in leaving the other nails so they all go and the biter is back to the beginning.

Having a set of artificial nails can often be the answer for several reasons. A skilful technician can make the nails and hands look so good that the client does not want to spoil them. Having paid for the service, the client is more likely to make sure the money is not wasted. The unconscious move to the mouth is immediately noticed as the teeth come across hard plastic instead of soft skin. Nails applied well need determination to bite off, although the biter who is determined will do it whatever it takes!

Preparation Although it is a challenge that will take the technician longer than usual, even the worst biter can have a set of very good-looking nails. The challenge starts with the preparation.

A biter will often have a very obvious layer of cuticle and a pronounced nail fold. The cuticle can be removed relatively easily, but the nail fold will take more time as it must not be forced. Manicures would help a great deal, but this may not be an option. If the nail fold cannot be lifted, it must be left to be dealt with after the artificial nails have been applied, either during homecare or manicures.

The remaining nail plate will be soft owing to the length of time it spends soaked in saliva. There may also be dents and crevices where bacteria can breed. Preparation must be efficient and thorough with the nail and surrounding skin very clean and the nail plate dehydrated as much as possible.

The skin around a bitten nail is usually puffy, again owing to the amount of time it spends soaked in saliva. The end of the finger is often slightly swollen from this puffiness, the sides of the nail plate hidden from view and the overall shape flattened. All this will change dramatically after a couple of weeks with artificial nails.

Applying the tips
Milder cases of nail biting need to have the tips applied in the usual way, remembering all the rules about leaving most of the nail plate exposed for the overlay bond and creating good curves. If the nail plate is bitten down past the hyponychium, the skin that is exposed will usually be swollen and higher than the nail plate and the tip will need a great deal of pre-tailoring before application. A tip, even with the contact area removed, when applied to this type of nail will point upwards as the skin will not allow it to lay flat.

A flat tip needs to be chosen and, if necessary, a wider one made narrow to provide the right 'C' curve (or lack of it). To find the right size, the skin at the sides of the nail must be pulled back very firmly with the finger and thumb of the technician so the full width of the nail plate is exposed. Like the fan nail, the width at the edge of the nail and the stop point must match exactly, regardless of any other part of the tip.

When the correct size has been chosen (or made) the contact area must be removed so that only a minimal amount of tip will be on the nail plate, leaving the maximum amount of nail plate exposed for the overlay bond.

At this stage the tip will still not sit on the nail properly, as the skin will push it up. The sides of the tip from the stop point down the sides of the free edge need to be carved out for the puffy skin to fit into (b). This will form a 'bridge' that will curve over the puffy skin and create a reasonable arch that curves down instead of up. This 'bridging' is necessary as, without it, not only will the nails look unattractive, but the skin that has been pushed down to fit the tip to the nail will push the nail upwards and make it very weak and liable to breakages.

When applying the tip with adhesive, it is advisable to use a much thicker adhesive than usual. With the skin in the way, the tip cannot be angled onto the nail and needs to be placed from the top. There is also usually an area around where the hyponychium should be that is lower than the nail and the skin. If using thin adhesive, it is difficult to avoid air bubbles when placing the tip in this way, which might allow a space where bacteria can thrive. A thicker adhesive will help to avoid the bubbles and fill up and cushion the area of the hyponychium.

The length must be very short, just to the end of the finger is ideal. The artificial nail will not be as strong as that on an unbitten nail and the client will be unused to having nails and will be clumsy for a few weeks.

Blending the tip on a small area can be tricky and if it is difficult to avoid the usually delicate soft tissue, it may be advisable to use a chemical tip blender. Although some people prefer an oval-shaped nail, a free edge that is slightly square usually better suits the wider fingertip of a nail biter.

The overlay will further improve the appearance of the nails and the homecare advice must be specific, as must the need for maintenance visits.

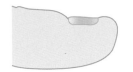
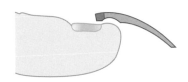
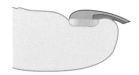

Bitten nails (a) badly bitten (b) side walls of tip removed to form 'bridge' over end of finger; contact area also drastically reduced (c) tip cut short and blended with overlay to compensate for poor shape.

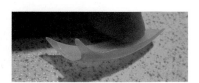

Tip pre-tailored for a nail biter

Alternative tips

French white tips

A **French white tip** is an opaque white, it is designed to create a quick and easy permanent 'French manicure' look. Although this tip can be used with any system, there are restrictions as to who can wear this tip. The tip must be applied to the end of the nail and not blended. The shape forms a perfect 'smile line' and the overlay will create the necessary strength. This tip is not suitable for:

1 A client who has a different 'C' curve from the tip (there are now several shapes of white tips available, so having a selection is worthwhile).

2 A short nail bed, as the extra white tip, when correctly placed, will make the nail look unattractive with too much white and not enough pink.

3 A client without any free edge; the tip's 'smile line' will need to be placed onto the nail bed instead of where it would naturally be and would result in an unattractive nail.

4 A natural nail that does not have an upper or lower arch that matches the tip.

There is a correct placement for this type of tip that can create a perfect French manicure appearance. There is also a wrong placement that can make the finished nail look very unattractive.

A client wearing this type of tip must have the growth of natural nail covered during maintenance treatments.

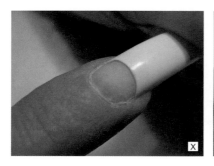
Wrong placement of French white tip and unsuitable natural nail shape

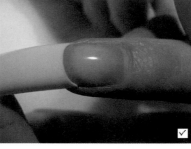
Correct placement of French white tip on suitable natural nail shape

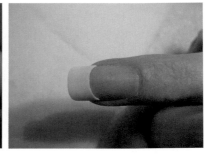
French white tip prepared for overlay

Clear tips

These are tips that are totally transparent and are usually used for various types of nail art. They are dealt with in exactly the same way as traditional tips. When they are blended in they will look dull and scratched, but as soon as an overlay is applied the dullness and scratches will disappear.

These tips should only be applied to nails that are very neat and without any free edge at all, as every irregularity will be seen through them.

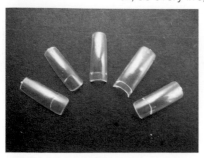
Various clear tip shapes

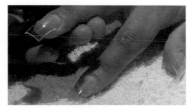
Clear tips applied to nails

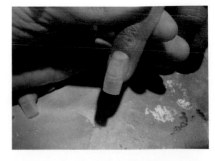
Clear tips blended and prepared for overlay

Designed tips

There are many pre-designed tips coming onto the market for quick and easy nail art. Some of them are in the form of tips with a small contact area and some have a larger contact area. Obviously these cannot be blended, as this would ruin the design.

The nail should be prepared in the usual way and the tips applied to the nail. There is usually no need to do anything else to the tip at this stage and the overlay can be applied directly over the tip.

Summary

This chapter has explored the stages in the process of lengthening a client's nails by plastic tip or overlay techniques – choice, application and safe removal – and how to cope with the many types of 'problem' nails that a client may present to the technician.

ASSESSMENT OF KNOWLEDGE AND UNDERSTANDING

1 What are the features of a plastic tip?

2 How is a tip type chosen to fit a client's nail?

3 Why is the correct width of tip so important?

4 How can any damage to the natural nail during blending be avoided?

5 How can tips be customized to fit various nail shapes?

6 Ideally, what is the maximum length of an artificial nail while still keeping the nail balanced?

7 What would you do if there is a bubble under the tip?

8 How would you apply a tip to:

   a. a nail biter

   b. ski-jump nail

   c. hooked nail.

9 When would you avoid using French white tips?

10 Why is it so important that the tip fits perfectly?

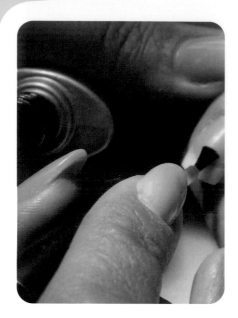

9
Applying overlays

Introduction

This chapter explains the differences in all the **overlay** systems available on the market today. It provides an unbiased information base and explains application techniques with ways to practise and perfect technique.

The perfect foundation has been created with the application of tips. Now is the time to create the perfect artificial nail that looks good and is very durable and strong. The tip has provided the required length, now the overlay on that tip will provide the required strength.

Wrap techniques

By overlaying a tip, a longer artificial nail is going to be created. The overlay can be applied to a natural nail that has some length but needs to be protected because it is weak. Some clients like to wear a **natural nail overlay** just to keep their nail varnish in perfect condition as it does not chip. This treatment is often known as a **nail wrap** or natural nail overlay (NNO for short). This term probably came from a technique that was used many years ago by manicurists before the products and techniques we know now were available. If a client had split a nail or had weak nails, a piece of tissue was placed on the nail with a clear varnish. Several more coats of varnish were applied to smooth the surface. The tissue was sometimes wrapped slightly under the free edge, especially if there was a split. This is where the term 'wrap' came from and this procedure is probably the forerunner of the fibre system. Fibre users will now sometimes wrap the fibre mesh under the free edge to seal and strengthen it.

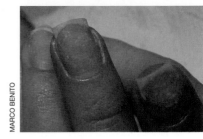

Weak damaged nails ready for overlay

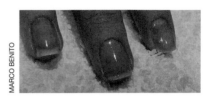

Nails protected by overlay

Overlay systems

This aspect of artificial nail work can sometimes be the most confusing for the beginner. There are several different 'systems' and many different companies, all insisting that their system and brand is the best. Some companies sell all systems, others sell only one of them. For help with choosing the best system see Chapter 7.

Many clients and technicians believe that the end results of the systems look very different. This is often the case, but it does not need to be. A beautifully applied set of nails should be a perfect shape and look natural whatever the system. One system need not look thicker or more natural than another. Colours and finishes can make a difference, but the skilful technician can even overcome this with some little tricks of the trade!

TOP TIP

NB application is the same for a NNO and a nail with a tip applied and blended.

The systems in use

All products in artificial nails belong to the acrylic family of chemicals. Acrylics are a vast family of various types of plastic. The word 'system', when it is related to artificial nails, describes the specific method and type of acrylic that produces the overlay.

Each system has a specific collection of various components and it is this collection and the application method that differentiates the systems. The tip application remains the same for each, although various brands may recommend specific preparation products. It is worthwhile taking these recommendations as, although cheaper options are often available, specific branded products have been developed to work with the system products to help achieve a better result. Introducing different or additional products or chemicals into the system can lead to problems.

Liquid and powder

This system is probably more commonly known as 'acrylic', although the term is strictly inaccurate as all the systems are based on acrylics. The system (usually referred to as L&P) was arguably the first to be used for artificial nails using materials from the dental industry and the term 'acrylic' has stayed since then (see Chapter 1). It uses a liquid monomer and powder polymer (see Chapter 7) that cure to form a solid polymer. Its versatility in the hands of a skilled technician is immense and it is generally considered to be the trickiest to learn. It is sensitive to many external conditions, application techniques, and the time available to get it right before it hardens is limited. It is, however, a very popular system and is the favourite in the UK and US.

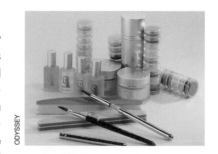

Liquid and powder products with coloured powders

It has many advantages in that any shape can be sculpted onto a tip or a free form (see Chapter 10); it can easily be used to correct difficult nail shapes; powders are available in different colours to allow the technician to create permanent French manicures or enhance natural skin tones. The overlay can be built to create the strongest structure and the strength within the overlay is excellent.

Its main drawback is the fact that the monomer is quite volatile and has a strong odour. Many technicians do not like the smell, or strong odours may be inappropriate in a beauty salon. Working cleanly, correctly and hygienically can minimize this problem. There are some products on the market that are classed as '**low odour**'. This usually means that the evaporation rate is lowered. The newer versions of this type of product can work very well and, if odours are a problem and a technician prefers a liquid and powder system, they are certainly worth considering.

A version of this system is the **UV light-cured** liquid and powder system. These are applied in a very similar way to the traditional acrylics; the main difference is that they do not polymerize until UV light is applied as the catalyst. This can be very beneficial for beginners as they have plenty of time to apply the overlay in the correct shape. For experienced technicians, both hands can be worked on, which avoids any additional time for curing. These monomers are in the low-odour category and therefore can be more user-friendly if odours are a problem. The overlay that is produced is as versatile and strong as traditional acrylic but, with some brands, has a characteristic that must be dealt with carefully: many UV-cured materials do not achieve a total cure and a sticky residue is left on the surface where oxygen has inhibited the cure. This residue is unpolymerized monomer, which is a skin irritant. It must be filed off during the shaping stage but continual contact with the skin for either the client or the technician can result in an allergic reaction.

Most brands of L&P have powders in several colours. This gives the technician the ability to create very natural looking artificial nails that suit the client's preferences. The most usual combination of colours available are:

- *Clear*. Used for either the entire nail or over the nail bed. Suitable for a nail bed that has a good colour.

- *Pink*. A powder that has a slight pink pigment added to it to enhance the colour of the nail bed. Used in the same way as clear. There are some brands that produce different shades of pink, so the shade best suited to the client can be chosen. Some pinks can be a little 'violent' and, if there is only one choice in the brand, take this into consideration when choosing which brand to use.

- *Bright white*. This is a heavily pigmented powder for use on the free edge only. It will create the very specific appearance of a French manicure. The application of this needs lots of practice as it is essential to achieve a perfect smile line for it to look good. This is also used during maintenance to put the smile line back to the right place.

- *Natural white*. This has less pigment than a bright white and will create a more natural looking nail. The application of it on the free edge still needs care but the smile line is not so sharp. Even if this is not used during the first application of artificial nails, it is very useful to cover up the natural nail growth at the free edge. This growth of nail visible through the overlay often prevents wearers from having their nails varnish-free as it does not look attractive. When choosing brands, check that the natural white is dense enough to do this job.

- *Natural*. This is not so common in modern brands now, but is a milky version of clear. It was very common in early liquid and powder systems as a good clarity in the overlay was difficult to achieve and the milkiness hid imperfections. Some clients still like the look of a milky nail, but it should never be used to hide poor workmanship such as visible lines from previous maintenance treatments.

- *Natural colours*. These are opaque powders in skin tones that can be used as they are or mixed to exactly match the skin tone. The advantage of these is that they can cover imperfections e.g. a nail biter, or can be used to extend the natural nail bed for a more aesthetic appearance.

- *Coloured powders*. There are many brands that have introduced multi-coloured powders. These are for use either as a 'permanent' colour instead of varnish or they are used to create nail art designs. The preparation and application is the same, but various colours may be applied in different sequences rather than following the order indicated. See Chapter 13.

TOP TIP

A word of warning when using opaque coloured powders on the nail plate: lifting of the overlay or the beginning of any other problem cannot be seen due to the opacity of the overlay. Care must be taken during maintenance services to make sure there is no lifting that could be harbouring bacteria.

The liquid and powder systems are applied with a brush made of natural hair, usually sable or the better quality Kolinsky sable, by dipping the tip of the brush first into the liquid monomer and then into the powder polymer where it picks up a bead of the material. This bead is then applied to the nail and pressed into place. Polymerization either occurs within a few minutes or when placed under a UV light if it contains a **photoinitiator**.

UV gel

The UV gel system could be considered to be a 'pre-mixed' system, as there is only one material that is applied. The only other necessity is a UV light source. The gels are available in many different versions, all with different features and benefits. The main differences that will be immediately noticed by a technician is the viscosity (thickness) and how it flows. Some gels are very runny, others are very thick. Some thick gels will eventually flow, others will stay where they are put. Gels are available coloured, or clear.

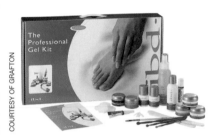

UV gel system products

All gels are applied to the nail and moved around with a brush before being polymerized under a UV light source. As with all systems, there are many application techniques developed by various companies to suit their gels, but there are two basic application methods: one of them is probably the easiest method of applying overlays of all the systems; the other requires a little more skill, but allows a nail to be sculpted onto a tip for maximum strength.

Another benefit of this system is that it is virtually odour-free and therefore may be more suitable for use in areas where stronger odours are a problem. In addition, the gels can be very flexible and therefore move more with the natural nail.

The disadvantages of the UV gel system are that some gels and their application methods cannot produce an overlay that is as strong as the liquid and powder systems and are therefore suitable only for those clients who are not too hard on their nails. Many of the gels on the market can be removed only by buffing and not by soaking off with a remover. Some consider this to be a benefit, others consider it to be a disadvantage (see Chapter 11).

Following cure, most gels have a sticky layer on the surface. This is uncured monomers and needs to be removed with care and not allowed to touch the skin. Most brands have a specific product to do this job but an alcohol-based solvent or varnish remover can be used.

Gels are available in a range of colours in the same way as liquid and powder systems and their use on the nails is the same. Multi-coloured gels for nail art designs (see Chapter 13) are becoming popular, but the same warning for opaque overlays in the liquid and powder system applies to gels.

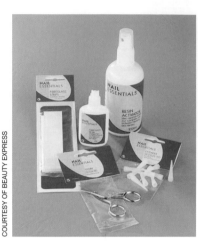

A fibre system

Fibre

The third main system involves the application of a fibre mesh (usually silk or fibreglass) with a cyanoacrylate resin. This is polymerized or activated with a spray or paint-on chemical. This system is quite gentle on the natural nail, as the overlay produced cannot be very thick and remains quite flexible. It needs very little equipment and the starting costs for trainees are usually relatively low. Odours are kept to a minimum and are negligible if a paint-on activator is used in preference to a spray.

This system is very popular as a natural nail wrap, as it is quick and fairly easy to apply and never produces thick, clumsy-looking nails. For manicurists, it is ideal as a natural nail repair. The overlay is easy to remove.

The disadvantages include the fact that the overlay cannot be built up to create a maximum-strength structure and imperfect natural nail shapes can be corrected only by tip application, not a combination of tip application and overlay. As the overlay is quite thin, the artificial nails are not as strong as the structured nails of other systems. Some technicians find the application techniques a bit too 'fiddly', but others love it.

Choosing a system

All the systems have their advantages and disadvantages: it is the technician who makes the difference. Some will hate a specific system and think it does not work at all; another technician will love that system and produce wonderful results. When, as a beginner, the choice of system is a problem and all the marketing and advertising make the choice even more confusing, the best way to choose the right system to learn with is to try them all. (See also Chapter 7 for help in choosing a system.)

Learning a new skill is easier when the task is enjoyable. It can be more frustrating if the tasks are unpleasant. Unfortunately, trainees tend to be under the impression that applying artificial nails is really easy, which is how it looks when a skilled technician does it. But trainees often discover it is not quite like that. It is not enough to watch the various systems being applied; the best approach is to try the different systems yourself to get the feel of how easy (or not) each system may be for you.

A liquid and powder system is not ideal for the person who immediately cannot stand the smell; a UV gel is to be avoided if the 'stickiness' is annoying; fibre should be left alone if handling the fibre suddenly produces clumsy fingers. No one system will be immediately easy but, hopefully, one will stand out as being the one that may become easier more quickly.

Beginners are advised to choose a system to learn with, and stay with that system until all the various skills are mastered. At this time, when the technician is very confident in their work, another system can be added. Whatever the system, it should be easier to learn, as the outcome now will always be a beautiful set of artificial nails.

The structure of the overlay

The three zones

When applying an overlay, it will help to think of the nail with its tip in terms of three different **zones**:

1 **Zone 1** is the free edge where the overlay needs to be thin on the edge so that the finished nail does not look artificial.

2 **Zone 2** is the area beside the smile line and onto the nail bed where maximum strength is needed. This is the area of the nail that receives the most stress. It is

often called the 'stress area' and should have a highest point that is called the 'apex'. The strongest natural structure is a curve (pressure is dispersed along the curve and is not concentrated over one point). The apex should be where two curves, the upper arch and the 'C' curve, come together at their highest and thickest part. This will create maximum strength for the whole nail without putting any stress on the natural nail, the nail bed, or the matrix.

3 **Zone 3** is the area near the base of the nail. Like Zone 1, this should be thin so that any ridges on the nail bed are avoided and, by being thin, it will be more flexible and able to move with the softer natural nail in this part of the nail plate.

If these zones are always kept in mind when applying an overlay, the correct shape and strength will be easier to achieve.

The application procedure

The steps in the application procedures listed below are general and, although they will be appropriate for many brands of products, it is advisable to check with the manufacturer or distributor their recommendations for application techniques. Always follow the manufacturer's instructions when using nail products and always avoid mixing system products from different brands. Polymerization chemistry is carefully balanced and mixing potentially hazardous chemicals could be dangerous and could cause problems.

Liquid and powder *Practising product control*: Picking up the product with a brush in such a way that it can be applied to a nail is one of those things that looks very easy. It does, however, take a little bit of practice! For a beginner, picking up the perfect 'bead' can sometimes seem impossible.

- Some liquid and powder brands need a specific ratio (this is the amount of liquid to powder), others are less sensitive. There are some brands whose manufacturers recommend that a dry ratio is used in Zone 1 (more powder means harder), a medium ratio in Zone 2 (combination of **hardness** and flexibility) and a wet ratio in Zone 3 (maximum flexibility over the softer part of the nail).

- Usually the bead that needs to form on the tip of the brush needs to look smooth and glassy.

Practising product control for a little while is time well spent for a beginner. Understanding how the product behaves and practising picking up various beads will save a great deal of time, especially if these first attempts are placed on a nail and either have to be removed or buffed into shape.

- To do this, get a piece of unwanted plastic or glass, dappen dishes with monomer and powder (use coloured powder as well as clear or pink as they behave differently owing to the density of pigment), a brush and some disposable towels.

- Dip the tip of the brush into the liquid and wipe it on the sides of the dish expelling any air bubbles, dip the tip of the brush into the surface of the powder (not deep), hold it there for about 2 seconds and lift it out. It should have a bead of wet product on the tip.

- If the bead is so wet it falls off, there was probably too much liquid still in the brush, so it would need to be wiped on the side of the dish a bit more. It may be that the brush needed to be in the powder a bit longer to pick up a bigger bead.

- If the bead that is picked up is rough, with obvious powder on the surface, the ratio is much too dry. Maybe there was not enough liquid in the brush or the brush was left in the powder too long and picked up too much powder.

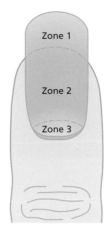

Zones of the nail

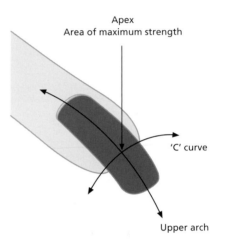

Curves of the nail

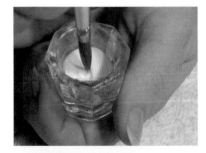

Dipping a brush in powder

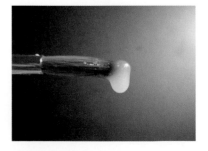

Bead too wet

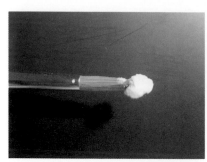

Bead too dry

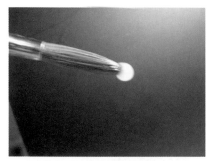

Perfect bead

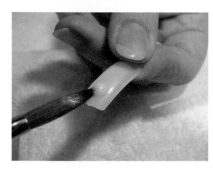

Too little on tip

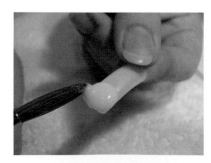

Too much on tip

Practise this a few more times until a bead can be picked up that is smooth and glassy in appearance and does not fall off the brush. Different methods of dipping the brush into the liquid can be tried, such as sliding the brush down the side of the dish, noticing how far the brush goes into the liquid, squeezing both sides of the brush on the sides. As a brush is made of natural hair and many brushes are handmade, each one is going to have its own characteristics. One brush may hold much more liquid than another.

Picking up powder: There are different methods of picking up powder: little circles can be drawn in the surface of the powder or the brush can be drawn through in a line. The brush should never be dipped in further than the tip and there should be sufficient powder in the dish to avoid the brush touching the bottom. If this happens, the bead sticks to the dish and is difficult to get out. It is also worth tapping the dish on the desk to smooth out the surface of the powder. A smooth surface makes picking up a bead much easier.

Bead control: When a bead can be picked up confidently, it is worth moving on to 'bead control'. This will demonstrate what the ratio of the bead is and the trainee technician can determine if this is correct.

- This is done by picking up a bead and gently placing it on the plastic or glass. If the bead is on the very tip of the brush it should come off the brush onto the surface with ease. Once the bead is on the surface, it should start to melt. How it does this demonstrates if the ratio is correct. By melting, the bead loses its shape and eventually becomes flat.

- All brands are slightly different but, as a general guideline, if the bead melts in less than 3 seconds it has a wet ratio, if it takes over 5 seconds, it is dry. A medium ratio, which is usually the one to aim for, should hold its shape momentarily and then start a slow melt.

- Doing this a few times, using the various ways to pick up a bead, will show the trainee how to pick up a bead of the right ratio.

This can now be taken a step further. Nails are different sizes and so are the zones on each nail. Now the right ratio can be achieved, it is time to practise picking up a bead that is not only the right ratio but also the right size! A step further again: the right ratio of the right size in a different colour, for example white-tip powder. Coloured powder usually needs more liquid owing to the colour pigments present, so this should be tried out first to get the right ratio.

After that, different-sized beads can be picked up to see how much liquid is needed in the brush, how long the brush should be kept in the powder, and so on. After this has been practised, it is worth deciding beforehand what the bead is going to be for. For example, a Zone 1 white tip for a little finger with a short free edge (very small) and then a Zone 1 white tip for a middle finger with a medium-length free edge (considerably bigger), and so on.

Determining how big the bead needs to be before it is picked up will save time later and is part of the way towards creating a good structure with a brush and not correcting a bad structure with a buffer.

Condition of the liquid: During this little exercise, the condition of the liquid should be noted. If it is looking cloudy or if there is powder at the bottom of the dish, it is badly contaminated. If this liquid was used on a nail with a clear or pink overlay, it would look cloudy and mottled. This contamination must be avoided during working and is easily achieved. When working, the brush should be occasionally dipped into the liquid and taken straight out without wiping it on the sides of the dish, but then wiping it on a disposable towel or tissue. This, if done a couple of times, will remove the build-up of powder that accumulates in the hairs and then goes into the liquid. When using white-tip powder, the brush should be cleaned in this way after each nail. This is because the powder will remain in the brush and the next time the brush is dipped in and pressed on the side of the dish, the powder will be left in the liquid and the nails will become more and more cloudy. Some technicians even have a separate dish of liquid just for white-tip powder to prevent this happening.

Application on the nails: Once a certain amount of product control is achieved, the application onto the nails can start. This procedure is the same as that for a natural nail overlay.

Creating the perfect shape: One of the most important aims of applying overlays is to create as close to the perfect shape as possible with the brush and not rely on correcting mistakes with a buffer afterwards. This obviously takes practice. Liquid and powder overlays continue to polymerize for quite some time after they become hard enough to buff. Too much buffing can interrupt the polymer chains being formed and create weak spots. Also, buffing away what has just been applied can waste a great deal of time. It is much easier to try to apply it correctly in the first place and the buffing as a refinement stage.

Application using white-tip powder

1 The nails should have the tips perfectly blended, the dust removed and be clean and oil-free. One hand is worked on at a time from start to finish.

2 Apply primer (if instructed by manufacturers) very sparingly around the base of the nail. Make sure the primer is dry before applying overlay.

3 Clean the brush first by dipping it into the liquid, taking it straight out and wiping it on or between sheets of disposable towel. Discard the towel in a metal, lidded waste bin.

TOP TIP

Have a small lint free pad dampened with your nail dehydrator by you. Use this to wipe your brush clean and change it often. This will help to keep down vapours from the monomer.

ALWAYS REMEMBER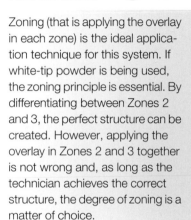

Zoning (that is applying the overlay in each zone) is the ideal application technique for this system. If white-tip powder is being used, the zoning principle is essential. By differentiating between Zones 2 and 3, the perfect structure can be created. However, applying the overlay in Zones 2 and 3 together is not wrong and, as long as the technician achieves the correct structure, the degree of zoning is a matter of choice.

EQUIPMENT LIST

clean terry towel on desk	tip cutters
three layers of disposable towels	liquid monomer in clean, covered dappen dish
tissues or disposable towels	powder polymers in clean, covered dappen dishes
hand sanitizer	
nail sanitizer	primer (if required)
nail dehydrator	clean sable brush
cuticle knife	files of 240 and 180 grit
cuticle nippers	oil
tips	buffers, such as a white block
adhesive	three-way buffer or block

4 Start with the little finger, pick up a bead of white-tip powder that is approximately the right size and place it in the centre of Zone 1 closer to the smile line than the edge.

5 Wipe the brush on the towel. (With practice, this stage will not be necessary.)

6 Holding the brush at the same angle as the upper arch of the nail and with the tip of the brush, press the bead. Take part of the bead to one side wall and create the point of the smile line; take part of the bead to the other side wall and create the point of the smile line; create the smile line as neatly as possible with the tip of the brush and smooth the surface of the whole zone. If the brush is angled down slightly and the overlay is gently pushed up towards the smile line, a sharper line can be created and a thinner edge of the nail. If the smile line is uneven and needs straightening, the extreme tip of the brush (cleaned and dry) can be used to do this, making sure that the nail plate does not get monomer on it from the brush. Check the shape by looking down the barrel of the nail to make sure the overlay is even. The centre of this smile line will form the apex of the nail. (Some technicians like to apply white tip to each nail before Zone 2. This is usually to avoid contaminating the liquid. However, as the overlay starts polymerizing immediately, the bond between the overlay at Zone 1 and 2 may have a weak point in it as Zone 1 has polymerized too much to blend with Zone 2. A stronger overlay is achieved if the whole nail is completed and contamination is easily avoided.)

7 Clean the brush.

8 Pick up a bead of pink or clear of the right size and place it in the centre of Zone 2 next to the white tip.

9 Wipe the brush.

10 The bead will have started to melt while wiping the brush and will be ready to press into shape. Making slow and deliberate movements and keeping the brush parallel with the nail, press the bead and, like Zone 1, take part of the bead out towards the side wall, leaving most in the centre and blend over the white tip; take part out to the other side wall and blend over the white tip (4). Blend the whole zone over the tip. Check down the barrel for evenness and thin sides.

11 Pick up a bead for Zone 3 and place it in the centre of the zone.

12 Wipe the brush.

13 Press the bead and blend up over the whole nail.

14 With the brush flattened, press the overlay towards the nail fold, taking great care not to touch the skin with the brush and leaving a tiny margin of bare nail bed. With the flattened brush between the overlay and the nail fold, gently press the overlay to thin the zone and create a good bond with the nail plate.

15 Check shape from both sides to make sure the upper arch is in place and the overlay is smooth. Check overlay from down the barrel.

16 Repeat process for each finger. Polymerization has occurred when the overlay can be tapped with the handle of the brush and a 'clicking' sound can be heard. If the click sounds dull, it is not sufficiently cured. Discard the towel that has been used to wipe the brush.

17 When all the nails on one hand are finished, go back to the little finger with a 240 grit file. Gently buff over the whole surface to smooth out any bumps and ridges. Carefully blend the edges of the overlay making sure the tiny margin of exposed nail plate

TOP TIP

Wiping a small amount of oil onto the nail after step 19 will show up any flat areas as the overlay will appear slightly shiny. This helps in creating a good shape before the finishing glossing.

is not buffed. Check overlay from all angles to ensure a perfect structure. Refine the free edge to make it as thin and even as possible.

18 Repeat for all nails.

19 Return to little finger and buff whole surface with a white block as this will start to refine the surface ready for the final stage.

20 Repeat for all fingers.

21 Using a three-way buffer in the correct sequence (usually black, white, grey) buff all nails to a high-gloss shine without any dull spots (dips in the overlay).

22 Remove all the dust, including that which has collected under the nail and discard layer of disposable towel with all the dust.

23 Apply oil to each nail and massage into nail and cuticle.

24 Repeat the whole process on the other hand.

25 When both hands are completed, tidy desk by cleaning brush thoroughly and storing flat and away from dust, discard any unused monomer onto the disposable towel remaining on the desk. Make sure powder dishes are covered. Wipe the surface of the desk with a cloth dampened with a mild disinfectant and prepare for next client with clean towels, etc.

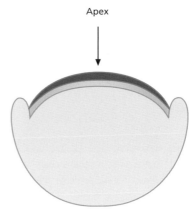

Apex

View of even overlay by looking down barrel of nail

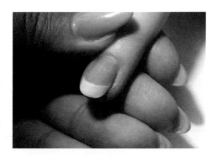

Overlay before finishing

If the overlay is being applied without white tip, it should still be applied in zones, but it would not be necessary to create a smile line. Otherwise the process is the same.

Troubleshooting: If the overlay looks powdery in Zone 3, it is usually because the client's hands are very cold or the liquid monomer is cold. This hinders the rate of polymerization leaving unpolymerized powder on the surface. This can be corrected by warming the client's hands before application or making sure that the monomer is at room temperature before using. If it is an emergency, for example, the first client of the day in a salon that has not yet warmed up, the covered dappen dish with the monomer can be placed in a bowl of tepid water (not hot) to bring it to room temperature.

If the brush was not cleaned properly after the last use and has a lump of product in it, soften the product in some monomer (nothing else) and use a paper towel to try to remove the debris. Do not use your fingers as a sensitivity to the product may result. An orange stick can be used to dislodge the debris, but this will usually result in damaged hairs and a brush that does not work very well. Discard the monomer that was used. Do not be tempted to use any type of brush cleaner. This will introduce a chemical into the system that is not meant to be there.

Remember to clean and store your brush correctly when you have finished the service.

Step-by-step: Application using white-tip powder

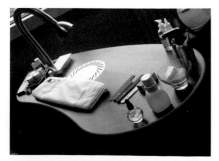

A desk set up ready for an L&P overlay. Notice there are two points of extraction: downward to remove dust and upward to remove vapours.

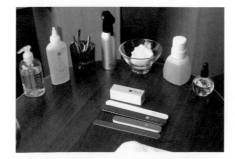

One side of the desk has all the preparation products.

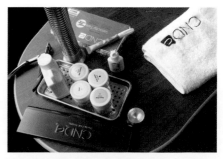

The other side of the desk has all the overlay products ready to bring across when ready.

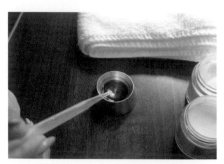

Using a pipette, place a small amount of monomer liquid in a dappen dish that has a lid. Do not put too much in the dish. It is easy to top up. A shallow dish like this one makes it easy to expel bubbles from the brush.

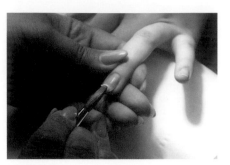

Apply a primer to nail plate if necessary and allow to dry. Pick up a small bead of white powder with brush and place in the centre of zone 1.

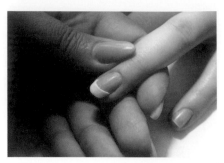

Using small pressing movements, take some of the bead out to one side and create a sharp smile line with a pointed 'dog ear'. Repeat the process on the other side. Make sure the 'C' curve is even and the extreme edge is thin. Tidy up the smile line if necessary.

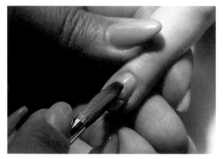

Pick up a medium bead of clear or pink powder and place in the centre of Zone 2 close to the smile line.

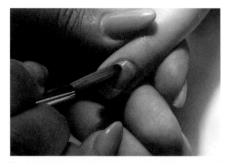

Using small pressing movements take some of the bead to either side of the nail, angling the brush to create a thin and even overlay at the side walls. Blend the overlay into Zone 1 for a smooth finish. Check the 'C' curve and side view for the correct structure.

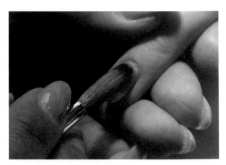

Pick up a small bead of clear or pink powder and place in Zone 3. Angle the tip of the brush and, using some pressure, move the bead into Zone 3 and create a clean and tidy edge. Blend into zone 2.

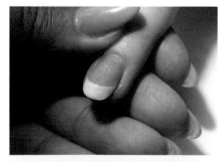

Make sure the overlay has cured sufficiently by tapping with the handle of the brush. It should 'click' and not be a dull sound. Ideally, the nail should need minimal refining at this stage.

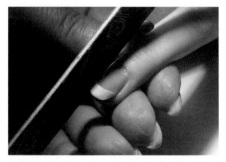

Using a thin file, refine the side walls. Then, with a 240 grit file, refine and smooth the overlay. Check from all angles to make sure the structure is correct. Make sure there are no dull or flat spots.

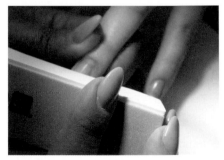

When the overlay is a perfect shape, use a glosser or three-way buffer to shine the surface.

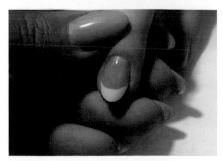

Massage nail oil into the nail and surrounding skin.

UV gel

Versions of this system is often considered to be one of the easiest for a beginner to learn. This is possibly true as, once the tips have been applied, there is a very straightforward method of applying UV gel as an overlay. The artificial nails produced by this method are not always very strong, as it does not create a structure with the curves that produce a strong nail. This method would be suitable for those who will wear their nails quite short or who are used to having long nails and are therefore unlikely to break them.

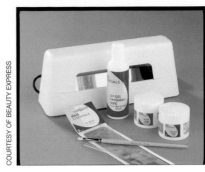

A UV gel system

There are many different types of gels on the market now and the technology of this area has advanced a great deal in the last few years. The range of gels now available will allow a skilled technician to do everything with gel that can be done with a liquid and powder system.

The gel 'system': Gels now come in all colours and the gel 'system' can comprise a single component – that is, one type of gel – or it can comprise several gel components, all of which are recommended as being needed to create an artificial nail. Like all other systems, the choice is down to personal preference and cost.

Gels are 'pre-mixed' system, needing UV light to polymerize rather than another chemical. There are two distinct types of gel in use: self-levelling and non self-levelling.

The bonds in gels are very strong and this usually makes them resistant to solvents. If this is the case, the overlay cannot be 'soaked' off and requires buffing to remove it. This can be seen as a benefit or a hazard – a solvent-resistant overlay is also resistant to damage and discoloration from nail varnish and remover.

Soaking nails in a solvent to remove them is very drying to the nail plate and the surrounding skin, and the nail plate especially takes time to recover from this major dehydration. If artificial nails are not being replaced, oils and moisturisers can be used after removal to help this recovery. Occasional rumours arise in the industry suggesting that this method can be damaging to health. All chemicals are damaging to health if an individual is overexposed, and the overexposure level to the solvents used in this industry, such as acetone, is very high (see Chapter 4).

Removing artificial nails by buffing needs skill and this can be achieved only by practising on real fingers. At first, it can be time-consuming and, when done improperly or excessively, can cause severe damage to the nail plate. Ideally, the removal of nails should be a rare occurrence and take place only when the client does not want artificial nails any more. There are gels on the market now that can be removed with solvents so widening the choice for technicians and clients.

A word of warning about coloured gels (and acrylics): an opaque overlay could be hiding a problem! If lifting has occurred or if the nail plate or nail bed has become infected, this will not be visible. The only way to ensure this is not happening is to remove the overlay at regular intervals that, in itself, could cause a problem. Belief that the overlay will not lift is not sufficient, as a client may be resistant to any overlay, or may become resistant at any time owing to a change in the nail plate.

With a one-component gel system, the gel is applied to the nail in one or more layers to build up strength. In a system with two or more components, there is usually a gel that acts as a bonding layer; it is compatible with the nail plate and also with the next layer of gel; next there is a thick gel that can build an overlay with the required structure, that is curves, and then a sealer gel that provides a high-gloss shine and protection. The manufacturer's instructions should always be followed.

EQUIPMENT LIST

clean terry towel on desk	gels
three layers of disposable towels	UV lamp
nail wipes	primer (if required)
hand sanitizer	clean brush, either nylon or natural hair
nail sanitizer/dehydrator	
cuticle knife	finishing wipe (if required)
cuticle nippers	file of 240 grit
tips	oil
adhesive	buffers, such as a white block
tip cutter	three-way buffer (if required)

Application to the nails Both hands are worked on at the same time with this system.

1   Both hands, with tips applied, must be clean and totally dust-free (gels are very susceptible to dust as it causes a lumpy overlay).

2   Apply primer to Zone 3, if required, and allow to dry.

3   Open gel and, with a clean brush, apply a thin layer of gel to each nail, taking care not to touch soft tissue (remove with an orange stick if this happens). The gel is applied in this method in the same way as nail varnish, but bring the brush to the edge of the nail and wipe downwards off the edge. This will help to seal the edge and prevent any shrinkage of the overlay. If a 'whole-hand' lamp is being used, include the thumb, otherwise just apply gel to the four fingers.

4   Turn on lamp and ask client to place fingers under the lamp, making sure that the fingers are correctly placed and all are exposed to the UV light. This usually takes 2 minutes, but refer to lamp's instructions.

5   While the first hand is under the lamp, repeat the process on the other hand.

6   Remove the first hand and replace with the second.

7   If a small lamp is being used, the thumb will need to have the overlay applied now, and then it can replace the second hand after the cure time.

8   Repeat for thumb of second hand.

9   Apply second layer of gel to nails of first hand while second thumb is under lamp and cure.

10   Repeat until all fingers of both hands have had second layer.

11   If the nails are long or are likely to be subject to heavy use, it may be necessary to add a third layer in the same way.

12 When all nails have had sufficient layers applied and they have been cured, replace lid of gel and clean brush with nail varnish remover, or equivalent, on a tissue.

13 Gels have a sticky surface layer of uncured monomer. This must be removed and most brands have a product that will do this job efficiently without damaging the gel. The monomer must be kept off the skin. Using a nail wipe with the remover, start with the little finger and wipe from the nail fold towards the tip. By doing this there is little chance of the monomer touching the skin. If the same wipe is used on a larger nail than a small nail, monomer from the previous nail will come into contact with the skin and the client will develop a sensitivity and become unable to wear the artificial nails. The monomer must be thoroughly removed, as any remaining will be in the dust created at the next stage and will touch the skin of both the client and the technician.

14 It is possible to leave the nails exactly as they are now if they look a perfect shape; however, there are often small imperfections in the surface and sometimes the gel will have shrunk slightly so that the extreme tip looks more rounded than it should.

15 If the nails need refining, a very soft file should be used or a white block, as the surface of a gel is usually quite soft. The shape should be checked from all sides.

16 At this stage there are two options: the nails can be buffed with a three-way buffer which will produce a natural shine (not a high shine as the surface is usually too soft) or, after the sticky layer is removed, a thin layer of the gel can be applied, and cured to produce a high gloss. If the second option is chosen, all the dust created by the buffing must be carefully removed with the finishing wipe on a tissue and the paper towel where all the dust that has collected removed.

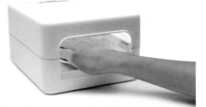

Cure for recommended time

17 Apply oil and massage.

18 Clean desk and prepare for next client.

Structuring method with a thicker gel

1 Both hands, with tips applied, must be clean and totally dust-free (gels are very susceptible to dust as it causes a lumpy overlay).

2 Apply primer to Zone 3, if required, and allow to dry or apply bonding gel if appropriate and cure for recommended time.

3 Open gel and, with a clean brush, apply a bead of gel to the centre of the nail where the apex should be. Take part of the bead to the side wall at the stress area and take part of the bead to the other side wall at the stress area. Ease part of the bead down towards the nail fold, taking care not to touch the skin. Bring part of the bead with the brush to the edge of the nail and wipe downwards off the edge. This will help to seal the edge and prevent any shrinkage of the overlay. The gel should now have a thin layer at the free edge in Zone 1, a thicker layer at the stress area in Zone 2 and a thin layer in Zone 3. The surface now needs gently smoothing over with feather light movements of the brush until the shape is right from all angles. If a 'whole-hand' lamp and a gel that does not run is being used, include the thumb, otherwise, just apply gel to the four fingers.

4 Turn on lamp and ask client to place fingers under the lamp, making sure that the fingers are correctly placed and all are exposed to the UV light. This usually takes 2 minutes, but refer to lamp's instructions. It is possible that a heat reaction may be felt by the client. Polymerization is an 'exothermic' chemical reaction (gives off heat) and the reaction in a gel is usually very fast. If the gel layer is thick or if the client has

thin or sensitive nail beds the heat may be felt. The client should be warned that this may happen and to help avoid it, the fingers should be placed under the light for 5 seconds, then removed for 5 seconds. This should be repeated at least once more and the heat sensation, if it is going to happen, may be avoided. If the heat is felt, and it is usually quite sudden, tell the client to remove her fingers and press them on the desk very firmly. This will stop the reaction and then the fingers can be replaced. (Many modern gels have been formulated more accurately and should only be used with the recommended UV lamp. If all instructions are followed the 'heat spike' should be avoided.)

5   While the first hand is under the lamp, repeat the process to the other hand.

6   Remove the first hand and replace with the second.

7   If a small lamp is being used or a gel that can run, the thumb will need to have the overlay applied now and then it can replace the second hand after the cure time.

8   Repeat for thumb of second hand.

9   When all nails have had sufficient layers applied and they have been cured, replace lid of gel and clean brush with the finishing wipe, or equivalent, on a tissue.

10   Many gels have a sticky surface layer of uncured monomer. This must be removed and most brands have a product that will do this job efficiently without damaging the gel.

11   The nails now need refining as there are often small imperfections in the surface and sometimes the gel will have shrunk slightly and the extreme tip look more rounded than it should. The structure should also be checked to make sure it is correct and the same on each nail.

12   A very soft file should be used as the surface of a gel is usually quite soft. The shape should be checked from all sides.

13   At this stage there are two options: the nails can be buffed with a three-way buffer which will produce a natural shine (not a high shine as the surface is usually too soft) or a thin layer of the gel can be applied and cured to produce a high gloss after the sticky layer is removed. If the second option is chosen, all the dust created by the buffing must be carefully removed with a finishing wipe on a tissue and the paper towel where the dust that has collected removed.

14   Apply oil and massage.

15   Clean desk and prepare for next client.

Step-by-step: UV gel

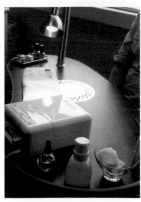

Desk set up in readiness for a UV gel application.

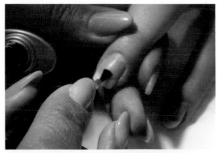

Most UV gel systems have a bonder layer or primer. On a nail that has had a tip applied and has been prepared (see Nail Preparation), apply a very thin layer of bonder gel to each finger on the first hand making sure the whole nail is covered and the gel does not touch the skin.

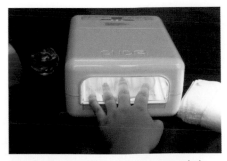

Cure for the manufacturer's recommended time. While the hand is in the UV lamp repeat for the second hand. NB it may be necessary to cure the thumbs separately.

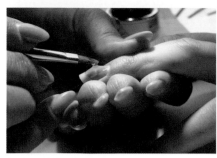

Apply a thicker layer of the builder gel. Notice how the brush is used to build an apex in the centre of the nail. At the free edge pull the brush down to seal the edge. Cure in the UV lamp for the recommended time. NB depending on the viscosity of the gel, it may be necessary to 'fix' the layer on two nails at a time to prevent the gel from moving while you apply a layer to the next two nails. Alternate the hands so one hand is always under the lamp.

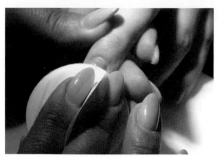

Using an alcohol-based product, remove the inhibition layer from each nail, wiping from the cuticle to the free edge.

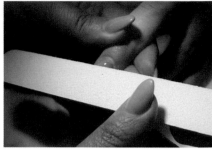

Using a 240 grit file, refine the shape of each nail looking at it from all angles to make sure it is even and has a good structure and a thin free edge. Remove all traces of dust with a cotton pad dampened with an alcohol-based product.

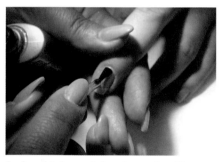

Apply a thin layer of gloss top coat making sure the whole nail is covered, the edge is sealed and the surface is smooth. Cure for the recommended time in the UV lamp.

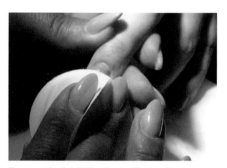

Remove the inhibition layer. The nails are now finished and ready for massaging in some nail oil.

Step-by-step: UV gel nails with a white tip

The steps are for a straightforward gel overlay. If a client would like a pink and white gel nail, the white tip product should be applied after the nail has been refined and before the gloss top coat.

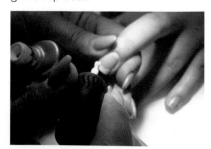

When all the dust has been removed from the nails, apply the white-tip product just as if painting a French manicure. The smile line can be sharpened by using a clean gel brush. Cure in the UV lamp for the recommended time. Then apply the gloss top coat.

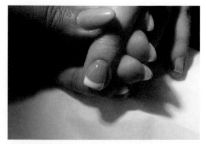

Finished nail.

TOP TIP

To make sure your gel brush is clean and will not create dips in your overlay, prime it!

Take a plastic backed remover pad, pick up a little gel and work it into the plastic. This will make the brush pliable and straighten out the hairs ready for application.

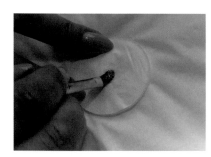

Prepare the brush

EQUIPMENT LIST

- several layers of disposable towels
- nail wipes or cotton wool
- hand sanitizer
- nail sanitizer/dehydrator
- cuticle knife
- cuticle nippers
- tips
- adhesive
- tip cutters
- fibre scissors with a very fine and very sharp blade
- fibre mesh, silk or fibreglass, kept in a plastic cover or box
- resin with long nozzle
- activator, spray or brush-on
- 240 grit file
- white block
- three-way buffer
- oil

The fibre system

This is a relatively easy system, but it relies heavily on the skilful application of the tips. Owing to the nature of the products, it is not possible to create any additional curves in the overlay, as can be done with a liquid and powder or a thick gel. Therefore the shape of the finished nail relies on the shape of the tip. It is possible to build in a little extra strength with the fibre, but this is minimal.

There are fewer actual brands of this system on the market – that is, a collection of products that make a full system under one name – than for the other systems, but the individual components are readily available.

Mesh and resin: Silk or fibreglass can be used as the mesh. The resin used in this system is sometimes called a **no-light gel**. This should not be confused with a UV gel. A no-light gel in this system is a cyanoacrylate resin that is slightly thicker and therefore more like a gel in consistency. (It is, however, possible to use fibre with a UV gel to give added strength or for free-form sculpting.) There are also two different ways of activating the resin: a spray or as a brush-on. Both are effective and usually contain similar chemicals. It is a matter of choice, but a brush-on activator will obviously put fewer chemicals into the air, which will help to avoid any sensitivity developing in individuals.

Application

1 One hand is worked on at a time from start to finish.

2 The nails with tips must be clean and dehydrated. (This system does not require any primer and the rough surface of the nail plate is enough to hold the overlay.)

3 Using the scissors and avoiding handling the fibre too much, cut a piece of fibre that is the approximate width of the nail to be overlayed.

4 Remove the fibre from its paper backing and use the backing to hold the fibre while it is put in place.

5 Place the fibre onto the nail close to, but not touching, the nail fold. Use the backing paper to press the fibre onto the length of the nail (1). Avoid touching it with your fingers as they will leave behind a small amount of moisture and this will prevent the resin from soaking into the mesh. Trim the sides if necessary by sliding the blade of the scissors

down the side wall and cutting away the excess. Trim the excess length of fibre by angling the scissors backwards on the nail tip so the fibre is cut slightly shorter than the tip (2). This allows the end to be sealed with the resin. (If the artificial nail needs extra strength, a strip of fibre can be placed across the stress area. This can either be a strip placed on the nail before this stage, or it can be a double layer of the fibre.)

6   Repeat this for all the fingers, excluding the thumb.

7   Apply a very small amount of resin down the centre of the nail (3) and, with the side of the nozzle, use little circular movements to spread the resin over the nail and work it into the mesh. More resin can be applied if necessary but, at this stage, the pattern of the mesh should still be visible, but very wet.

8   Repeat for all fingers.

9   Go back to the little finger and apply a very small amount of resin down the centre of the nail and spread it over the whole nail with side of nozzle. (It will not need spreading if a brush-on activator is being used.) Take great care not to touch the skin and to leave a tiny margin of bare nail around the edges. Seal the tip of the nail with the side of the nozzle. (If too much resin is applied, it will run into the side walls.)

10 Repeat for all fingers.

11 If a spray activator is being used, hold it at least 30 cm away from the nails and spray once (ensuring the aim is right!) (4). The resin needs only minute amounts of spray activator. If too much is sprayed or it is too close, a sudden heat reaction will occur that is very painful for the client and can ruin the overlay.

12 If a brush-on activator is being used, have the brush cleaner at the ready. (Brushes used with this product can get stuck with polymerized resin and must be put in a solvent between uses to keep them clean. It is usual to have another bottle of a similar size containing the solvent and a spare brush so they can be alternated during applications.) Spread the resin with the activator brush to cover the nail while keeping the product off the skin and leaving a tiny margin around the edge (8). This will mix the activator into the resin and speed up the polymerization process. (This activator is usually much weaker than the spray-on version, so the process is slower.)

13 Repeat for all fingers, putting more activator on the brush for each finger. Replace brush in activator bottle.

14 Apply another layer of resin to all fingers and either spread with nozzle or leave for brush.

15 Activate in the same way as before.

16 Repeat the whole procedure from Step 3 on the thumb.

17 Another layer of resin may be applied if more strength is required.

18 If a brush-on activator is being used, remove the spare brush from the solvent and wipe it on a paper towel to remove most of the solvent. Wipe the brush that has just been used on the paper towel and place it in the solvent. Put the spare brush into the activator bottle ready for the next use (9).

19 The overlay should be relatively smooth and should need minimal buffing to refine and smooth the surface. If the activator has been sprayed too close, there may be pits in the surface that will need buffing out. (If this happens and by removing them the overlay is made too thin, the nail should be cleaned of dust and a layer replaced.)

20 Refine the surface further with a white block (10).

21 Bring the nails to a high shine with a three-way buffer (11).

22 Remove all dust and apply oil.

This nail system is not solvent resistant at all. If nail varnish is to be worn then a very gentle remover should be used otherwise the surface will be destroyed. If varnish is repeatedly removed, the whole nail may be undermined.

Step-by-step: Applying the fibre system

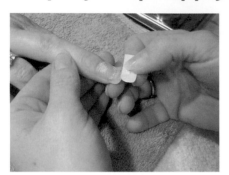

(1) Apply fibre to nail.

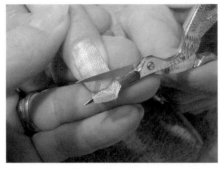

(2) Cut excess fibre with scissors and wet fibre with resin.

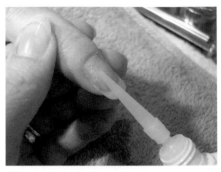

(3) Smooth resin with nozzle.

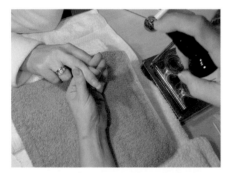

(4) Activate resin holding spray away from nail.

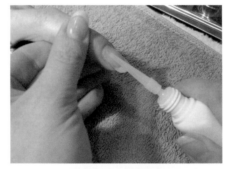

(5) Apply second layer of resin and smooth.

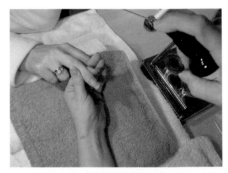

(6) Activate resin holding spray away from nail.

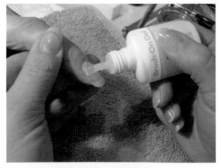

(7) OR apply brush-on resin/gel.

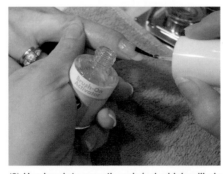

(8) Use brush to smooth resin/gel which will also activate it.

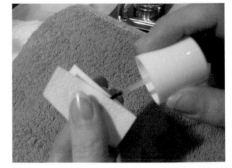

(9) Wipe activator brush before replacing in bottle.

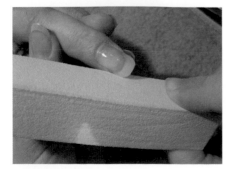

(10) Refine surface.

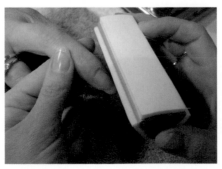

(11) Buff nail.

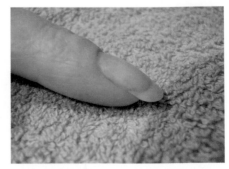

(12) Finished nail.

Creating the natural-looking nail

A nail correctly applied in one system should not look widely different from one applied in another. The white tip that can be used in an acrylic system may look different from others, but there are white gels available and the fibre system can use French white tips.

The finish can sometimes look different and a gel with a high gloss looks different from the high shine achieved by buffing an acrylic. However, if a client who wears acrylic nails prefers the high gloss, the gloss gel can be applied to an acrylic to give it that effect.

When applying nails, the most important aim is to create a natural-looking nail that suits the hand and is the strongest structure it can be. A technician is only as good as their last set of nails. No one can create perfection every time and a beginner needs to be able to look at their results and recognize what can be improved. An eye for balance and symmetry is not always a natural skill and needs to be learned. A trainee technician who has natural skill is very lucky; most do not have it and need to develop it. Many are not even aware that they lack this skill and send clients out with very strange shapes on their fingers.

Problem shapes

Following on from the problem shapes encountered in Chapter 8 on tip application, there are some shapes that can be improved using overlays.

Ski-jump nails

If the tip is put on at the correct angle for a ski-jump nail, the lower arch will be good but the upper arch will be very strange. This can be very easily corrected by careful structuring of the overlay to create a good upper arch and a strong nail (see diagram).

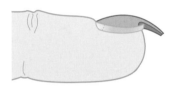

Tip blended and overlay applied to correct poor upper arch

Bitten nails

Still the most difficult problem to overcome, like the ski-jump, the bitten nail can be further improved by the overlay. The overlay only has a tiny nail plate to hold on to and the length must be just to the end of the finger, but, the overlay can be applied so that the upper arch can look quite natural. The nail really needs to be covered with coloured varnish to hide the lack of a smile line but, if this is done, the finished nail will look very good. Alternatively, natural opaque powders or gels can be used to disguise the lack of nail plate.

Tip cut short and blended with overlay for bitten nails

NB keep the artificial nail very short! There is not enough nail plate to hold a long nail and a nail biter will not be used to having nails so will very easily knock them off.

Twisted nails

If natural nails were allowed to continue growing, they would curve down and twist in a clockwise or anticlockwise direction. These twists may not start until the nail has reached a decent length, but they may start on the nail bed. This can be seen if the shape of the barrel is viewed from either the tip looking towards the hand or from the hand looking towards the tip. It is difficult to see if the nail plate is very short, but the longer the nail is the more obvious the twisting becomes. Once a tip is applied and blended, a twist may become obvious. The lower arches will be uneven with one side dipping down more than the other. This can be easily rectified during the blending of the tip by matching both sides of the lower arch. The twist of the barrel can be rectified by placing slightly more product on one side than the other and making the 'C' curve of the nail even. The additional amount of product is minimal and it is very easy to overcompensate. The easiest way to see this is by turning the client's hand around and looking down the nail from the hand down to the tip.

Creating artificial nails using a 'nail form'

Nail forms are relatively new to the professional nail market. They are most definitely NOT an easy way to apply an overlay for those who have not perfected their skills! They are a very useful addition to the nail technician's service offerings for the client who wants artificial nails but does not want to spend an hour and a half or more in the salon. Using this technique it is possible to apply a full set of L&P or UV gel nails in 40 minutes. This will also be invaluable for the salon who is trying to compete with a competitor who is a 'discount salon' and offers 40 minute full sets.

In practical terms, the most useful way to use nail forms is to apply a clear or pink overlay. It is possible to apply a pink and white nail but this does take longer and therefore takes the application time up slightly. If the tip has been applied properly or the client likes to keep her nails painted there is no reason why a set of these are not perfect for a busy client.

As with all nail services, this takes practice! The various brands of nail forms are slightly different. Some have an 'upturn' around the edge that you may find advisable to remove in order to create a thin edge in Zone 3. You will need to practice and try ways that suit you and create a perfect overlay.

Procedure

1   Prepare the nails and apply tips.

2   Dehydrate the nail plate and apply primer if required by the system.

3   Choose the correct nail form for each finger and set them out ready to use. (If a form is slightly too big, it can be trimmed to fit perfectly.)

4   Starting with the little finger, take the nail form and place a bead of L&P or UV gel into the centre. Move it around until it goes to the sides of the form and as far up the form as will cover the tip you have applied to the finger. Use more L&P or gel if necessary.

5   Turn the nail form over and place on to the prepared nail and very gently press over the nail plate. Hold this for about 10 seconds for L&P.

6   Repeat with all nails on one hand. If using UV gel the fingers will need to be placed under the UVC lamp for the recommended amount of time followed by the thumbs if it is a small lamp.

7   Check that the overlay on the first finger has cured by tapping with your brush.

8   Holding the end of the nail form, pinch the edges together to break the seal and twist the nail form off the overlay. Repeat for all fingers.

9   Using a fine file, tidy up the free edges.

10   The overlay will be shiny and perfect so there is no need to refine and buff. Just massage some nail oil into the nail and surrounding skin.

Step-by-step: creating artificial nails using a 'nail form'

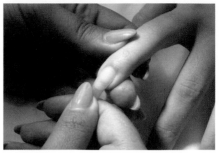

(1) Select nail form
After applying and blending tips, preparing the nail and applying primer if required, select a nail form that fits the nail perfectly. If there is not a perfect size the choose one that is slightly too big and trim with curved nail scissors. Make a mental note on the length of the nail within the form so you know where to place the l&p.

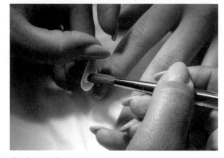

(2) Apply l&p
Pick up a medium sized bead of l&p and place it inside the form.

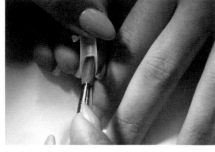

(3) Spread
Move the bead into the form until it covers the form from side to side and at the cuticle end. Place another bead to get correct length if necessary. Remember where the length of the nail stopped within the form (there are usually marks on the outside of the form to help).

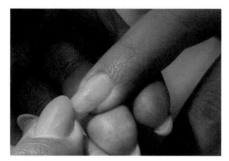

(4) Apply to nail
Turn the form over and place accurately on the prepared nail.

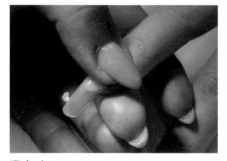

(5) Apply pressure
When the form is in place apply a slight pressure over the nail plate for 10–20 seconds. Move on to the next nail.

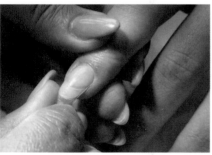

(6) Pinch
When the overlay is cured (check this by tapping with the handle of your brush and there should be a clicking sound not a dull sound), pinch the end of the form to release it from the overlay.

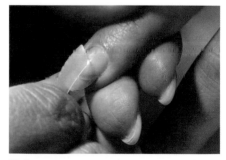

(7) Remove
Gently lift away the form from the nail by slightly twisting it so one side comes away first.

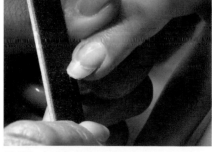

(8) Tidy
Tidy up the free edge taking care not to touch the top of the nail as this will spoil the shine. Apply nail oil and the nail is finished!

Toenails

It is becoming a more popular service to overlay (or rebuild) toenails. Not many people like the appearance of their feet and a nail technician can help this situation. Both L&P and UV gel can be used for this. Some clients like to have a pink and white overlay that makes their toes look clean and healthy and they can apply and remove polish if preferred. Some like to

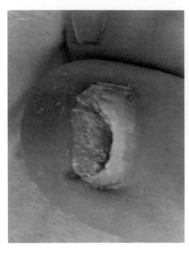

Damaged toenail before

use the semi-permanent colours. (As with fingers, take extra care that there is no lifting! Toes are even more susceptible to infection!)

All the same rules apply when enhancing toenails but you must remember that feet are very often the perfect environment for infections and toenails are often 'wetter' than fingernails.

Big toenails are the most common nail to suffer damage. This may be due to tightfitting shoes or a client who plays a lot of sport. Under these circumstances it isn't uncommon to lose a toenail because the base of it has been damaged due to leverage from shoes being put on the edge of the nail and therefore lifting it from the matrix.

Their susceptibility to infection can also lead to severe damage. No one likes to see an ugly toenail so it is a very good service to be able to offer. However, this does need specialist training! The before and after pictures are in this book as a demonstration of what can be achieved and NOT as a training aid.

Practice makes perfect

Applying artificial nails is not just about making nails longer. It is also a skill that can solve many problems and make imperfect nails look perfect. By understanding the systems and becoming skilful at creating shapes, a technician can do many things with artificial nails. It is possible to replace nail plates that have been lost through accident or illness. It is possible to rebuild nails that are deformed through damage or an hereditary factor. It is even possible to build a nail where one does not exist, such as where the tip of the finger is missing. (If any work like this is attempted with a client who has a medical condition, it is important to get approval from their doctor first.)

The secret of the true professional and successful technician is practice. No technician can practise too much, both in perfecting shape and product control and applying perfect nails to every client regardless of nail shape, condition and lifestyle. Nothing can replace the value of applying nails to a very wide range of people. Every nail is different and every lifestyle is different. Seeing nails that have been applied 2 weeks earlier will teach the new technician much more than just practising shape. Also, this is work that deals with people, so practising with people is essential. When practising, technicians should aim to apply a full set of artificial nail **extensions** in under 2 hours. This is acceptable for a client receiving a treatment from a technician, as opposed to a trainee. Every technician should aim to provide a full set of artificial nails in one and a half hours or less.

Some nail salons operate very well with every treatment being carried out in 1 hour or less. This is the choice of the salon and their clients and can be successful as long as all hygiene rules, working practices and client care are maintained. Other salons, on the other hand,

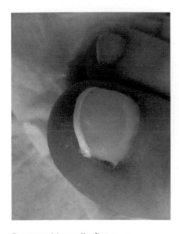

Damaged toenail after

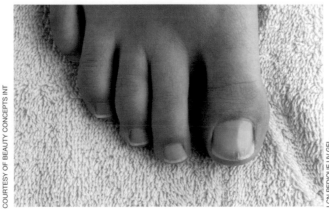

Damaged toenail before

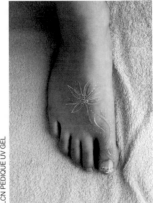

Damaged toenail with nail art

prefer to give their clients more time and a more relaxing treatment. The most important aspect of every treatment is safety and quality.

Aftercare advice

The following aftercare advice should be given to clients after every artificial nail treatment:

- Return for recommended maintenance treatments.

- If there appears to be discoloration under the artificial nail, return immediately.

- Do not pick off the overlay.

- Do not use nails as tools.

- Massage nail oil into the cuticle area every day.

- Do not file the surface of the nail.

- It is not advisable to shorten the nail as the thin layer at the free edge will be filed away to a thicker area.

- Use acetone-free varnish remover if necessary.

Potential retail recommendations

- nail oil

- varnish remover

- varnish

- hand cream

- top coat.

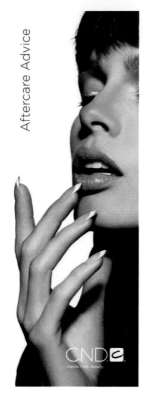

Aftercare

Summary

This chapter first examined the function and structure of overlays and then demonstrated step-by-step techniques for their application to create a natural-looking nail, whichever system – liquid and powder, UV gel or fibre – the technician has used.

ASSESSMENT OF KNOWLEDGE AND UNDERSTANDING

1 Explain briefly the application of: (a) powder/liquid, (b) UV gel, (c) fibre systems.

2 What structure creates the maximum strength for a finished nail?

3 What is meant by perfect shape and balance?

4 What is the purpose of zoning?

5 Suggest two methods of application that could correct or improve various nail shapes.

6 What conditions could adversely affect the application of overlays?

7 In a UV-cured material what inhibits polymerization?

8 Why is it important to provide treatments within commercially acceptable timings?

9 Why is it important to work with system products in the same brand and follow manufacturer's instructions?

10 What aftercare advice should be given?

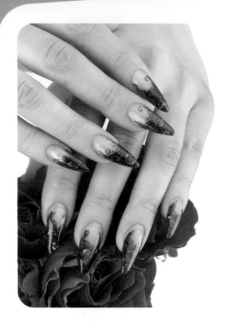

10

The art and skill of applying sculptured nails

Learning objectives

In this chapter you will learn about:

- **what a sculptured nail is**

- **how to fit a form in preparation for sculpting**

- **how to sculpt with each system**

- **remedial sculpting.**

Introduction

This chapter looks in step-by-step detail at applying sculptured nails.

Sculptured nails or plastic tips?

Many years ago, when only a few individuals were experimenting with dental products the plastic tips we are familiar with today were not available in their present form. The dental acrylics were strong enough to support themselves and the nail plate could be extended using just these products. If a 'platform' was placed under the edge of the nail, the product could be continued from the nail plate onto the platform to create a longer free edge. When the product had cured (hardened) the platform could be removed and there was a longer nail.

This method is generally called 'free-form sculpture' or **sculptured nails** and there are many different versions of specially designed 'platforms' that are called 'forms', the choice is a matter of personal preference. Many technicians learned how to do 'nails' in this way only and many still prefer this method to the method of applying plastic tips first. Applying artificial nails in this way requires skill, but then so does applying tips correctly. The method omits the tip application stage, but needs some time spent on placing the chosen form in exactly the right place. On balance, a technician skilled in sculpting nails can complete a set in a shorter length of time than a set using tips.

The results of the two methods rely entirely on the skill of the technician. For many, artificial nails with a tip will result in a stronger nail, but only if the tip is applied perfectly and there are no weak areas around the smile line, the blending or the side walls. A sculpting technician can also produce a perfect nail that does not have any of these weak spots. This can be difficult, as there will often be a step created where the form meets the nail plate and some product can seep under the free edge. If there is no natural free edge, there may be a step-up where the form does not meet the free edge. A sculptured nail must also have sufficient strength at the side walls without looking too thick, otherwise the free edge will snap off very easily. All of these features can be achieved by skilful application.

Systems and forms

Systems

The liquid and powder system is the one most commonly used to create sculptured nails, as its application and **curing** methods suit the way the nail is achieved. UV gel is also used as the thicker gels will stay in place on a form for UV curing to take place, and, with the coloured gels, a white tip can be achieved. The fibre system is rarely used in this way. It is possible to hold the fibre before the excess length has been removed and coat it with resin. This will result in extra length without a tip, but it will be very delicate and would not last very long. It would also be clear and would need coloured varnish to disguise it.

Forms

There are many different types of forms available. Most are *disposable* and are used from a roll. They have a sticky back that allows them to be held in place on the finger. Technicians have devised all sorts of inventive ways of shaping these to help produce the perfect nail. They are used for one nail and then discarded. They usually have a metallic finish of some description to reflect back the small amount of heat polymerization produces and ensures that the undersurface of the free edge is fully cured. With UV-cured materials, it is usually worth removing the form after curing and putting the fingers back under the light with the palm of the hand upwards to make sure the underside is cured. Alternatively, clear forms are available for light-cured products so the UV rays are reflected up to the underside of the free edge.

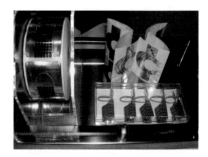

Various forms

There are also an array of *reusable* forms of different shapes and sizes. Like many things in the art of applying artificial nails, the decision about which one to use is a matter of personal choice. The forms, both disposable and reusable, are not expensive, so it is worth trying out as many as possible to see which is preferred. It is also worth having several types, as some will fit a specific nail shape better than others and this will make the fitting of the form much quicker.

Fitting a form

The choice of which form to use is for the technician to make. Technicians soon find a form that they are most comfortable with.

1   Many paper forms are supplied on a roll. A new form should be removed from the roll and the part to be fitted under the free edge as a platform for the artificial nail should be gently rolled between the thumbs to soften it and allow a curve to be easily created (1).

TOP TIP

If the form does not fit neatly under the free edge it may be due to the shape of the hyponychium or perhaps the nail dips down into the side wall. A small pair of curved scissors can be used to cut away part of the form that goes under the nail so a better fit is created. Take the time to do this otherwise product will leak through the gaps and create a lump that can trap debris.

2 The form should be held in both hands and fitted under the free edge. When it is under the free edge, look down the barrel of the nail to make sure the form fits securely without any gaps (2).

3 Gently attach it to the sides of the finger and check the form from all angles to make sure it fits the nail correctly. Then attach securely to the finger (3).

4 Look down the barrel of the nail to make sure that a 'C' curve has been created that is the same as the natural nail and that the curve of the form is straight (4). If there is any twisting of this curve on the form, a twisted nail will be created. The shape of the form usually allows this shape to be secured under the finger. If the natural nail is wide or particularly flat, this may not be possible, but it is important that the shape is not disturbed. If this happens, then use the part of the form that has been discarded (the hole where the finger goes) to hold this shape in place.

The nail is now ready to have a sculptured overlay applied.

Step-by-step: Sculpted overlay

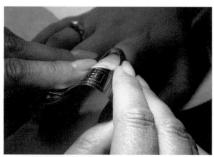

(1) Prepare the nail ready for an overlay. Take a form, bend it to create a curve and fit it under the free edge of the nail.

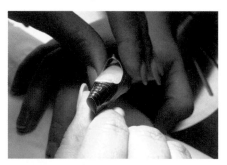

(2) Look down the nail and create a 'C' curve that suits the nail and is in line with the finger.

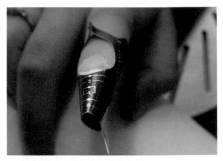

(3) When the perfect shape has been achieved and the form is tucked under the free edge and with a good fit at the side walls secure it by pinching together under the form and sticking it firmly to the sides and top of the finger.

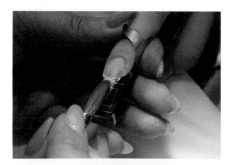

(4) Pick up a bead of white powder (the size will depend on the length of the nail to be sculpted). Place it on the form close to the edge of the nail. Gently press some of the bead out to one side wall and push up into a 'dog ear'. Press the other side of the bead out to the other side wall in the same way. Angle the overlay to create an apex and thin extreme edge of the nail. Look down the barrel to make sure it is even and with a good curve. Clean up the smile line with your brush.

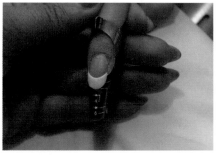

(5) The finished Zone 1 application should have good side walls, a good shape and a sharp smile line.

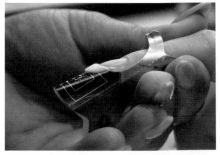

(6) Check the side view. There should be an apex for strength. A thin extreme edge and a strong and even 'C' curve. It is important to get this zone perfect as the other zones will follow its shape to create a perfect nail.

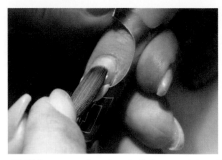

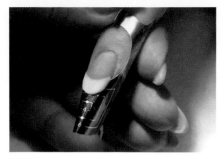

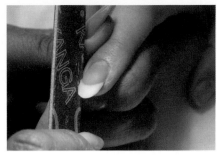

(7) Pick up a medium bead of clear or pink and apply to Zone 2. Press the bead to each side wall and blend with Zone 1. Apply to Zone 3 with a small bead, pressing it into the nail plate while creating an even edge.

(8) The overlay at this stage should look as close to the finished nail as possible.

(9) Remove the form and refine the nail with a 240 grit file. Look from all angles to make sure the structure of the nail has an apex and an even and smooth upper arch. The 'C' curve should have its apex and be even. Shape the free edge and refine to a thin overlay at the extreme edge.

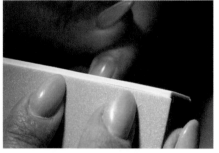

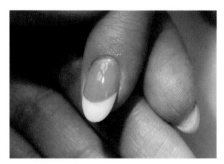

(10) Using a three-sided buffer or a glosser, buff the nail to a high shine then apply nail oil.

(11) Finished nail.

The application of a sculptured overlay is almost identical to that of an application over a tip. The main differences to remember are:

- With a liquid and powder system, the bead cannot be too wet as it will run down the form and be difficult to contain in the free edge shape until it starts to cure.

- While applying Zone 1, check the lower arch that is being created on the form and try to keep it as close to the finished shape as possible in order to avoid lots of reshaping when the form is removed.

- Make sure the side walls, particularly in the stress area, are sufficiently strong but without being thick.

- Check the 'C' curve and upper arch all the time.

- If the 'C' curve is too flat, it is possible to gently squeeze the form at the free edge before curing to increase the curve slightly.

- When using a UV gel system, the underside of the nail should be cured when the form has been removed. White tip gel is quite dense and the underside may not be completely cured unless replaced under the lamp or a clear form has been used.

A badly-shaped sculpted nail can often be put right with a file when the form has been removed but, with plenty of practice, a perfect shape must be strived for as the reshaping process is very time-consuming.

Many technicians believe this method is the quickest of all and those practiced and experienced in the technique may be right.

When the form has been removed, the artificial nail is finished in the usual way.

The maintenance of sculptured nails is the same as for those with tips.

Remedial sculpting

By using a form, a broken nail can be repaired, whether it be a natural nail or an artificial nail. Forms can also be used to lengthen a natural nail that has a good free edge but is a bit shorter than the other nails.

All the rules for application must be followed as usual.

The aftercare advice and retail recommendations for sculptured nails are the same as those for Chapter 9.

Summary

This chapter has demonstrated how to provide a sculpted nail, from fitting the form to the various techniques for applying each system.

ASSESSMENT OF KNOWLEDGE AND UNDERSTANDING

1 What is the difference between a 'free form' sculptured nail and a tip with overlay?

2 Why do many forms have a metallic finish?

3 Why is zoning especially important in a sculptured nail?

4 When applying a form, what are the two curves that must be followed?

5 Does the application of artificial nail products differ in any way from their application with a plastic tip?

6 Why should the 'C' curve be continually checked?

7 What extra step should be taken when sculpting UV gel and why?

8 When is remedial sculpting appropriate?

11
Maintaining artificial nails

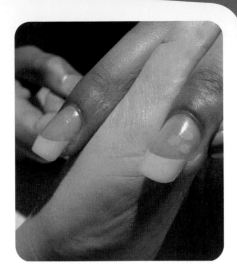

Introduction

Every client is a 'full-set' client once; after that, they become a maintenance client or a natural nail client. Skilful maintenance is as important as skilful application and will keep clients returning on a regular basis. This chapter explores in depth the value and techniques of a regular maintenance programme and examines the most common diseases and disorders the technician may have to deal with.

Value of maintenance

During training, maintenance is one of the most useful learning aids and it must never be dismissed or skipped over. Many hours can be spent on learning application skills, but every client is different and every set of circumstances is different. A trainee technician will learn nothing if they do not see the results of their application a few weeks later. The preparation of the nail may have been incomplete; the client may have a nail plate that is more oily than expected; the ratio of the product may have been wrong; the shape that looked good 2 weeks ago may now look horrible.

It is a fact that we often learn more from a mistake or something that goes wrong than from anything else. It is not enough for a trainer to explain what 'may' happen. It is essential that the beginner can see what has happened and try to work out why. If this is done with the help of a trainer then, when the technician is on their own with a client who has a problem, they will be able to work out why and will know how to put it right.

Like hair, nails are continually growing and what was put onto a nail near to the nail fold will be in a different place in 2 weeks' time. This is obvious if coloured nail varnish is worn for some time. There will be a gap at the base of the nail and that small area of exposed nail plate will probably have cuticle attached to it. Just as in hairdressing, when hair has been coloured or permed, the 'regrowth' is very obvious.

Need for regular maintenance

The appearance of an outgrown artificial nail is one consideration, but there are two more important reasons for regular maintenance treatments:

1 The technician will have explained to the client that they must watch out for any changes to the nail, and return immediately if anything is noticed. However, it is possible that there may be very slight changes that the client has not noticed, especially if coloured varnish has been worn. There may be some **lifting** of the overlay that is not very obvious. There may be a slight reaction to the products. There may be some minor nail separation owing to thin or dehydrated nail plates that was not evident before. It is important that the technician keeps a close watch on the health of the nails and skin as they should be aware of things to look for that may not be so obvious to the untrained eye.

2 After a period of natural nail growth, the structure that was created during application with the two curves (upper arch and 'C' curve) meeting at the apex or stress point of the nail to create the strongest nail possible will have moved.

Thickest

a

Thickest

b

Nail growth (a) Position of overlay at application stage (b) Position of overlay at 2 weeks' growth

The apex will have moved further away from the nail bed and could be on the free edge. This will unbalance the nail and make it susceptible to breakages. The smile line that was created either by the tip application or by a white tip overlay will also have moved and there will be a band of natural nail growth that will be a different colour to the tip.

Maintenance treatments

It is not recommended, under any circumstances, to maintain a set of nails that has not been applied either by yourself or the salon where you work. No technician can be sure of the procedures followed by another technician and the preparation may not have been as thorough as it should have been. There may be a problem that the nail is hiding. The products used previously may not be compatible with the ones you use.

If a there is an infection of some kind already under the overlay that is not yet obvious, when it does become apparent you may be blamed. Either suggest the client returns to their original technician for maintenance or, preferably, explain why you cannot provide a maintenance treatment and suggest that the nails are removed and a new set applied by you. Then you can be sure of the health of the natural nail and have confidence in the products used.

Infill or rebalance?

There are two types of maintenance treatments. One, called an '**infill**', is a short treatment that allows the technician to check for any problems and fill in the small area of growth to make the artificial nail look smooth without a ridge at the base (1). The other is called a '**rebalance**', as it removes the apex that has moved to the wrong place and replaces it in the right place, it fills the regrowth area at the base (2) and, if required, will put the smile line back to where it should be and cover the band of natural nail growth (3).

The decision as to which treatment is needed should depend on the rate of nail growth. If growth is slow to average, it is likely that an 'infill' will be required 2 weeks after the first application and a 'rebalance' 2 weeks after that. These treatments can then be alternated. If nail growth is average to fast, then a full rebalance may be needed every 2 to 3 weeks. Every client is different, but the general rule is 2 weeks between treatments. This must be shorter for a nail biter, who must be seen at one-week intervals for several weeks. Some clients may settle down to a treatment every 3 to 4 weeks if they have slow nail growth and are used to having long nails.

Assessment of client's nails

Before the maintenance treatment can start, the technician must look very carefully at the client's nails, especially on the first maintenance visit after application of a first full set. This is especially true for trainees and beginners and much will be learned from spending some time at this stage.

The aim for every technician is to see a set of nails return looking perfect except for the small growth area at the base and at the smile line. Experienced technicians will achieve this with the vast majority of new clients and all existing clients. Beginners will experience all kinds of problems that will need solving during their first year, but must never accept that this is part of wearing artificial nails. The saying of 'no pain, no gain' is most definitely not true in this case and, with skill and understanding, nearly every client should be able to wear beautiful and natural-looking nails without ever encountering a problem.

The incidence of an allergic reaction is probably the most worrying, but the chance of this happening to even the most sensitive client can be minimized, if not totally avoided, by good working practices.

Procedure to follow

As trainees can learn a great deal at maintenance treatments, it is a good idea to follow a set procedure. The differences between the systems at this stage are minimal.

What did the client want to achieve? When providing a maintenance treatment, always remember what the client wanted to achieve at the beginning. Did they want to grow their own nails as soon as possible or were they happy to have artificial nails for the long term? Did they want to grow the tips off and have natural nails with an overlay? European women, generally speaking, tend to prefer natural nails or, at least, artificial nails that look natural. They also tend to like to keep the option of reverting to natural nails open. In America, and occasionally in Europe, it is more acceptable to have artificial nails that look artificial. This is a very wide generalization, but many more women in America have their nails done. Products have improved from the harsh dental acrylics that were originally

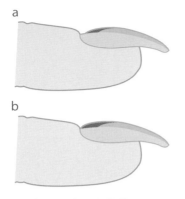

(1) Infill procedure (a) Buff overlay near cuticle (b) Replace overlay in shaded area

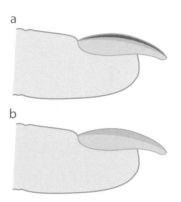

(2) Rebalance procedure (a) Remove most of overlay (b) Replace with complete overlay

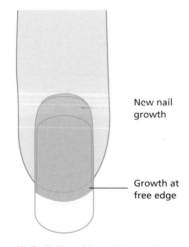

New nail growth

Growth at free edge

(3) Smile line at 2 weeks' growth

used and technical skills are improving as awareness of the industry grows. Now there is no excuse not to keep the natural nail perfectly healthy and in at least the same condition as when artificial nails were first applied.

Is the client happy? There should be discussion with the client as to how they are getting on and if they are happy with their nails. It may be that the original plan needs changing to achieve another goal. It is not unknown for a client to admit that they cannot cope with artificial nails or cannot afford long-term maintenance. If this is the case, the nails should be removed and a course of manicures suggested. The client should always feel that the choice is theirs and the technician's main aim is to provide them with what they want to take care of their natural nails, whatever the treatment may be. Many clients like the idea that their natural nails are growing healthily and protected under the artificial covering and, when the natural nail has grown to a good length, the artificial nail can be removed. This should be true for many clients if their natural nails are capable of growing in a reasonable shape. If this is the aim, the length of the nail should always stay the same as the first application, with infills and re-balances carried out. When the natural nail reaches the desired length, it is just a natural nail with an overlay (the tip has grown out). The overlay can be infilled, but thinned on successive visits until the overlay is as thin as possible or not needed at all.

Step-by-step approach At the start of each maintenance treatment, four steps should be followed, then nothing of importance will be missed out.

1 *Observation*: Look carefully at all the nails. A perfect, trouble-free set should look tidy. The only difference from when they were first applied should be the natural nail growth at the cuticle, leaving a gap, and at the free edge an obvious growth of natural nail. If there is anything more than this, there is a problem that needs solving and correcting and what is noticed should be noted on the client's record card. The shape of the artificial nail may not look as attractive as it did originally. It may look slightly bulbous at the sides or on the end. This will be due to the fact that the overlay was not applied in the best shape and was, perhaps over-thick at the side walls.

2 *Questioning*: The client must be asked how they have managed with the nails. If there are any broken, ask how it happened. If it happened easily then the structure may not have been strong enough. If it happened during a minor incident and was painful, the structure was strong enough, but maybe the nail was too long. If it happened during a minor accident, then any nails would probably have broken.

3 *Diagnosing*: If the nails are less than perfect, the technician needs to decide what the possible causes of the problem may be and discuss this with the client. The probable causes of the problem should be explained.

4 *Treatment*: Having followed the above steps, the most appropriate treatment can be decided upon and suggested to the client. If the nails are perfect, maintenance will be minimal. If, however, some are lost, broken or lifting, they will need to be replaced in such a way that the problem will not re-occur.

Putting right the problem

It is essential that the reason why the problem occurred is understood, and how to put it right. As a guide, some common problems have been listed, with their possible causes and treatment. It is impossible to list every problem as every client is different but understanding of the system, its basic chemistry and the anatomy and physiology of the nail should provide the technician with the tools to reach a logical conclusion. The solution to these problems is often termed '**contra-actions**' as they are actions taken in response to a condition or situation.

Broken nails (if some product is left on the remaining nail plate)

Reason	Solution
1 Too long	Shorten all nails
2 Weak	Rebuild stress area

Missing nails (nothing is left on nail plate)

Reason	Solution
1 Oil or moisture on nail plate (no damage to the nail plate)	Careful preparation
2 Client picking nails (damage to the nail plate will be obvious)	Discussion

Lifting in Zone 3

Reason	Solution
1 Cuticle on nail	Careful preparation
2 Oil on nail	Careful preparation, dehydrate twice or second coat of primer (if appropriate)
3 Overlay too thin	Add slightly more
4 Overlay too thick	Refine overlay in Zone 3
5 Overlay touching skin	Take more care in application

Chipping at cuticle

Reason	Solution
1 Overlay too thick	Apply smaller beads
2 Overlay too brittle	Use wetter ratio in liquid and powder system
	Use less activator for fibre
3 Client picking	Discussion

Chipping at free edge

Reason	Solution
1 Overlay too brittle	Use wetter ratio or less activator
2 Overlay too thin	Apply more, but taper

Discoloration of overlay

Reason	Solution
1 Contamination	Use fresh product and clean tools
2 Affected by UV light	Cover with UV-resistant sealer
3 Coloured varnish	Use base coat under varnish

Discoloration under overlay on nail plate: yellow–green	
Reason	*Solution*
1 Bacterial infection	If very superficial (that is very pale colour and small area), remove overlay, dehydrate, prime and re-apply; see client 1 week later. If more serious, remove overlay and refer to GP/pharmacist

Discoloration under nail plate: yellow, green, white

Reason	*Solution*
1 Possible infection	Remove artificial nail and refer to GP

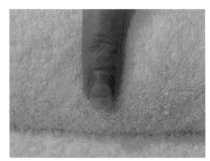

Missing nail – client damage

Sometimes, when a client returns, it is obvious that the aftercare advice she was given has not been followed, even if she says it has. It is usually obvious when a client has been picking off the overlay as some of the nail plate will have gone with it. If the overlay has gone and the nail plate is perfectly clean then there has been a problem with the preparation.

The following scenario is an example of many of these signs:

1   The recommended time for a maintenance treatment has been ignored. The new nail growth can be seen to halfway up the nail.

2   The remaining overlay has been picked off and the damage to the nail plate can be seen.

3   The length has been lost. This may be due to the artificial nail being out of balance and braking off or it may be due to more picking!

Some more examples of problems experienced at maintenance treatments and their probable cause:

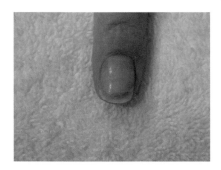

Chipping at the free edge and overdue for infill

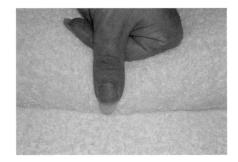

Nail needing a re-balance (notice growth in Zone 3 and nail growth at free edge, minimal lifting)

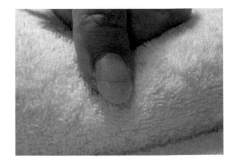

Slight lifting in Zone 3 (solution=prep)

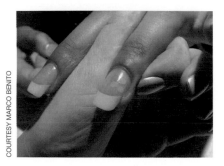

COURTESY MARCO BENITO

Localized lifting caused by thinned nail plate (probably from drilling), and tip too narrow

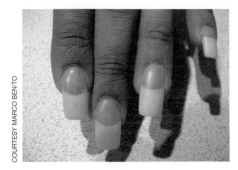

COURTESY MARCO BENITO

Overlay touched skin on fore and ring finger, lifting on middle finger (prep), cracking on fore-finger (no structure to overlay), all nails too long

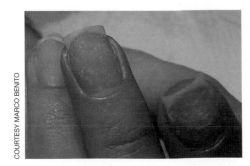

COURTESY MARCO BENITO

This nail plate has had an artificial overlay that has been picked off. Damage to the top layer can be seen and this is typical of this type of client damage

Discoloration under nail plate at free edge: white

- This indicates nail separation and may be due to a number of different reasons. The correct treatment would be to remove all products and, if the condition were very minor wait and see if it improves. However, with experience, it may be possible to decide whether it has occurred owing to a very thin nail plate that may have been caused by over-buffing previously (either by a bad technician or the client). A thinned nail can break the seal at the hyponychium and this can allow bacteria to enter under the nail plate. If the nail is kept clean and without product, the nail plate should re-attach itself in time and then artificial nails may be re-applied. A pharmacist should be able to suggest what will keep the area under the nail clean.

- A white area under the nail plate could also indicate nail separation that has allowed in bacteria or fungus. This must always be referred to a GP and the products removed.

- A further possibility could be a reaction to the products, either as an allergy or too much dehydration or as a result of a badly fitting tip putting too much stress on the nail plate. In all cases the products must be removed.

Skin reaction If there is any irritation of the skin, such as itching, swelling, redness or a rash anywhere on the body – but especially on the hands, fingers or face – the products must be removed immediately.

If this is done as soon as any slight reaction is noticed, the condition will stop. (It is very rare, but possible, that a severe reaction occurs suddenly without a warning.) The reaction will stop as soon as the irritant is removed. If acted upon quickly, the irritation will be mild and clear up quickly. If it does not stop within 24 hours or gets worse or if the reaction is more severe, then the client should visit a GP as soon as possible. This is an allergic reaction to one or more of the products or their ingredients. (If the reaction does not stop after all products have been removed, it is possible that it occurred as a result of another allergen that has nothing to do with the nails.) If the client wants to wear artificial nails after this (and many do) it is possible to slowly re-introduce some products by way of a patch test or a test nail to see which product or products must be avoided.

If a technician does not act responsibly and follow these guidelines, the condition may become serious and could result in permanent damage to the client's skin or nails. This could result in litigation, where the technician is held responsible if the correct advice was not given and the correct procedure was not followed. Public and product liability insurance will not cover a technician who has not acted in a professional manner and followed accepted industry guidelines.

The maintenance treatment

Once any problems have been addressed and notes made on the record card, the maintenance treatment can begin. The equipment required is exactly the same as for the first application. Any artificial nails that are missing will need to have a tip replaced in the same way as previously described.

Procedure for infills Deal with one hand at a time for liquid and powder or a fibre system and two hands for a UV-cured system.

1 Have the desk prepared and all tools, equipment and products ready plus the record card completed with notes from the consultation at the start of the appointment (1).

2 Sanitize hands.

3   Sanitize and dehydrate nails with appropriate product on a nail wipe or cotton wool by wiping the whole nail from the tip towards the nail fold.

4   With cuticle tool, remove any cuticle that is on the newly grown nail.

5   Using a 240 grit file, gently blend the edge of the overlay in Zone 3 (2). This will also remove the shine. If there is any lifting of the overlay in this area it will need to be buffed away, carefully and without over-buffing the nail plate. This can sometimes be time-consuming as more overlay can lift as it is being thinned out. There is no real safe short cut to this process. Many technicians use some short cuts such as nipping with cuticle nippers (this can lift away overlay that is bonded to the nail and take some nail plate with it) or getting adhesive to run under lifting area (this could trap any bacteria that may be present) or using a solvent in the expectation that it will deal with any bacteria or fungus (the solvent can get trapped and the area will still be unattached).

6   The shine should be removed from the whole nail surface (3).

7   Remove the dust with the dehydrator, taking care to clean around the side walls and nail fold, and apply primer if required (4).

8   Apply a thin layer of the product (liquid and powder, UV gel or resin) in Zone 3 as in the original application and blend it to the rest of the nail (5).

9   With a 240 grit file, shape the overlay as in the first application, checking from all angles that the structure of curves is right.

10   Refine surface with white block (6).

11   Finish with a three-way buffer or high-gloss sealant (after removing all traces of dust) (7).

12   Apply oil.

Step-by-step: powder and liquid infill

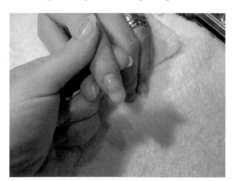

(1) Assess the nails

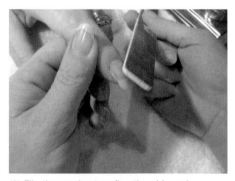

(2) File the overlay to refine the old overlay and remove any lifting

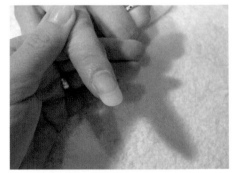

(3) Prepared nail after filing

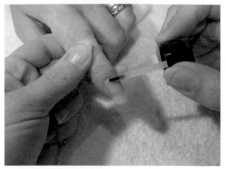

(4) Apply primer to exposed nail plate

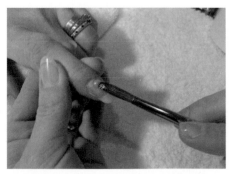

(5) Apply bead to Zone 3 and shape, blending into nail

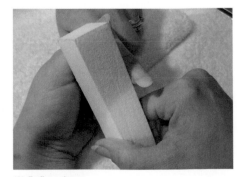

(6) Refine shape

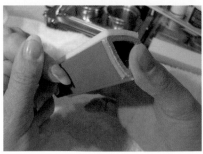

(7) Buff nail and apply oil

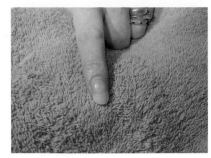

(8) Finished nail

Procedure for a re-balance

1 Follow steps 1–4 as above (1).

2 Shorten the length of the nail to the length and shape that was originally agreed.

3 Thin out the whole overlay, removing the apex so that the remaining overlay is a thin and even coating (2). Ensure that the tip of the free edge is very thin as, by shortening the length, the free edge will be thicker than the original tip and this will need thinning. (As the overlay is old, a harsher abrasive may be used to speed up the process, but care must be taken that the exposed natural nail is not buffed and the overlay is not buffed down to the nail plate by mistake.)

4 Clean nails with the dehydrator to remove all the dust and prepare the exposed nail. Prime if required (3).

5 Apply a new overlay in exactly the same way as the original overlay was applied (4) and (5). (If it is a fibre system and the original fibre has not been disturbed, it is not necessary to apply the fibre to the whole nail as it will get too thick as time goes on. A small piece of fibre placed in Zone 3 will be sufficient.)

6 Shape, refine and bring to a high shine as usual (6)–(8).

Step-by-step: Powder and liquid re-balance

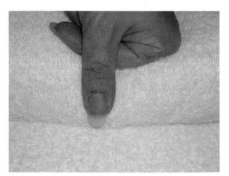

(1) Assess the nails

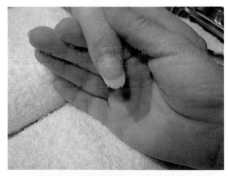

(2) Prepared nail with overlay removed to thin layer

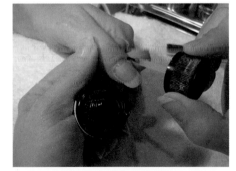

(3) Apply primer to exposed nail plate

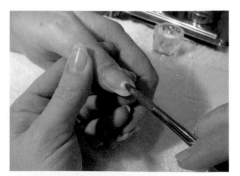

(4) Apply bead to Zone 1 and shape checking 'C' curve

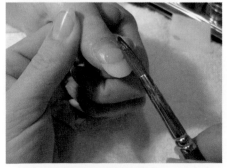

(5) Apply bead to Zone 2 and shape Zones 2 and 3 checking structure

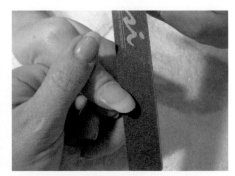

(6) Shape and refine the shape and surface

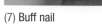

(7) Buff nail

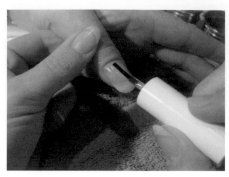

(8) Apply oil

Step-by-step: UV gel infill

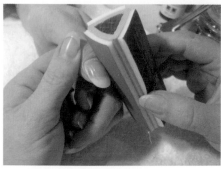

(1) Assess the nails

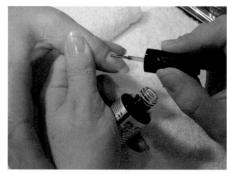

(2) Prepare nails and prime if required

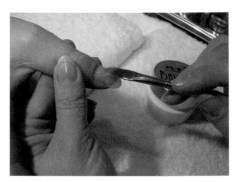

(3) Apply layer of gel

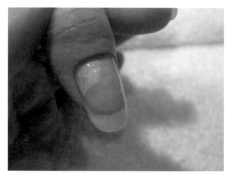

(4) Cure

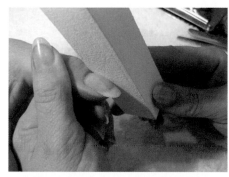

(5) Refine surface

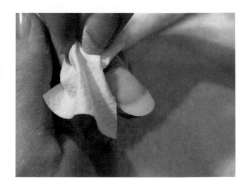

(6) Remove all dust

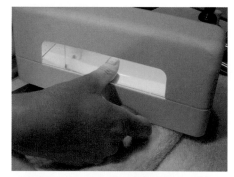

(7) Apply thin layer of sealant/gloss and cure

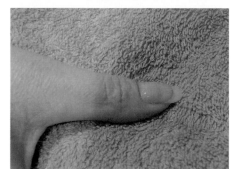

(8) Finished nail

Step-by-step: Fibre infill

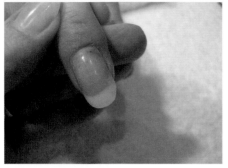

(1) Assess the nails

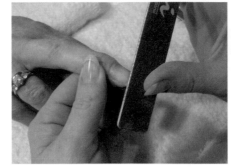

(2) File overlay

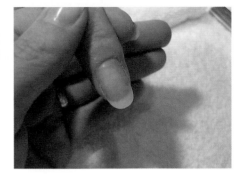

(3) Prepared nail

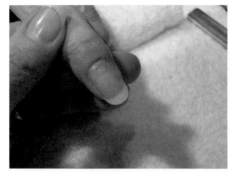

(4) Apply and smooth resin in Zone 3

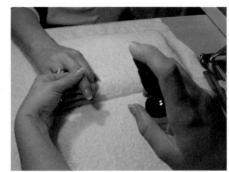

(5) Activate

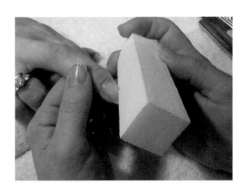

(6) Refine surface

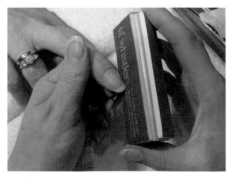

(7) Buff nail and apply oil

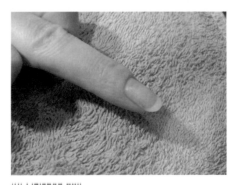

(8) Finished nail

Self-assessment skills

Opportunities to learn

It is at the maintenance stage that the trainee technician can learn a great deal. Obviously teaching and coaching by a good trainer are essential, but the beginner can continue to improve every time a client is seen without the trainer present. This can be done by self-assessment. A dedicated technician will carefully assess their work as there is always room for improvement, but this will probably be done in an informal and basically unstructured way.

Many professional and dedicated technicians enter competitions to help them improve their standards. A good person to assess 'nails' is an experienced technician who will study them from an objective viewpoint. At the end of any competition the judges are available for a 'critique' and the best technicians will take this opportunity happily. They do not go to 'argue about the score' but they go to find an objective opinion about their nails. They may agree or they may disagree, but there is a good chance that an experienced and objective judge may see something that the technician has missed, usually because the technician is looking too hard!

Good technicians will also go to the many workshops and seminars held by various companies and trainers. They may learn something new that will improve their skills, or an assessment on their performance may be available that will prove to be useful.

Beginners need to develop many skills and they also need to cultivate an 'eye' for balance and symmetry.

A beginner should never miss an opportunity to improve their skills and should see every client as an ideal opportunity.

A self-assessment programme

The following is a suggestion of how a trainee or beginner (or even an experienced technician dedicated to improvement) can carry out an effective self-assessment. The self-assessment should be used in conjunction with a record card, and it assumes that the first application is as good as the technician is able to achieve at the time.

First maintenance

- Describe each section of each nail (*Observation*):
    a. shape on looking down onto nail
    b. shape from sides
    c. shape of barrel
    d. smile line
    e. clarity of overlay
    f. Zone 3
    g. general.
- Client's responses (*Questioning*):
    a. How did the nails break? (If appropriate!)
    b. How have you managed with them?
    c. Have you followed all homecare advice?
    d. If not, what has been missed?
    e. Do you like the length and shape?
    f. Have they caused any problem?
- Correction of any present problems (*Diagnosis and treatment*):
    a. shape
    b. breakages
    c. clarity of product
    d. lifting
    e. chipping
    f. allergic reaction or infections.

● Finished nails (*this section does not need recording, just careful observation*):

a. free edge shape – each nail and in comparison with each other

b. upper arch – each nail and in comparison with each other

c. lower arch – each nail and in comparison with each other

d. 'C' curve – each nail and in comparison with each other

e. smile line – each nail and in comparison with each other

f. clarity – each nail and in comparison with each other

g. free margin – each nail.

Second maintenance As with the record of first maintenance, look at and ask all the same points. Compare results and determine if problems have been solved and results improved. If this is not the case, make a note of what is not right as before and complete a full self-assessment.

Nail diseases and disorders

There can be a great deal of confusion among technicians about the various nail diseases and disorders that may be seen on clients' fingers. Educators and information from various companies has been at best confusing, and at worst, contradictory. Even one of the most popular textbooks on the subject of nail technology contradicts itself in different chapters! How can technicians who want to do the right thing know what is the right thing to do?

There is one common and one not so common condition that technicians are likely to see during their career and available information can be confusing.

Green nails

This condition is likely to be seen by most technicians at some point but, hopefully, not too often. It is usually seen during maintenance visits or may come with a new client who has been going to another technician.

What type of 'green nails'? At this stage it is important to describe exactly what type of 'green nails' we are dealing with. Is there a yellow/green stain on top of the nail plate but under an artificial overlay of any description? This stain is always associated with an area where the overlay has lifted from the nail plate, usually in the cuticle or side wall area and sometimes on the free edge of the natural nail plate. This type of green nail is not connected with any discoloration under the natural nail plate on the nail bed, nor is it connected with a green nail plate that has never had an artificial nail applied to it.

The differentiation between these various conditions is essential and is often where the confusion lies. An important aspect of the nail technician's knowledge and practice is to recognize skin and nail conditions, but never to diagnose them. Technicians are not medically trained and dermatologists would have difficulty diagnosing genuine medical conditions without carrying out tests.

Confusion with these conditions always seems to involve the words 'bacterial', 'fungal', **'mould'** and **'yeast'**. The next confusion is whether a technician should treat the condition, send the client to a doctor, apply nails, not apply nails, take nails off, leave everything alone to let it go away of its own accord.

This condition, as described, will always be associated with a lifting artificial nail overlay. (If the discoloration is trapped under the overlay, it will usually mean that the client, or technician, has re-attached the overlay by letting nail adhesive seep under.) A lifted overlay provides an ideal environment for a certain type of bacteria to find a home, settle down and multiply! The environment is warm and moist with the water that has seeped in. It also has very little oxygen and does not get disturbed. As the first little bacterium starts to multiply it has a yellow 'metabolic by-product', but as more and more bacteria are created, the yellow colour darkens to green and, if left alone, it will eventually appear black. The nail plate can start to become soft and the nail bed can become tender as the bacteria colony breaks the nail plate down and eventually destroys it.

A good technician will make sure that clients are seen at regular and appropriate intervals. New clients should be seen no more than 2 weeks apart until the technician and client know exactly what to expect from artificial nails. The best technicians will sometimes experience a little lifting on clients' nails, especially new clients. If re-booking and client education is carried out properly then any sign of trouble will be detected before it becomes a major problem.

Treating a bacterial infection

If a client returns for a maintenance visit and there is a patch of yellow under a corner of the overlay, that is the beginning of a bacterial infection. It should never be any more than a pale yellowy-green if the client has returned for the correct appointment or understands that any change in the appearance of the nails needs an immediate return visit. The experienced technician can treat this condition, as it is mild and not necessarily infectious.

The artificial nail must be removed. If the natural nail is hard, very gently buff with a few strokes of a fine grit file. This may remove the colour but do not buff any more if the colour remains (it is safest to discard the file).

If the nail feels soft where the stain is, do not replace the artificial nail for a few weeks. After gentle buffing, dehydrate the nail plate with an alcohol-based dehydrator. This will remove the bacteria and take away the environment it needs to survive. A new artificial nail can now be applied. The yellow colour will probably remain slightly and grow up with the nail plate as it is a stain. If the stain changes in shape or colour, the bacteria is still active and the process was not carried out effectively and must be repeated more thoroughly.

Some technicians recommend that the stain is removed using a mild bleaching agent. As these are water-based it is better to leave the stain to grow out, as soaking the nail plate in water and another chemical may cause a further problem with lifting and soft nail plates as the water is trapped under the overlay.

This treatment should not be carried out if the technician is not totally confident that the cause of the problem is as described. Nor should it be carried out if the infection has progressed further than a pale green colour or the nail plate is very soft. If this happens, the artificial nail should be removed in a tip remover and not replaced. If the condition continues to spread or does not start to improve in a few days, the client should go to their doctor.

Other types of bacterial, fungal or yeast infections are very rare on the fingernails. They are more common on the toenails, as the toes spend a lot of their life in the warm, moist condition of a shoe. It is possible to have these conditions on a fingernail and, depending on the type, they can affect the nail plate, the nail bed and the soft tissue surrounding the nail. A technician must never diagnose any of these conditions and the golden rule is: 'When in any doubt, don't'. Only a dermatologist who has carried out tests can accurately diagnose a genuine infection and such infections are very rare. They also take a long time to clear once diagnosis has been made.

White spots on the nails

The second condition that a technician may see and is likely to be confused about is a fungal infection that creates white spots on the nails. It is more common on the toenails, but it can affect the fingernails.

I am sure every technician has had a client with a couple of white spots on their nails who says, 'I know this is a lack of calcium'. I hope every technician has also answered that it is very unlikely that it is a lack of calcium. It is most likely that they are little patches caused by trauma to the nail plate or matrix. The whiteness is caused by the nail plate layers parting slightly or the keratinization process being interrupted. If a client suffers from a lack of an essential mineral like calcium or zinc there are likely to be other symptoms and the last of their worries would be spotty nails!

It is possible, however, to confuse this very common condition with a more serious (but rare) fungal infection. If the nail has white spots or areas that appear soft and chalky on the surface of the nail, it is possible that the client has a fungal infection called leuconychia mycotica, and this can be easily spread by buffing. This condition does not always appear on every nail and can run along a ridge rather than be a spot.

As for all conditions, the technician must not diagnose but should recommend, without scaring the client, that they should see a doctor. In the greater scheme of things, this infection is not serious, but it is contagious and can spread to other nails, the technician and other clients. It is also not very pleasant for the client who has gone to a technician to improve the appearance of their nails. They want nice nails, not white crumbly ones (or green ones), and it should be within the expertise of the technician to point them in the right direction to achieve their aim.

The removal of artificial nails

There are many occasions when it is appropriate to remove artificial nails, for example:

- the client wanted long nails for a short time only
- the natural nail has grown to a length the client is happy with
- the regular maintenance required is not possible for the client
- the client has had a set of nails applied by someone else
- there is a problem with the nails, e.g. allergic reaction, infection, etc.

Liquid and powder and fabric nails are removed in the same way:

- Remove any coloured varnish.
- Pour enough acetone into a small metal bowl (or one suitable for solvents) to just cover the nails.
- Place bowl in a larger bowl of warm (not hot) water.
- Make sure the client is seated comfortably, preferably at a desk (holding bowls of acetone on laps can result in accidents!).
- Ask the client to place their fingers in the acetone and cover the bowl and the client's hands with a towel to prevent vapours escaping.

HEALTH & SAFETY

Always dispose of the used acetone safely and always have the room well ventilated.

TOP TIP

Applying oil or a barrier cream to the skin around the nails will help prevent the extreme drying effect of the acetone. This effect is very temporary and moisture will be replaced immediately but the skin does look unpleasant following the removal.

HEALTH & SAFETY

Always follow the manufacturer's instructions.

- Liquid and powder nails will take approximately 30 minutes to come off (see Chapter 7 for an explanation of the process). This time may be longer due to the thickness of the overlay and temperature. Artificial nails that have MMA as the monomer will take a lot longer.

- The resin used in the fabric system will take only 10–15 minutes.

- Do not remove the nails before the process is complete, as the product will harden immediately and then take longer.

- When all the product has gone from the nail, remove the fingers and dry them.

- Apply nail oil to the nails and fingers as they will look very white and dry.

- Buff the nails to give them a shine.

- If artificial nails have been worn for a long time, the natural nail may feel a little weak. Two or three layers of a strengthening top coat (not hardener) will help protect them until they become stronger, which will take a couple of days.

UV gel nails are removed as follows:

- Many UV gels are not affected by acetone, so the only way to remove them is by buffing the nails off.

- Great care must be taken when doing this, as it is very easy to buff the nail plate without realizing.

- Remove any colour first.

- Using a course grit file, but taking great care when near the skin or new nail growth, remove some of the overlay.

- Before the overlay gets thin, use a fine grit file.

- When the overlay is thin, keep wiping the nail with varnish remover. This will show up overlay as shinier than natural nail and thus prevent buffing the nail.

- When the overlay and tip have gone, buff the nail for a shine and apply oil.

- The natural nail may need some protection from a strengthener.

If the gel used is a type that can be removed with acetone, the procedure for liquid and powder can be followed after breaking up the surface of the gel with a coarse grit file.

There are a number of electronic devices available to aid removal. Some use a very gentle heat to keep the temperature of the acetone warm to speed up the process; others use ultrasonics to keep the acetone agitated. Only use equipment that is designed for this purpose. Do not use heaters that are meant for any other purpose as they may get too warm and cause the acetone to evaporate into the atmosphere quickly. Do not use ultrasonic equipment for cleaning jewellery, as the frequency may be dangerous for living tissue.

A general critique of problem nails with suggestions and recommendations

The following selection of pictures are of artificial nails that have been 'presented' to nail technicians at a (mostly long overdue) maintenance treatment. These are all relatively common problems and the comments may help learners to understand what has gone wrong and what to avoid during the original application! (With thanks to Aet Kase)

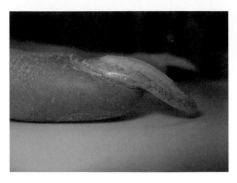

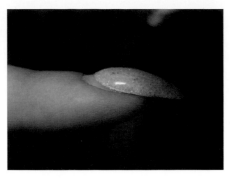

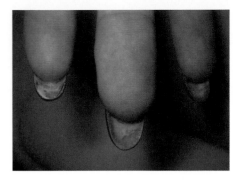

1. The original nail was applied with a lower arch that was far too downward sloping for the nail. This has been further encouraged by adding a high arched overlay. It may be that the natural nail had a distinct downward curve but this should have been corrected. There also appears to be some sensitivity to the products on the skin as it is very dry and flaky. It may be necessary to change products for this client.

2. It is difficult to tell if there is any lifting of this overlay as it is opaque but there is some cracking of the edge which would suggest lifting. The overlay is much too thick and arched. The client should be encouraged to return more often for maintenance as this is longer than 2 weeks and the nail is seriously out of balance!

3. This is a very common problem. The edges of the natural nails have curled away from the overlay and become stained and unsightly (and on one finger broken off). This can be avoided by making sure the overlay on a natural nail encases the edge to prevent this plus the client should be strongly encouraged to use nail oil daily including under the free edge as this will keep the nail flexible. If the client does not want to have the nails removed and a new set applied, it is possible to tidy up this area by using an e-file (see Chapters 3 and 15).

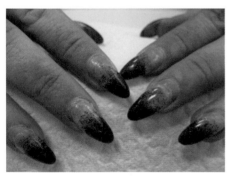

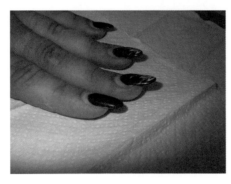

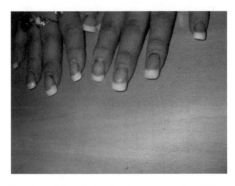

4. This picture shows a lot of problems with prep and application (plus a client who should have had an appointment sooner!) There is a great deal of lifting on most nails. The overlay in this area seems to be brittle and thin and broken away in some places. On the middle and ring fingers on the left of the picture there is lifting down the side which suggests that the overlay was touching the skin here and not pressed into the nail to create a good seal. This looks like an L&P that has the wrong ratio and is applied too thinly in Zone 3. it also looks like a client who never applies nail oil which is essential for L&P as it helps to keep it flexible.

5. Another long overdue appointment! This is a good example where the tip that has been applied (or the form for sculptured nails) was much too narrow. This can be seen clearly on the middle finger. Also there is no structure to the overlay. It is completely flat and had thick and rounded edges instead of thin and sharp edges.

6. This set of nails is showing some minor lifting around the edges where red polish has seeped in. The overlay is far too thick on all of them and an ugly downward curve can be seen especially on the forefingers. All of these problems could be improved by a good maintenance treatment. Most of the overlay needs removing to thin it out and the lower arch can be filed away.

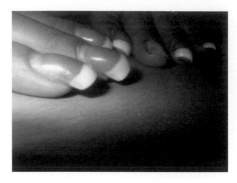

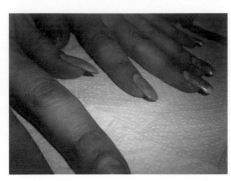

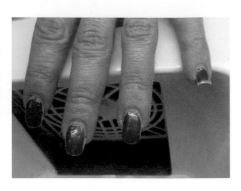

7. A shocking example of a thick and badly structured nail! Again, they needed maintenance at least 1 week before and were probably a bit too long for the client as can be seen by the missing nail. However, this could have been caused by the nails being seriously out of balance!

8. The main comment to make about these is that they are too flat. There is no structure in them at all except for one nail and that has its apex in entirely the wrong place!

9. A very poor application of coloured gels. The gel has shrunk away from the sides and base leaving the artificial nail uncovered.

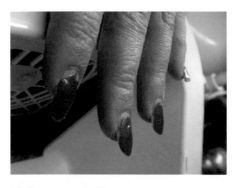

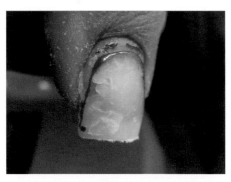

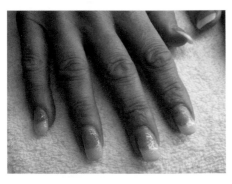

10. The same nails. They appear to be tips (that are lifting at the sides) with a thin overlay or perhaps just the coloured gel that has not provided any strength. A bizarre shape of the little finger can be seen which suggests this was a ski-jump nail that has not been corrected by the tip application.

11. This may be the same nail with the colour removed and what appears to be a fibre and resin overlay. The overlay is extremely brittle and has cracked away from the nail. This would suggest that too much activator was used and the overlay was too thin.

12. These nails appear to have a UV gel overlay that has a very lumpy application and uneven application with no shape refining. If the gel had been applied accurately to the edges then refined and smoothed before applying a top coat they would have looked a lot better.

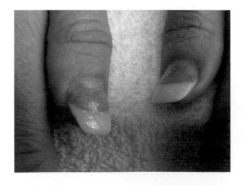

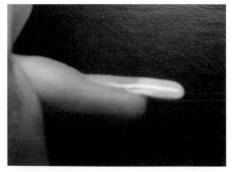

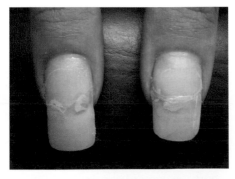

13. A perfect example of an uncorrected ski-jump nail. The tip was too narrow and it was applied following the upward tilt of the nail instead of at a downward angle to compensate for the nail growth. This started the problem but in addition there is no structure to the overlay to provide more correction to the angle.

14. Although out of focus, it can be seen that there is no structure at all to this nail. It is completely flat (probably a paint on UV gel) and very ugly. The tip has been applied flat instead of with a curve. Even a paint-on gel can be applied with structure by keeping more at the apex and then refining the shape.

15. These are quite bad stress fractures caused by the overlay having no strength at its weakest point and the nails being too long for the wearer.

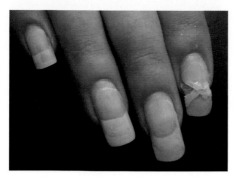

16. As before but lifting can also be seen on the side of the ring finger where the overlay has touched the skin.

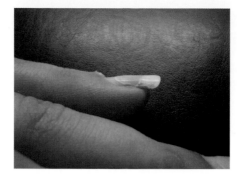

17. This nail, again, has no structure and a bulbous edge. The sides are breaking away and lifting as there was no bond created there with the thin overlay. There also seems to be a wart on the skin which is a contra-indication as warts are contagious.

Summary

This chapter has demonstrated the value of a regular maintenance programme for the health of a client's hands, and outlined how the technician should approach some of the more common diseases and disorders that may be encountered with a client. 'Maintenance' of the technician's expanding skill base is no less important, as the self-assessment exercises make very clear.

ASSESSMENT OF KNOWLEDGE AND UNDERSTANDING

1 How is the structure of the artificial nail affected after 2–3 weeks' growth?

2 What is the difference between an infill and a re-balance treatment?

3 Why is it important that clients return for regular maintenance treatments?

4 Name four reasons for the overlay to lift in Zone 3.

5 Why is effective communication important during maintenance treatments?

6 Why is homecare advice essential and what are the main points to be covered?

7 What would you do if discoloration was noticed under the overlay?

8 Under what circumstances would you remove artificial nails?

9 Why are maintenance treatments an excellent time for learning?

10 How would you remove:

   a. liquid and powder nails?

   b. fibre nails?

   c. UV gel nails?

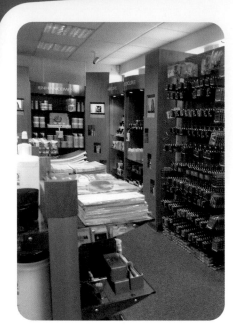

12
Business matters

Learning Objectives

In this chapter you will learn about:

- methods of contributing to an effective business

- how to deal with time management and appraisals

- some business promotion ideas

- how to investigate a business idea

- if you want to work as a freelance technician

- basic finances

- some basic business evaluation.

Introduction

Becoming a nail technician is not just about sitting at a desk 'doing nails'. It is a professional career and whether you are employed in a salon, working freelance or plan to open your own business, there is the massive area of commerce to consider.

As a professional, commercial effectiveness is an intrinsic part of your work and understanding the basic concepts of 'business' is essential. You may not be planning to open your chain of nail salons but if you want to be a successful and employed nail technician you need to play an important role in your place of work.

You may be familiar with the term 'entrepreneur' who is a person who sets up and grows a business. There is a newer term 'intrepreneur' which, in the spirit of an entrepreneur can work within an existing business to help strengthen and grow it. Starting a new business is not for everyone but being successful should be central to your career.

The nail industry is growing at a very fast rate. It is one of the service industries that has a very large percentage of 'micro-businesses', that is a business, often unregistered, with fewer than five employees. Probably one of the most popular career routes for nail technicians is to be self-employed and working within a salon on a rental arrangement or from a 'home salon' or as a mobile technician.

This route does seem to be popular with newly qualified technicians and can result in a successful business or lead onto bigger and better plans. But, whether it's a small, single person business or a salon with several employees, it is still a business that needs careful planning.

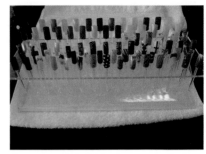

Great way to display nail art

Contributing to an effective business

As a member of staff, a true professional will not just do their required job and go home. They will want to be a part of the success of the business. This is not only a way to maximize an individual's income (as so many technicians are working on a salary plus commission basis) but will also promote and project that individual's importance within the company and increase the possibility of promotion. Taking on internal projects are useful additions to a CV.

Project

Scenario The owner of the salon in which you work has read about a new professional brand for manicures and pedicures. They are interested in looking into it to see if it is a good idea to introduce into their business. They already use an effective and popular brand but realize that it is important to provide the best up-to-date services for their clients. They do not have time to spend on finding out about the new brand and ask you to do it for them.

Methodology Create a project plan that will provide them with all the information they need to make a decision on the new brand. Make a list of the sections within the project and give yourself a timescale for the completion.

Examples of sections:

- All product information and marketing material.

- Product costs and opening order.

- Service costs (i.e. the cost of products used for each service).

- Cost of training staff to use the products.

- Comparison with the existing salon brand both in cost and effectiveness.

- Suggested changes to services offered by the salon.

- Retail opportunities with the new brand.

- Suggested stock levels that meet with the salon's existing procedures.

- Suggestions on how to phase in the new brand in the most cost-effective ways, e.g. a sale of the outgoing brand or a timescale of phasing out the old brand and phasing in the new brand.

- Suggestions of some promotional activity to introduce the brand to the clients.

Time management

If you are employed and part of a team or running your own small business, you know the saying: 'Time is money'. Efficient use of your time is of huge benefit to you whether it is your 'money' or your employers. You will be less tired and enjoy a satisfying working day if you have control over your time and use it efficiently.

Some days or periods of time there can be just too much to do or think about.

Prioritize. Make a list of tasks that need to be carried out then rearrange them with the most important or most urgent at the top.

If you come up against a problem that seems too difficult and you keep putting it off then:

- *Actively problem solve*. Just taking the first few steps towards solving the problem makes it seem like a much smaller problem! A few small steps will often lead to the complete solution.

- *Carry a notebook* with you all the time. When you think of something or there is something you need to remember, put it in your notebook as then you can always look back.

Most people lead such busy lives with work, learning, socializing and 'downtime'. Don't rely on your memory. Keep a *diary* and be disciplined at writing every event, appointment and target in your diary. Plan as far ahead as possible and remember to look ahead before you commit yourself to more appointments or tasks.

Those who are really good at managing their time always have their personal '*to do lists*'. Keep a weekly and daily list in your diary or notebook and tick off each task as you do them. Make sure at the end of each day/week that you have, at the very least, achieved the important tasks and transferred those remaining to the next list.

Appraisals

When working in a salon with your own list of appointments it is important that you work efficiently and effectively. It is also important that you increase business for both yourself and the salon.

Your line manager should be giving you regular appraisals with regard to your performance. These appraisal meetings should benefit both you and the business and should not be a one way discussion.

Take on the responsibility of your work performance and targets

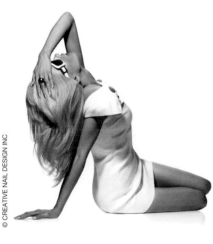

- Keep a record of all your appraisals.

- If you are given performance targets take them seriously and monitor your progress,

- Give yourself your own sales challenge e.g. aim to retail something to 75 per cent of clients on a specific day.

- Evaluate your skills and decide which areas you need more training.

- During an appraisal meeting suggest a training course that you could go on to improve your skills.

- Set yourself a target of re-booking 80 per cent of clients.

- Find ways of encouraging your clients to try a different service or 'up-selling' a treatment, e.g. from a basic manicure to a luxury manicure.

- Discuss ways of improving sales with colleagues.

When working in a salon environment there may be plenty of clients coming through but when they sit at your desk it is your responsibility to provide an excellent service and keep that client coming back!

Promoting the business

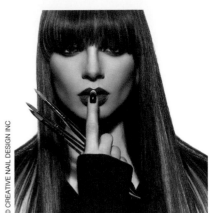

© CREATIVE NAIL DESIGN INC

Whether you are employed in a salon or nail bar, starting your own freelance business, introducing a new product or range or just wanting to give business a boost, there are many ways this can be done. As with most business activities, planning is essential.

Planning and carrying out a promotion is hard work and usually a lot of fun. However, lack of planning will make the whole exercise a waste of time. Thorough planning will guarantee a measure of success.

Whatever the scope of the activity, from the smallest (e.g. placing a small advert in a local paper) to a major event (e.g. taking part in a fashion show or having a big salon open day with demonstrations) the organized approach is the same.

The main objectives must always be to enhance the image of the business and/or to increase the turnover of the business. However, there are many elements within this that must be considered.

To be more specific, what do you want to achieve from your promotional activity?

- increase your client base?

- introduction of a new brand?

- introduction of a new service?

- increase your retail sales by:

  - trying something new?

  - supporting the salon treatments by homecare products?

  - buying seasonal products?

- establish and reward client loyalty?

- offset the competition?

A promotional activity is about effective communication so you must decide how you are going to do this depending on your specific objective. For example:

- advertising

- a sales promotion

- an event

- marketing.

Advertising and marketing

These two activities are closely connected and usually confused. Choosing the right one to match your objective is important. Advertising is a part of marketing and it is all about effective communication.

Marketing in this context is targeted and often free. It could be a press release to the local media (newspapers, radio) in the hope they will make you a news story in their beauty pages. Or it could be posters strategically placed for your target market (e.g. the local gym, playgroups, clothes shops, etc). It could just be a fabulous window display using marketing material from your product brand with some creative props that focus on your specific promotion.

Advertising, part of a marketing strategy, is often a paid for, impersonal communication about your products and services. This could be in the form of advertising in a local paper, a mail shot, local radio, etc. Within the media methods, advertising and marketing often go hand in hand so you will get a news story on the beauty or local services page if you place an advert.

The decision on which to choose will be based on your target market and your budget.

Sales promotions

A sales promotion can be a relatively easy activity if resources are limited and can have a whole variety of objectives depending on the type of promotion.

Examples of sales promotions:

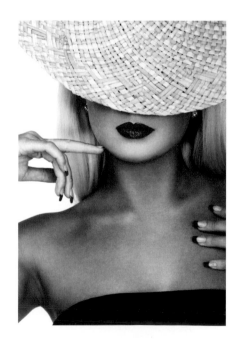

- sample giveaways (maybe your supplier would be willing to support this)
- buy a specific product and get an associated product at a reduced price
- book a certain number of treatments and get the last one free
- introduce a friend and get a reduced service or product
- loyalty card scheme.

Whatever type of sales promotion you decide upon you must also decide how you are going to communicate it. This is where some advertising and marketing can come in.

Events

As with any promotional activity, the type of event will be dependent on a lot of factors. For example: budget, target market, resources. But the scope is huge.

Examples:

- an open evening
- sponsoring a local social or business event
- attendance at a bridal fair
- a local fashion show
- a 'by invitation only' salon presentation
- a sponsored event for charity (e.g. sponsored walk etc.).

When you have decided on your main objectives and the type of promotional activity you want to do you need to look at it in more detail before you start the real work of organizing it.

Smart objectives

This is an accepted way of evaluating a chosen activity before time and money is spent on it.

The appropriate activity must be:

- Specific – decide exactly what the activity is to be and who the target is (e.g. new clients, a specific age range, etc). Be precise about what you want to achieve.

- Measurable – both in budget terms and the degree of success (i.e. the increase in business through new clients and/or increase in retail sales).

- Achievable – able to happen with the resources available. Don't attempt too much.

- Realistic – the type of activity and expected results are realistic. Do you have the resources to make the objective happen?

- Timed – have a timescale for the:

  - planning stage

  - the activity

  - the expected results.

Once you have reached this stage the research and organizing must start in earnest. There are lots of areas that must be taken into account.

Examples (in no particular order):

1 The budget for the activity.

2 Resource requirement.

3 Areas of responsibility for all those taking part.

4 The requirements and restrictions of the venue.

5 Contractual restrictions of the venue and possibly suppliers.

6 Local bye-laws that may affect the activity.

7 Health and safety issues before, during and after the activity.

8 The identification of any potential hazards and, if necessary, carry out risk assessments.

9 How the evaluation will be carried out.

ACTIVITY

Using all of the pointers given in this section and in collaboration with others if possible, plan a promotional activity.

- Create a folder with all the information and records of all ongoing analysis of the decisions made.

- Demonstrate the reasoning behind all main decisions.

- Include the budget and all costings.

- Show the research into every aspect of the activity.

- Draw up a timetable of planning deadlines and one for the event itself.

- Detail the roles and responsibilities of all those involved.

- Carry out the event and include a scrapbook of images and marketing material (where appropriate).

- Evaluate the activity for effectiveness.

- Measure its success in line with the main objective.

Working for yourself

There is a saying/proverb: 'He who fails to plan, plans to fail'. This is very accurate and a commercial approach is not always highlighted in the training provision in this sector of the industry. Some basic knowledge is a good starting point for those who are hoping to start their own business. This chapter is a starting point that will help to direct individuals to the right places that will help with their fledgling business ideas.

Fail to plan? Then plan to fail

However small your business idea is there are some basic plans that are needed to help you make a good start. It may be that you need to look at the possibility of a business loan from your bank. You certainly need to look at a business idea from a financial perspective. Then there are some activities that are essential to help make the business become a success and grow including how to market your business and let potential clients know you are there.

This chapter doesn't have all the answers as every individual set of circumstances will be different. What it will do is cover a variety of topics that need to be considered and suggest methods and places to look in order to find the appropriate answers.

There are a series of projects that are based on research specific to the individual. No one can know the answer to everything but knowing where to start looking is sometimes all that is needed. Legislation may change or may be very specific to geographical areas.

Investigating a business idea

So many nail services trainees will have dreams of, one day, owning a salon. Many will have very specific plans to finish training and start a freelance career. So, whether this is your first business idea, a career move away from an employed position or you think it is time for growth, this first important project is for you.

The project is quite large so has been broken down into smaller activities, all of which will come together into an extensive research document that will help you evaluate your idea at each stage. The finished project will be useful in a final business plan for the purposes of a business enterprise loan or similar. It will also open areas that require more specific and detailed research and planning once you have decided that your idea is potentially viable.

Describe your business idea

In a few paragraphs that are not too long, describe your idea.

- Explain the basic concept in general terms, e.g.:
  - a mobile nail service
  - a home salon
  - renting a space in an existing salon
  - opening a salon.
- Try to identify at least one unique selling point (USP), e.g.:
  - only one in the area
  - unique collection of services
  - personal skills or achievements (nail artist, award winner, etc.)
  - new nail service offered
  - new brand in area.
- Describe your target market, e.g.:
  - age groups
  - working people, full-time 'mums', groups.
- How you will operate, e.g.:
  - mobile with a car
  - new salon (business premises or home)
  - evenings/weekends for working people
  - party plan.
- Business name.

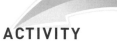

ACTIVITY

Create a project that looks at the market in which you want to start your business idea. It is essential that you understand the commercial market you hope to enter and become a part of.

If it is a small business you are planning, your immediate environs are the most relevant but it is also important that you have a basic idea of the market sector in general. For example, you don't want to enter a market that is on the decline in the public interest so you will need some general information on the growth of the industry.

Collect Information

As a guideline, these are some of the areas you could research and gather information from:

- Local competition in nail services:
    - salons in your immediate area and further afield
    - mobile services
    - home salons.
- Collect price lists for information on service menus and charges.
- Collate all the brands, both professional and retail that are available.
- Make a note of the 'USP's' of each of the competitors (if there are any!).
- Find some statistics on the growth of the professional market plus retail sales of nail products. (Detailed market research reports are available but are expensive to access. Use trade magazines, newspaper reports, etc. that can be found on the web. You are looking for general trends not an in-depth statistical report. Quotes could be useful but make sure to make a note of who the quote is attributed to and where you read it.)
- It could be a good exercise to critically evaluate your main competitors by looking at what you like about their service offering and what you don't like or believe you could do better.
- If you live in a small town or village, look at the population in comparison to the nail services on offer. Compare this to a nearby community and comment on how busy the salons appear to be.

Evaluation

When you believe you have collected sufficient information on the market that will directly affect your business write an evaluation of your findings. Include in this:

- What you believe to be a gap in the market.
- How you think you can fill it.
- How you can be as good as or better than local competition.
- How, in general terms, you can get this across in your marketing approach, e.g. how you can emphasize your USP's.

Conclusion

In a few sentences, sum up the findings of your research and suggest how your business idea could successfully fit your own specific market.

NB try to be objective! Just because you want your business idea to work doesn't mean it is the right idea. You need to make your conclusions as if you were convincing an outside person who knows nothing about the industry.

TOP TIP

Remember, clients are willing to travel to receive a fantastic service! It is usually a fantastic skill, not price, that is promoted by word of mouth. Make sure you are the best around! Ongoing learning is almost always the key to this plus keeping abreast of new products and techniques.

Working as a freelance technician

So, your business idea has been compared favourably to your local competition. Now is the time to start looking at the idea in a little more detail.

Your skill and knowledge are the two most important aspects to your business. At this stage the next most important aspect to look at for professional nail services are the products and brand you will be using. The industry has come a long way from the early days and now there are many excellent products available.

When starting and running a business, it is important to choose the right products for you and price should not be at the top of the list. You will have learned your nail skills using product brands and many newly qualified technicians go on to use these in their professional life. These brands may be the right ones for you but it is a mistake to just assume this without looking at the market.

There are ranges for natural nail treatments, foot treatments, enhanced nail brands and systems, nail art products and retail lines. It may be appropriate to have different brands for the different services but, specifically with the enhanced nail brands, it can be very important not to mix brands within the service areas. The choice is down to the individual technician but always bear in mind how the product lines within the different brands can work together. For example, nail preparation products pre enhancements may work during a manicure but manicure products will probably not work to prepare the nail for enhancements. Therefore additional products may be needed when the same will work for both.

TOP TIP

If you are planning to work as a mobile technician, the number and sizes of products are important! Too many make your kit far too heavy. Too few could result in a less than perfect service. For health and safety purposes, every container must be correctly labelled. You cannot decant products into a smaller container unless it has the full manufacturer's label on it. To economize in product costs, purchase the smallest size and the largest size. Then the small container can be kept topped up. NB remember to follow hygiene and product safety guidelines when decanting.

Some reasons for researching the market:

- Try different ranges as there may be one that you like more for a variety of reasons.

- The supplier may provide excellent support.

- Marketing materials and other resources (e.g. good product information) may be excellent.

- Opening orders as a new customer suit your budget.

- Reordering procedure suits your business methods.

- Your clients will expect you to be aware of the market.

- Clients may ask you how another range compares with yours.

- You may want to simplify ordering and a specific brand may have every range you need for your business.

- You may be able to take advantage of special offers that cross over ranges within the same brand.

- The supplier may offer free training.

- A specific polish range has the range of colours you require.

- You want good retailing opportunities.

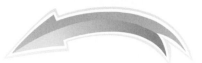

ACTIVITY

Product Research Project

Brief: research at least five different brands for each of the following services:

● manicure

● pedicure

● nail enhancements (preferred system or combination of systems)

● colour

● nail art (optional).

(If one brand has a range for several of the services it can count as one for each one it covers.)

Organize the collected information in the following sections:

● Brands with price lists and product information.

● Breakdown of each service costs for each brand, e.g. cuticle remover: £0.05 per service; mask: £0.12 per service; hand cream: £0.14 per service; base coat: £0.20 per service, etc.

● Choose one service , e.g. manicure, and create a product comparison chart with characteristics such as cost per service, your personal score for the range of products, feel and fragrance of skincare products and effectiveness, availability of product information, supplier support, marketing material, etc. NB it would be good practice to do this for each of your services but for the purposes of this project one of them will suffice.

● List the total cost for an opening order for each service for each brand. Where a brand is relevant for several services, list them together and show a total expenditure.

Evaluation: using all your collected and compared information, evaluate your findings logically. Point out the positive and negative characteristics for each brand. Include in here some information on your potential competition and the brands they are using.

Conclusion: based on your evaluation, write a few sentences with your decision on the best product range for your business idea with your reasons.

TOP TIP

Consider this: look at the busiest salon in your area; what brand do they use? Do you want to choose a different brand as a point of difference with a competitor? Or do you want to use the same brand as clients in the area are familiar with it and your marketing can then focus on your skills?

TOP TIP

In the year or so after you have started your business it would be a worthwhile exercise to look back on this project and re-evaluate your conclusions and decisions to see if your results have matched your expectations. If you have been disappointed, reading this through will help to avoid future mistakes. If a new brand, product line or new technique in the market looks interesting this will be a useful reminder of what you need to consider before deciding to take it on.

Your BUSINESS IDEA is now beginning to take shape. So far you have explained what your business idea is and have demonstrated that you are capable of investigation and researching important commercial decisions.

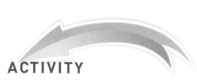

ACTIVITY

Choose the scenario that closely fits your BUSINESS IDEA. Using the appropriate list from those that follow, create a file of information. Start the file with a **Checklist** of each of the pieces of information you need and tick each one off when you have gathered the information.

You have the core of your business. Now you need to start building out from the core by adding more and more information until you are in a position to decide if your BUSINESS IDEA is a viable commercial proposition.

The 'logistics'

The basis of your BUSINESS IDEA will determine the size of this section.

We will look at three main scenarios and the type of information needed to progress with your IDEA.

The lists following are just guidelines. Depending on your type of business, geographical area and many other details you will need to include additional information specific to you. The notes provided do not give the answers but give a brief explanation of the requirement and suggested places to find the required information. Much of the information can be found on-line. If you use this resource, print the information and add it to your file. Not only will you need it when completing your business plan it will also be a very useful reference in the future.

Scenario 1: a freelance mobile nail technician

Your IDEA involves you offering your nail services to clients in their own homes or places of work. This scenario assumes you will be using your own form of transport as, unless your work radius is within walking distance or has easy public transport routes, the transportation of a professional kit can be problematical.

1 *PAYE, NI, VAT*

As a freelance technician you will be responsible for paying your own tax and NI as a self-employed person. Every working person needs to complete a yearly Self Assessment for Her Majesty's Revenue & Customs (HMRC) and a self-employed person must also complete the relevant section.

PAYE (Pay as you earn) is the method you use to pay the tax due on your income (Income Tax). It is very important that you let HMRC know that you are self-employed as soon as possible or there may be penalties to pay.

You must pay your National Insurance (NI) contributions. The Class payable varies with your income and there is an exemption if your income is very small.

VAT (value added tax) is a tax that must be paid on 'taxable supplies' (and nail services and retail items fall into this category) when your **turnover** has gone over the 'VAT threshold'. It is unlikely that you will need to register for VAT for quite some time but you do need to be aware of the threshold and the general process. Registering for VAT when turnover is under the threshold is voluntary. It should, however, be considered as VAT paid on equipment, products and petrol for example can be reclaimed. Your charges on services will also be subject to paying VAT to HMRC so the current VAT level will need to be deducted from your income.

Leaflets for all these topics are available at your local Tax Office and there is a vast amount of information available on the following websites:

www.hmrc.gov.uk

www.direct.gov.uk

It is absolutely essential that you keep careful records of all records associated with your business.

2 *Professional insurance*

When working on clients, even friends, it is essential that you have a professional indemnity insurance. At the very least you must have 'public and products liability' cover that will protect you from the (unlikely) risk of funding lawsuits and other claims arising from your services.

There are additional areas that are very seriously worth considering:

- Accidental damage. When working in a client's home accidents with product spillages, for example, can easily happen.

- Product/equipment insurance.

- Loss of earnings due to illness or incapacity.

- Also working in your own home.

Insurance is available to qualified technicians from all insurance companies. Some ready-made packages specifically designed for nail technicians are also available from several professional associations and insurance experts:

www.professionalbeauty.co.uk

www.beautyguild.com

www.babtac.com

www.salongold.co.uk

www.comparethemarket.com

3 *Car insurance and costs*

It is not enough to have a general insurance for your car. You must have business insurance for it otherwise you are not sufficiently covered when driving to and from appointments. Get this information from your current insurer.

If you are working as a mobile technician, your car and its associated costs play a big part in your overheads (see glossary). Not only does it impact on your service costs it will also play a part in your Tax Return as to how much you can claim as a genuine business expense.

This expense is an important overhead as it takes the place of the costs involved when working on your own premises.

4 *The Sale of Goods Act 1979 (as amended)*

You will be selling your nail services when you start your business and this is covered by this act for the protection of your clients. This will also apply to products you may sell. You have a responsibility in this area and must understand the important points of this legislation. A clear explanation of this Act and other relevant links is on:

www.businesslink.gov.uk

Other links are on this site that will help with understanding Trading Standards, Office of Fair Trading, Supply of Goods and Services.

5 *Health & Safety*

Issues concerned with health and safety are extensively covered elsewhere in this book. Print all relevant information from the sites recommended in that section and add to your file.

ACTIVITY

List all the costs of running a car (business insurance, road tax, MOT, services, petrol, wear and tear and depreciation). Break this down into how much a mobile service costs per hour of your working day.

ACTIVITY

Collect information on:

- Sale of Goods Act
- Distance Selling Act
- Trade Descriptions Act
- Consumer Protection legislation.

Create a file of this information. Take each piece of information you have collected and write a short explanation on the relevant points and how this legislation affects you in your business. Even if some of it (e.g. Distance Selling Act) does not apply to you, it is very useful to have a general idea of how consumers are protected.

HEALTH & SAFETY

When working as a mobile technician your personal safety must be paramount! Visiting strangers' homes alone is potentially dangerous. Make sure you leave your up-to-date schedule with details of times and places at home where it can be found. If you are out all day, have someone who you can check in with by phone every few hours so they know you are safe. If you are in a client's home and there is anything that makes you uncomfortable make an excuse and leave! (An excuse could be that you are feeling unwell.)

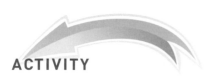

ACTIVITY

Having read the information on Promotional Activities (and possibly carried out the project associated with it) adapt the information for the promotion of the launch of your new business. Collect all the information in a folder:

- List your target markets, e.g. mums with young children, working people, elderly people, older teens, offices, etc.

- Decide on your method of communication, e.g. advert, mail shot, etc.

- Decide on your marketing material, e.g. price lists, appointment cards, homecare advice, posters, mail shots, etc.

- Research the cost of design and printing.

When it is time to launch your new business all the necessary information will be ready to go!

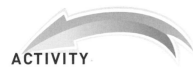

ACTIVITY

Draw up a complete list of every tool, consumable and product you need to start your business. Add their prices and where you need to buy them from.

It is inadvisable to purchase unnecessary items at this stage as you may find you change your mind once you start or find products and tools better suited to your mobility issues.

Larger sizes do often save money but this is not always the case. If you are buying products using mail order, see if there is a level of spending that gives free delivery.

(Continued)

6 *Data Protection*

This relates to any data connected to identifiable living people. It is mostly concerned with information collection on a far bigger scale than a mobile nail technician; however, it does apply to client record cards. Be aware of it and collect the relevant information for your file.

www.ico.gov.uk
www.businesslink.gov.uk

7 *Mobility*

Finding and using the right equipment for your business is essential! So much time and effort will be wasted using the wrong choices of kit bag, mobile desk (if appropriate, but strongly recommended) and other ways of storing and transporting your products and tools.

It is worth spending some time researching the various options of kit bags, trolleys, portable desks, lamps, etc. in an attempt to spend money on the right one from the beginning.

There are many sites that sell a variety of equipment, for example:

www.beautyexpress.co.uk
www.beauty-boxes.com
www.roosalon.com

8 *Marketing and promotion*

An essential part of your business is making sure people know you are there! There is a separate project that looks at this subject but the information from this will be very useful to keep in this file.

9 *Products, tools and stock*

In an earlier activity you have researched and decided upon the products you will need to carry out your mobile services. Now you need to list all the products and tools you will need to purchase to start your business.

One of the decisions you will have to make at this stage is what products, if any, you will be retailing to your clients. Retailing to clients can boost your income significantly but, being mobile, you need to plan carefully as you cannot carry vast amounts of retail lines. Clients often make 'impulse purchases' especially when their technician has done a good job in homecare education.

You will need to set aside an area in your home where stock can be safely stored until you need it.

10 *Business policies*

When running a business that involves services to clients you need to have clear policies from the beginning. These can range from cancellation charges, booking fees through to complaints, presence of children, smoking and mobile phone use during services.

From the outset you need to make your business policies clear but avoiding 'frightening' potential clients.

When visiting clients' homes it is very difficult to control your working environment. There are several important health and safety issues that you can address before you arrive for your booking (and it is much easier to do this at the time of booking that when you are in your client's home).

Smoking: not only is it dangerous to smoke around many nail products, while you are in your client's home it is your place of work and smoking is not allowed. You need to make this clear to your client but focusing on the danger of smoking around volatile products is an easier option.

Ventilation is essential when working. Do not work in a room that doesn't have very effective ventilation (e.g. a window wide open).

Children and pets can be a serious problem when working in a client's home. It is not acceptable or safe to have young children around when providing a nail enhancement service.

Your client must agree to a time commitment. It is not acceptable that your service is held up for telephone calls, attending to children and other domestic occurrences.

11 *Service fees and timings*

Every commercial service needs to conform to a 'service timing' (i.e. a 30 minute manicure must take 30 minutes). A working day needs to follow a strict timetable in order to avoid clients being kept waiting and to keep to commercially acceptable hourly rates.

A mobile technician has the additional cost of travel time. This is a non-productive time with the additional cost of travel and must be built into hourly income. There is an activity later in this chapter that looks at hourly overheads. It is very important that this exercise is carried out and added to this file.

Scenario 2: a home salon

Create you own checklist with all points from Scenario 1 (where appropriate) and add:

12 *Permissions*

If you are planning to convert an area in your home or create a purpose-built out-building you will need to get planning permission from your local authority.

A residential property cannot have a business being run from it without this permission unless it is just a home office that doesn't involve visitors on a regular basis.

Your business will obviously involve as many clients as possible! This could have an impact on neighbours and car parking.

Any purpose-built structure or, for example, a garage conversion will need local authority planning permission. A structure, such as a log cabin may not need permission to build but will need permission to be used as a business.

It is essential to contact your Local Authority and find out about your specific requirements. Every Local Authority has its own website and this is a good place to start but it will only provide you with guidelines.

13 *Business insurance*

Running a home salon as a business cannot be integrated into your usual home insurance. You must take out an insurance that specifically describes the business you intend to carry out.

Cash and Carry's often have special offers or VAT paid/free days.

Trade shows often have special deals available from exhibitors.

Take all of this into account when making this list so you can plan to take advantage of any savings you can.

Then create a complete stock list that you will use to help you keep a realistic stock level and organize re-ordering.

Decide what the stock level of each product needs to be for you to provide an efficient service. Planning smart and cost-effective buying will help you avoid spending more than you need.

If you are going to be retailing to your clients you will need a separate stock list for retail lines.

There is very useful stock control and inventory information and advice available. This is more applicable to larger businesses but the basic principals apply.

www.businesslink.gov.uk

ACTIVITY

Write a 'terms and conditions' document that could be provided for each of your clients setting out your business policies. Include:

- Your booking deposit (if appropriate).
- Cancellation fee and details.
- Complaints procedure and time-scale (e.g. if a client is unhappy with your service they must notify you within x number of days and you must observe the problem before comment).
- Working conditions (e.g. ventilation, smoking, children, etc.).

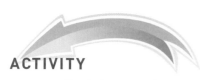

ACTIVITY

Choose the room within your home that you are gong to use as a 'home salon'. Draw a floor plan to scale. Research the wall, floor and window decoration that you like and will project a professional image. Create a 'mood board' of colour swatches. Research furniture and place the furniture in your scaled view of the room.

Create a spreadsheet of expenditure needed to convert (or build) a 'home salon' room. List all the resources needed to create a professional home salon from décor to flooring; from client chair to wash basin; from soft furnishing to electric sockets.

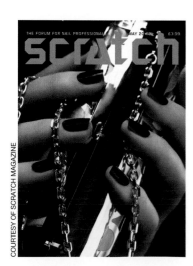

Scratch cover May 2008

Call your existing home insurers and get quotes for a home salon. Plus get quotes from other companies for a comparison.

14 *Health & Safety*

All the H&S issues for a salon apply to a home salon. See Chapter 3 for more information. Many of the requirements apply to an establishment with a minimum number of employees. This is a legal requirement but a salon of even one nail technician still has all the same health and safety issues.

A home salon is no different from a salon in commercial premises. Insurance requirements will be the same as will local authority environmental health requirements.

It is very good practice and a demonstration of a professional approach if a home salon approaches health and safety as if it were a far bigger salon.

Compile all the paperwork and information as required for a commercial salon and address it for your home salon.

It is essential that both you and your clients are in a safe environment. See Chapter 3 on Preparing the work area.

15 *Décor and furniture*

As a BUSINESS IDEA it is not enough to just decide to 'do nails at home'. If you intend to bring strangers into your home and want to be viewed as a professional nail technician, it is important to project a genuine professional approach.

Your 'home salon' needs to have the 'feel' of a commercial salon and not just the 'front room' or 'back bedroom' of your home.

Think about a décor that feels hygienic, professional and, above all, comfortable. Bare in mind that there needs to be convenient hand washing facilities for your 'home salon'. There also needs to be access to a toilet for clients.

16 *Stock and display*

Your home salon should function like a commercial salon, it should also look like a commercial salon. Small, attractive displays of products (e.g. polishes), product marketing material and nail associated posters and pictures are easy options. Even a collection of covers from a trade magazines such as *Scratch* can look very effective.

When choosing home salon decoration, take into consideration the fact that your clients will be sitting with you for fairly long periods of time. During this time they will be looking around. It is a good idea that products and marketing material catch their eye and instigate a conversation about the products. This is an easy way to retailing. A client sees an interesting product/piece of marketing and asks you about it. You have the opportunity to explain all the features and benefits of the product in relation to the client. The client may then consider that this product is a 'must have' and there has been no 'hard sell' involved.

Some salons occasionally sell associated products for the benefit of their customers. For example, small items of jewellery etc. This can be a good idea and creates a bit of interest. It is, however, important to keep a good level of professionalism in the salon environment and not make it into a shop (that is unless this is part of the BUSINESS IDEA where nail services are ancillary to a retail idea).

Scenario 3: rent a space/desk in a salon

Adapt all of the lists above to suit your scenario. Then add:

17   *Rental agreements*

There are several implications here. For tax purposes you need to show that you are trading independently otherwise you may be considered as an employee of the salon.

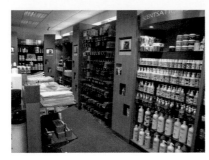

Well stocked professional wholesalers

For your protection and the understanding of rents for commercial properties, research the various types of agreements and their impact on the lease holder. In this scenario, the lease holder will not be you but an understanding of rental agreements will be very useful in the dealing you have with the salon owner.

You need to have a written agreement from the salon owner that makes every aspect clear.

Look at very clear rental agreements for your space/desk with regard to:

–   Rent e.g.:

o   Is there a percentage of income to be paid as 'rent'?

o   Is there a flat rent?

o   Who provides products?

o   What is the ceiling rental (i.e. maximum rent)?

o   Is there a 'start-up' period where no rent is due?

o   Is there a sliding scale of 'rent?

o   Does the rent include any marketing and promotion?

o   Does the rent include 'consumables' such as refreshments, laundry, etc.?

o   Does the rent include reception services?

o   What is the space available within the agreement?

o   Where and how can the services be promoted within the salon?

o   Does the rent include all other costs, e.g. taxes, heating, lighting, etc.?

–   Responsibilities:

o   Who books appointments?

o   Who promotes the service?

o   Who provides marketing material?

o   Who advertises and promotes your services?

o   Who 'owns' the clients (this is often a problem! What is important is to get this issue agreed at the beginning)?

o   Who keeps the client details?

o   Who does the client pay?

o   What are the VAT arrangements?

o   What days are you expected to be in the salon?

o   If there are other technicians in the salon, how are clients booked?

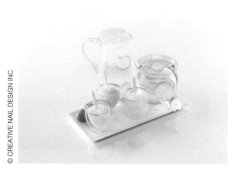

- ○ Who provides the furniture?
- ○ What are your holiday arrangements?
- – Legalities:
  - ○ Is the leaseholder entitled to 'sub-let'?
  - ○ What is the term of the primary commercial lease?
  - ○ What is the term of your 'sub-let'?
  - ○ What restrictions are there in the primary lease?
  - ○ What period of notice is there for the primary lease and the 'sub-let' lease?
  - ○ Does the rent include a proportion of the council tax and other financial requirements?
  - ○ Who and what is licensed for your services?
  - ○ If you leave under the terms of the lease are there any trading restrictions?

There is no definitive answer to any of these questions. The only answer is to research some general situations on websites such as:

www.knowledge.hsbc.co.uk

www.smallbusiness.co.uk

www.businesslink.gov.uk

As far as possible, research various situations, note the scenarios and compare the best solution.

A good forum to investigate good and bad situations is: www.salongeek.com

The financials

When you are self-employed with your own business, even if it just involves you, you have a responsibility for the control of your finances.

Before you start a business and as part of your business plan you must look at a medium range financial plan. If you are planning on taking out a business loan or applying for a start-up grant this is a required exercise. If you are funding your business yourself it is also very good practice as it will help you budget, spend wisely and, hopefully, have contingency plans in place for unexpected or unforeseen situations.

Cashflow

The flow of cash into and out of a business is the 'life blood' of it. Sometimes, what flows out doesn't balance with what is flowing in. This may be alright if it is for a short time but can be disastrous if the situation continues.

Creating a 'cash flow forecast' is a very useful (and essential) exercise before starting a business. It will demonstrate what income is needed on a monthly basis; it will highlight any periods that may have cash problems and is a very useful tool to monitor the growth (or otherwise) of the business.

From all the exercises you have carried out in this chapter so far you should have almost all of the information you need to chart your overheads and outgoings into a spreadsheet.

These will roughly fall into two main categories:

- Start-up costs – all expenditure you need to launch your business. These should be one-off payments and shown in the first column.

- Overheads – these will be ongoing costs of rent, car, telephone, stock, products, PAYE, NI, VAT (if appropriate), printing, etc. These may be monthly payments and some will be quarterly or of other frequencies.

Ideally, these should be calculated on a monthly basis (although a very small business may prefer a weekly spreadsheet to begin with). These will have a monthly total and are unavoidable payments.

The other part of a cash flow forecast is your estimated income. This is the hardest part of all! You need to estimate your income and it must be based on some solid assumptions.

You will have decided on your pricing structure by now so you need to estimate the number of clients you will have in each month (or week). In an ideal situation, these should slowly grow as the months go by. They will also be seasonally affected. For example, Christmas should see an upturn in clients. Summer holiday time usually means more pedicures etc.

The best way to create a cash flow forecast is using a computer spreadsheet such as *Excel* in *Windows*. This way the sums are automatically calculated for you. If you are unable to do this yourself, ask someone who can to create a template for you so you have one you can adapt. If neither is possible, you will just have to use a paper and pencil! Pads of spreadsheets are available from office supplies.

The upper part of the spreadsheet is where you put your income subtotals for each month with a total at the bottom of this section. The lower part of the spreadsheet is where you list all your outgoings with a total at the bottom.

Below this is a 'running total' of income minus expenditure. This is bound to be in the minus (red) figures for a while as your start-up costs will be accounted for.

Each month the final total is carried forward to the next month as a starting balance. This does not necessarily relate to your bank balance. What it does show is how the flow of cash through your business is working. If it is done as accurately as possible it should highlight any problem areas where outgoings far exceed income, e.g. during quiet months, or when you need to order more products or have a large overhead to pay.

When you have completed your spreadsheet and it is accurate and realistic it is good practice to compare your estimates with actual figures when your business is launched. You will soon see if your predictions are right or, if not, where they need tweaking!

By keeping actual figures alongside your estimates you will have a good idea on when and how to budget for your overheads and business development costs. If you need a 'top-up' business loan any lender will expect to see your careful and realistic financial planning.

Record keeping

As a self-employed and freelance person, it is your responsibility to keep financial records. In large business this is a full-time job that needs qualifications and experience. For a micro-business it just needs some basic knowledge and organization.

Even a micro-business will benefit from the services of an accountant if only for advice on your tax return. However, even with the services of an accountant, basic book-keeping is essential. It is required by law to keep financial records that relate to your business. It is also required by law that you must keep your financial records for 6 years.

ALWAYS REMEMBER

With this exercise it is essential that you are realistic and DO NOT base your assumptions on what you would LIKE to happen.

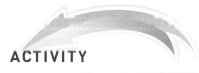

ACTIVITY

Create a cash flow forecast for your BUSINESS IDEA. Do this either on a PC spreadsheet or as a hard copy (paper). Keep careful notes on your assumption reasoning.

Analyze your spreadsheet making notes of problem areas and how you plan to overcome them in a cost-effective and business-like way.

For further information go to www. businesslink.gov.uk

Whether you keep records electronically (on your PC) or on paper, they must be kept accurately and filed accordingly. There are many inexpensive accounting programs available for small businesses and this is probably the easiest method of keeping your records.

If you decide to use the services of an accountant they may have a preferred computer program. They may even provide you with the software to do this. Whatever you decide you do need to have a basic understanding of the process.

If you are a micro-business that just involves you and has no employees, there are two sets of financial records that you need to keep. If you are employing people there is a great deal of additional information you need to keep.

As a general rule you need to keep records of every transaction in your business. As so much banking is done online these days you do need to keep an accurate record of the financial status and movements within your business.

You must file and keep all relevant bank statements.

A rough division of these is:

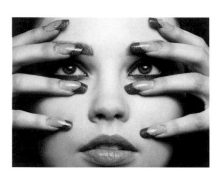

- Receipts (Sales Ledger) – it is unlikely that you will issue invoices to your clients! However, every time a client pays you with cash, a cheque or a credit card you must record it. If you are VAT registered it must be recorded with the VAT separated out.

- Payments (Purchase Ledger) – every time you make a payment on the business you must record the payment and file the receipt. (Regular payments such as rent just needs a filed copy of the payment schedule.)

(A nail technician providing nail services in the scenarios described in this chapter will receive a payment immediately. Other career routes may involve chasing late payments.)

For this type of business it makes sense to keep weekly records. A very simple method is to record:

- Receipts – as a daily total on a spreadsheet (do not use clients' names) or in a notebook to transfer to a weekly spreadsheet.

- Payments – record the details of every payment and make a note of where the receipt can be found. This may be a paper receipt (e.g. petrol, equipment and stock purchases). Give this a number that is noted on the record and then file it in date order. If it is, for example, a direct debit (e.g. rent, NI) it will be shown on your bank statement. It makes tracking easier if payments of this kind have a reference to the item on your statement.

Invoices Invoices are rarely required for the type of business we are describing in this chapter. However, there may be occasions where a special job (e.g. a wedding party, a corporate event) requires you to submit an invoice as they need to record their payment in their records.

As a business you must supply a correct invoice. This needs to have:

- Your name and contact address, telephone number or email address (do not put your address if you are freelance working from home but a contact method must be provided).

- The details of the person or company you are invoicing.

- The date of the invoice.

- Details of the services and/or products offered.

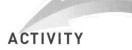

ACTIVITY

Decide on the book-keeping system you intend to use and set it up. If it is computer software, enter all the relevant details and go through the tutorial that will be with the software. If you are using a paper accountancy system buy your chosen system (there are several available in an office supply shop) or use the one recommended by your accountant or financial advisor. Enter all the information you have so far.

- The date of the service.

- The details of the services and/or products being sold.

- The subtotal or the services and/or products.

Purchase orders Purchase orders are issued from the buyer to the seller and constitutes a legal offer to purchase products or services. This may be useful for a freelance technician if you are providing your services at an event for example. You can ask the organizer who is booking you to provide you with a purchase order that will put in writing all the details. This would include the fee to be paid, the time you are required, etc. It is a binding agreement and very useful in avoiding misunderstandings later!

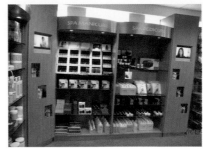
Wholesalers

Evaluate your business

Whether you are just starting on the beginning of an idea or you have a small business up and running, it is a very good idea to evaluate the business and try to look at it impartially. It is hard to do this but there is a very good 'tool' to help you in a 'SWOT analysis' as a guide.

Draw four squares on a page and label them:

STRENGTHS

WEAKNESSES

OPPORTUNITIES

THREATS

Strengths and weaknesses are internal factors, i.e. specific to you and your businesses.

Opportunities and threats are external factors, i.e. how other people or situations can or do affect your business.

Strengths could be:

- your skills

- your unique offering

- location

- your dedication to ongoing learning

- keeping abreast of the market

- pricing structure and menu.

Weaknesses could be:

- lack of experience

- poor quality products

- no planning

- no experience in marketing.

Opportunities could be:

- appropriate training courses

- new and exciting products

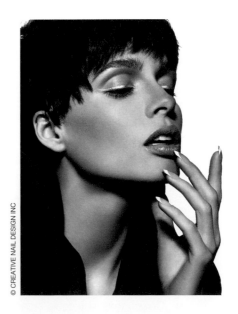

- developing a new market (e.g. via a website)
- a joint venture (e.g. renting space in a busy hair salon).

Threats could be:

- strong competitors with a good reputation
- local pricing structures (NB you do NOT have to be the cheapest)
- competitors with a new and exciting product/ technique
- location.

Think hard about each of these areas and be realistic. Be specific and avoid any grey areas. Enter your thoughts into the relevant box.

You will see there are two negative boxes and two positive boxes. Look at the negatives and find ways to turn these into positives. Look at the positives and use these to make your business even better.

There are many easy tools such as a SWOT analysis explained on the web.

Business Matters has been a guide for a technician planning to start a small business or to work as a freelance artist. It is just a beginning and covers several areas that need careful thought and lots of planning. There is so much help available from organizations today so try to use as many as possible.

Summary

Now you have read this chapter, you should have completed almost enough research to write an effective business plan. There is a generally accepted format for these and some ideas or templates are available from banks and business link. To start a small business most of the sections in these templates need to be completed but the level of information will be nothing like as detailed as for some of the examples that are used.

Good luck!

ASSESSMENT OF KNOWLEDGE AND UNDERSTANDING

This chapter has been concerned with you carrying out your own research and discovering answers to situations relevant to you.

Ask yourself these questions to assess how your knowledge and understanding has developed:

1   Do you have some ideas on how you can help the business you are employed by?

2   Are you an effective and efficient member of a team?

3   Have you got ideas on business marketing and advertising?

4   Do you think you could organize a simple promotional activity?

5   Can you look at the choice of salon products objectively and come to realistic conclusions?

6   Are you confident that you can devise a service menu and realistic pricing?

7   Do you have a better idea on a variety of freelance opportunities and how to start your own business idea?

8   Are financial issues still a mystery or do you understand the basics?

9   Will you be able to impartially evaluate your business?

10 Can you create a thorough business plan?

13
Nail art, basic and advanced

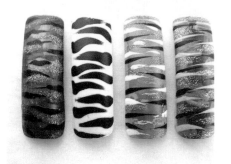

Introduction

Nail art is a very important part of the technician's skill. Just painting colour on nails is nail art! Many technicians do not master this art and assume that they can do it naturally. Not true! It takes practice and a very good eye for detail, as this chapter will show, demonstrating both basic and advanced airbrushing techniques.

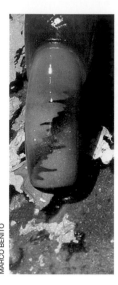

MARCO BENITO

An airbrushed design

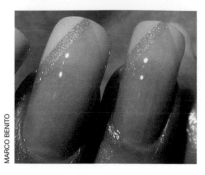

MARCO BENITO

An airbrush design

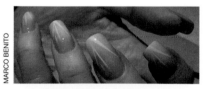

MARCO BENITO

An airbrush design

The nail art skill starts when a 'French manicure' is applied, as this is actually two colours painted very accurately. The skill becomes even more advanced when other colours and actual designs become involved. A technician does not need to be a great artist in order to create quite stunning and very commercially acceptable designs. A natural artist will obviously find this aspect of the work easy, but a 'struggling' artist can generate just as much income with some easy shortcuts.

There are many products available on the market today that, with a few guidelines and hints, can create stunning 'masterpieces' at minimal cost and effort. The real effort is practicing! This cannot be skipped. Nail art is visual and there are a relatively small number of basic techniques that, using readily available products, can be demonstrated in a few step-by-step pictures. Every newcomer to nail art has found that, with the right direction and range of products, a few ideas will lead on to many, many more. Technicians should aim to create their own masterpieces; it is very difficult to copy another person's work but it is easy to be inspired by ideas.

Although some more unusual designs are included, the aim of this chapter is to provide the knowledge, understanding and practical skills of the various techniques of nail art and, hopefully, spark plenty of creative ideas. The level of nail art here is that which is practical in a commercial salon or mobile situation.

Most of the techniques included here could easily be incorporated into a commercial salon if its clientele were interested. three-dimensional and **cut-out** designs are the least likely to be commercially viable because, for a client, they are impractical. Most employers of technicians would welcome the additional skills involved in simple and effective nail art. However, skills in the more advanced forms of nail art will not necessarily make a technician more or less employable. Understanding the basic skills, health and safety and the materials being used is by far the most important.

Nail art for your clients

First, remember that all the health and safety rules apply, as do full client consultations and an understanding of nails and all their problems. This is still a professional service and you are charging for it!

Not every client is a nail art devotee. Most will not be in the slightest bit interested, some will wear a form of nail art for special occasions and some will want the biggest, the best, the most unusual, the most bizarre all the time.

Your skills as a nail artist are obviously important in this subject, but so are your skills at understanding what people want. A suggestion of a subtle or sophisticated piece of nail art may spark the interest of an uninterested client, but pushing a full set of extravagant nail art could scare them away for ever.

If a client shows an interest in nail art the next step is careful questioning and showing them examples of designs. Make sure you understand what your client is saying and that you are clear about the degree of 'statement' she is interested in making. For example, a client usually known for her conservative taste in clothes and natural nails with sheer or delicate colours, who is interested in nail art for a special occasion, is only likely to be interested in a very subtle design. Alternatively, a client who likes to try out new ideas, such as the latest fashion trends, may be open to a more interesting suggestion such as rhinestones or some airbrushing. The client who is an individual and likes to make a strong statement of image will like lots of original (but practical) ideas. They may have a good idea of what they want and bring in a picture of a design, or they may like to let you decide for them.

> **❝❝ ANECDOTE**
>
> Many years ago I knew a client who was in her early 80s and a wonderful character, coming in weekly for nail art. Her nails were long and natural, although sometimes with a little help from an overlay. She would wear the outfit that she wanted her designs to match. This could be tartan or leopard skin or diamante. Her 'toyboy' of 70 loved her style and so did we. On one occasion, this lady had a fall and damaged her ankle so she was visited at home to have her designs done. But that situation did not last for long. Out she came into the town with her heavily bandaged ankle and walking sticks. Her doctor had told her to wear a slipper on the other foot. She did exactly as she was told. Only her slippers were fluffy mules with a stiletto heel!

Bold characters are quite rare in a traditional salon and not many technicians will be required to create 'masterpieces' very often. Masterpieces are not very practical in day-to-day salon work because (a) the time taken and material used would make the cost to the client prohibitive for such a temporary decoration, and (b) elaborate designs would be very difficult to live with on a practical basis.

However, the various advanced techniques included in this chapter are very useful for sparking ideas and creativity and many of them are effective and can be produced quite quickly and therefore be relatively cost-effective for clients. The truly elaborate designs seen on trade magazine covers and in competitions are created by very artistic technicians who love to express this type of art form. It shows how the various techniques used by technicians can be extended and manipulated to demonstrate how versatile the material is and how a simple nail can become a work of art. In the real world of the salon, with its paying clients, the images created are there to amaze and enjoy and to bring attention to the skilful and visual art of the nail technician.

Some technicians will be better at nail art than others. For those who are not so artistic there is no need to think that they will not be able to provide a nail art service for their clients. There are many, many easy techniques and products that allow the most 'artistically challenged' technicians to produce some stunning designs. For those able to create the more imaginative designs, always keep in mind the practicality of providing the design in a salon or mobile setting – that is the time and cost factor.

On a practical level of offering the service to clients, the very best approach (after lots of practice on tips and real fingers) is to make a display of your own designs. Organize these in sections depending on the cost. To calculate the cost, the exercise in Chapter 3 is very valuable. On top of this, don't forget to add the cost of the time it will take.

Some designs are very quick and use little product, for example a flick of paint with a nail art brush or a simple **marbelling**. Other designs are very quick but use more costly products, for example polish secures that are fast to apply, but cost much more than a flick of nail art paint or a couple of 'blobs' of varnish.

Nail art is very tricky to price. If it costs too much clients are unlikely to want it as it will only last a short time. However, you must be realistic in your pricing and the most favoured designs are bound to be those that are quick to apply but look stunning. The simplest designs are often the most effective and may appeal to a wider client base.

On your display board have designs in two or three colour ways to demonstrate that a design can be customized to suit the client and how different colour combinations can

TOP TIP When allowing for time in costing a design, use an average time that the design would take. The client should not be penalized for a slower or less experienced technician taking 30 minutes where a faster technician would take 10 minutes.

TOP TIP Create your own display board as you may not be able to copy another technician's design and make it look the same.

TOP TIP Practice all designs on a tip and then a real finger. The appearance and application is different.

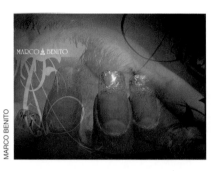

MARCO BENITO

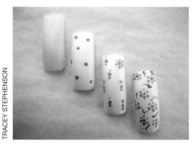

TRACEY STEPHENSON

(1) Steps: Base colour, flower centres, flower petals, finished design with stems added

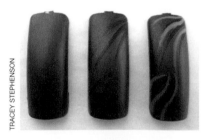

TRACEY STEPHENSON

(2) Steps: Base colour and stripes

change the design dramatically. Start the display with the simpler and less expensive designs and progress to the more elaborate and more involved designs.

Although designs look effective displayed on quite large plastic tips, remember that the design will look very different on a much smaller nail on a finger and some designs are much easier to apply on a tip than a real nail as the surrounding skin can get in the way!

One of the best forms of promoting the nail art service is by wearing it.

The basic techniques

All the basic techniques are easy! All they need is some ideas, a bit of imagination and the right equipment and products.

The paints used are different from nail varnishes. They are usually water-based acrylic artists' paint, as this gives a very dense colour, can be mixed and is easier to use for fine detail. There are lots of effects that can be achieved with paints, a selection of nail art brushes and a 'marbling tool'.

Nails need to be painted with a base colour that will be part of or enhance the finished design. This is usually a nail varnish that should be touch dry before painting any designs.

- Very simple but effective designs can be achieved by placing dots of colour. Use either a very small round brush or a 'marbling or dotting tool' to apply the dots (1). Care needs to be taken on the size and regularity of the dots as this can spoil a good design.

- A very long, thin brush dipped in paint can achieve fine stripes and create quite sophisticated designs (2).

Abstract patterns or marbling can look stunning with a good choice of colour combinations. Flicking the colour from side to side with a fine brush or placing spots of colour on the nail and mixing them together with the 'marbling tool' achieves this effect.

- Those who are not so good at hand painting designs can use stencils. The types that are readily available have a sticky back to keep them in place. These are applied to a dry nail and painted over. When the nail paint is completely dry they are removed, leaving the chosen design behind.

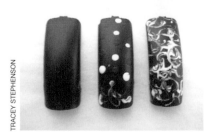

TRACEY STEPHENSON

Steps: Base colour, add two or more different coloured dots, swirl together

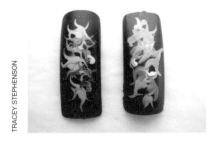

TRACEY STEPHENSON

Designs using marbling

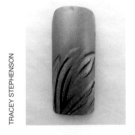

TRACEY STEPHENSON

Design with brushes

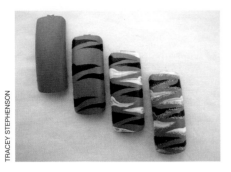

TRACEY STEPHENSON

The steps for hand painted designs

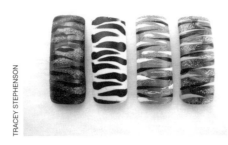

TRACEY STEPHENSON

Designs with brushes

- Pictures of all sorts can be painted on a nail with a steady hand, a good imagination or an easy picture to copy. (Most nail artists keep large numbers of pictures to copy onto a nail or just to give them inspiration to create an original design.)

- Buy or find a palette. This can be any plastic surface that can be easily cleaned with water. This can be used to place nail art paints on for use or mixing. Have a small water spray to hand then, if your paints start drying out, give a small spray of distilled water to keep them workable.

Nail art paint is water-based and any mistakes can be easily removed with a wet nail wipe, or a cotton bud will remove a small part.

In all nail art, sealing the design is very important and, when the paint is dry, a sealer or topcoat must be applied to fix the paint and also bring out the colour. The manufacturer's recommended sealer should be used, as some topcoats may react to the paints. Clients should be advised to re-seal the nails every couple of days to keep them fresh looking and avoid any chips.

Nail art brushes

There are many brushes specifically sold for nail art purposes but also remember that art shops sell many shapes and sizes too. A small collection of brushes is necessary to the technician in order to create a wide range of styles and these can be purchased relatively cheaply from suppliers and, with care, will last a long time.

Brushes

- *Detail brush*. This is the smallest brush and is used for hand painting details or placing dots.

TOP TIP

Old CDs are excellent mixing palettes.

TRACEY STEPHENSON

Designs using brush techniques

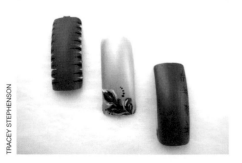

TRACEY STEPHENSON

Hand painted designs

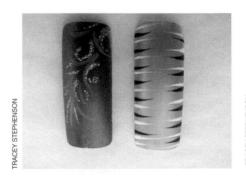

TRACEY STEPHENSON

Hand painted designs

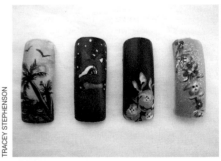

TRACEY STEPHENSON

Hand painted designs

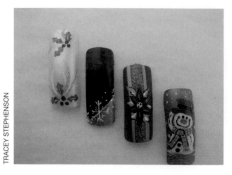

Hand painting with a theme

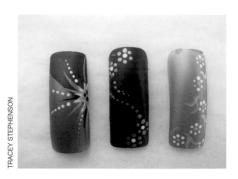

Designs using dots and hand painting

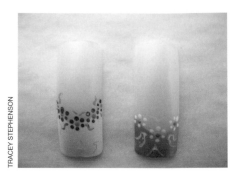

Designs with French and dots

TOP TIP

If you have a very long striping brush, try placing three or four dots of different coloured paint next to each other on a plastic palette (or similar). Lay the brush in the dots and turn it so all the hairs are coated. Then lay the brush on the nail and lift off. An attractive multi-coloured stripe will be left behind. Try different colours and techniques of applying to the nail and see what happens.

TOP TIP

Put dots of two different colours on your palette. Dip one corner of a flat brush in one colour and the other corner of the brush in the other colour. Then apply to the nail turning the brush in a circular motion. See what happens!

- *Striping brushes*. These are available in different sizes. Their length and the number of hairs are relevant. A shorter brush with several hairs will produce lines that are thick. The longer and thinner the brush, the finer and longer the line they produce. It is worth having at least two of these: a medium one for lines and flicks and a very long one for fine stripes.

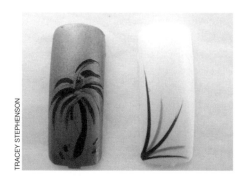

Designs using striping

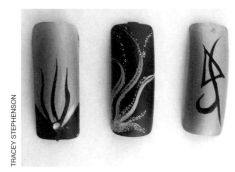

Designs using striping

- *Flat brush*. This is a brush with a small flat head that can create several effects and is used to fill in colours. It can shade and smudge and create swirls.

- *Fan brush*. This brush can create texture and blend colours together. It is probably not as versatile as the others but worth having.

Foiling

Foiling is another very easy technique that uses various designs of a foil supplied on a roll. This is almost instant nail art, as some foils have designs on them and just need applying to a painted nail.

- Nails should be painted before using foils. They can be painted with a base coat, but it is worth spending the extra time to paint a colour, as this will enhance the effect.

- Foils are supplied with a special adhesive that should be painted onto the nail in a very thin coat. The adhesive is usually white and needs to turn clear before the foil is applied; this takes a very short time. The foil is then applied to the tacky adhesive, pattern side uppermost, gently pressed onto the nail with either a finger or a cotton bud and the backing pulled off leaving the foil behind. It is not necessary to cut any foil from the roll, as it will only stick to where the adhesive is.

- This is an amazingly quick process that can have spectacular results. As the foil only sticks to where the adhesive has been applied, patterns or pictures can be drawn with the adhesive. The foil needs a special sealer, as most topcoats will destroy the delicate layer. Several layers of sealer are also needed, as with all nail art, to keep it intact.

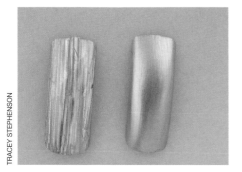

Foiled nail

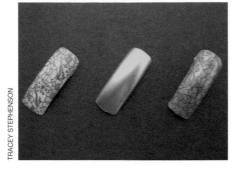

Same foil but silver polish under one

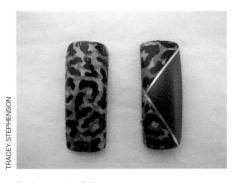

Designs using foil

Polish secures

As the name suggests, this technique requires polish to secure the design. Many different products are available for this easy technique. **Polish secures** are the term for small stones or shapes with a flat back that are placed into the wet nail varnish and held secure when it dries. The products that fall into this category sometimes have different brand names. Most of them are available in different sizes and, although it depends on the design, the smaller versions are usually the most effective.

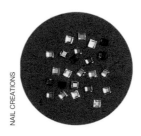

Polish secures – square rhinestones

- *Rhinestones* (or *diamantes*). These are clear or coloured stones that look like precious or semi-precious stones. They are usually made of glass or crystal and cut with facets to reflect light. They can be used to encrust a design or a judiciously placed single stone can bring a simple design to life. In relative terms they are not cheap and the designs utilizing them should reflect this cost. Good quality rhinestones will not dull or lose their sparkle if sealed with a topcoat and this will ensure they stay on the nail for the maximum time, especially if the client re-applies a topcoat. Although stunning, even the smallest rhinestone stands quite proud from the nail.

- *Flat backed beads*. These, like rhinestones are usually coloured glass but they are rounded rather than cut with facets. Applied in the same way to wet polish, they look like beads on the nails.

- *Flatstones*. These are a less expensive version of rhinestones. As the name suggests, they are quite flat and usually very small, but they sparkle well. They can, however, lose their sparkle under a topcoat. If this is the case, then apply a thicker layer of topcoat than usual and push the stones into the wet polish. This should hold them in place without the need to seal them.

- *Pearls*. These are flat backed plastic shapes coloured to look like pearls. Although white is the obvious colour, they can be obtained in pastel colours, such as pink or lilac. They can look very pretty, especially in a design for a bride. Again, take account of their size.

- *Stone shapes*. There are some interesting shapes available now, such as flower made of coloured glass.

- *Foil shapes*. These are tiny pieces of shiny or holographic plastic cut into different shapes that can look very effective incorporated into a design. The shapes may be circular, stars, moons, hexagons, even tiny hands and dolphins! These are applied in the same way, but care must be taken with the topcoat. They need to be sealed as edges that are not covered by topcoat can catch and be pulled off, although some topcoats have a solvent that is too strong. This will cause the colour to be affected and it will often streak.

- *Metal studs*. A very effective and less 'glitzy' polish secure are metal studs. These are available in gold or silver colours and different sizes.

- *Fimo canes*. These can be bought in ready cut or in long 'canes'. There is a vast variety of designs that can be laid on the nail once a very thin 'slice' has been cut. Some of these can be partially transparent.

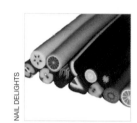
Fruits fimo canes

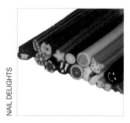
Fimo canes

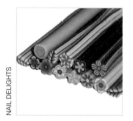
Flower fimo canes

- *Crushed shells*. These are available in many colours and can be applied as a base for other decorations to go on top or can be used alone or with colour variations. They have an opalescence that can look spectacular.

Flowers and shells

- *Dried flowers*. Various tiny dried real flowers and leaves are available and applied in the same way.

- After the base colour has been applied (or other design) a topcoat or sealer must be painted. While this is still wet, the 'secures' can be placed on it. The easiest way to pick up 'secures' is with a wet orange stick or with a small piece of Blu-Tack on the end of an orange stick. The Blu-Tack can be shaped into a point to make picking up the tiny shapes easier.

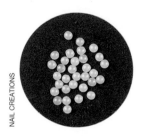
Polish secures – pearls

- When all the shapes have been placed, the whole nail needs to be sealed with a thick coat of sealer or topcoat. Make sure your topcoat does not affect the colour of foil shapes.

- Recommend to your client that they re-apply a topcoat every 2 to 3 days to keep the design fresh and avoid damage to or loss of stones.

Alternative application methods:

1 Use a spot of nail adhesive to place the decoration on the nail

2 Embed in a UV gel topcoat before curing

3 Place on the nail and apply a layer of clear L&P or UV gel over the whole design.

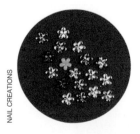
Polish secures – flower beads

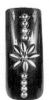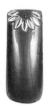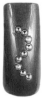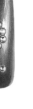
Designs using studs

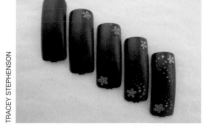
Base colour, apply secures

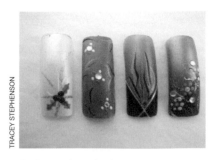
Designs using mixed techniques

TOP TIP Never put an orange stick in your mouth to wet it! If Blu-Tack is not available, dip the stick into varnish remover or a small dish of water to wet it.

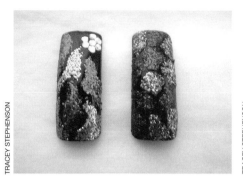

TRACEY STEPHENSON

Designs using glitter dusts

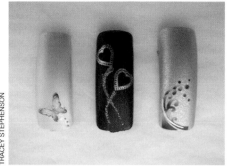

TRACEY STEPHENSON

Designs using transfers

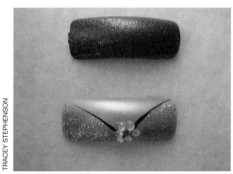

TRACEY STEPHENSON

Designs using glitter polish

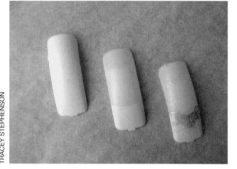

TRACEY STEPHENSON

French with a transfer

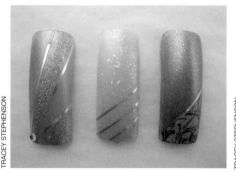

TRACEY STEPHENSON

Designs using striping tape

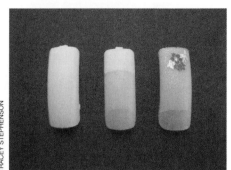

TRACEY STEPHENSON

French with a transfer

Glitter dusts

Glitter polishes and glitter dusts are a very versatile range of products to create or enhance nail art. Obviously, glitter can be applied to the whole nail, but it can also be used to make patterns or designs; a well-placed highlight on a painted or airbrushed design can make a simple piece of nail art spectacular.

- Glitter polishes can be painted straight from the bottle with either the brush supplied or a fine nail art brush. Glitter dusts can be used to create more specific designs by picking up the dust with a brush dipped in sealer, as this will give an effect that is denser than glitter polish. The dust will also stick to wet sealer, so the tip of a nail dipped into the pot will collect the dust on the tip only or where the sealer is wet.

- Like all nail art, glitter dusts need sealing. The sealer must be painted on thickly and gently to avoid moving the dust.

Transfers and tapes

There are many transfers are available to apply to nails. These are ready-made nail art and can be very effective. Some need to be soaked off their backing with water (place a few drops onto the backing paper to soak through and then the transfer slides off) or they peel off their backing and stick straight on to the nail.

Tapes are also available in many plain colours and patterns. They have a sticky back and must be placed on the nail and then trimmed with a small pair of very sharp scissors.

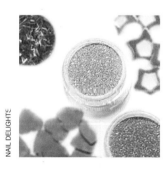

NAIL DELIGHTS

Glitter and shapes

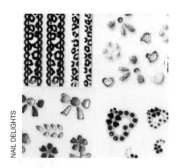

NAIL DELIGHTS

Stickers

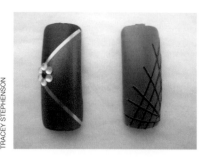

TRACEY STEPHENSON

Designs using striping tape

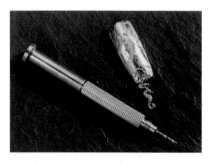

Nail peircing tool

Nail jewellery

Many different types of nail jewellery are available.

- Some of the designs are applied to the nail as a 'polish secure', that is stuck to wet varnish. These can only be very light and small. Larger designs can be applied to the nail with nail glue. Both of these are reusable, as they can be removed with nail varnish remover.

- Other types of nail jewellery involve making a small hole in the free edge of the nail. This can be done with ease using a specially made tool that has a very sharp but tiny drill. There is no problem at all piercing an artificial nail, but care must be taken when piercing a natural nail:

  - A natural nail should be strengthened with a coating of resin as used in a fibre system.

  - The free edge must be long enough to provide a space for the hole without being too close to the hyponychium. If the hole is made on a nail that is too short the seal at the hyponychium could be damaged.

- There are two types of jewellery that require a pierced nail. One has a post that is put through the hole and secured with a tiny nut on the underside. The piercing tool has both the drill and the socket to tighten the nut. The other type has a clasp or ring that is attached to the nail through the hole. The first type usually sits on top of the nail plate and the second hangs from the edge.

To pierce the nail:

1 Make sure there is sufficient free edge to safely pierce.

2 Turn the finger over so that the underside of the nail is visible and the nail and finger are resting on a soft surface, for example, a piece of cork or several layers of tissues.

3 Place the tip of the drill on the nail, not too near the edge but also in the right place for the jewellery to fit on the nail (not too far away from the free edge for a pendant or ring).

4 Gently turn the drill until a neat hole is made; withdraw the drill by turning in the opposite direction.

5 Turn the finger over and smooth the surface of the nail with a white block.

6 Apply the nail jewellery.

7 If a pendant has been applied, advise the client to remove it while dressing, doing housework, washing hair, etc., as it is possible to catch it and split the nail.

These are some basic instructions for starting off in the realms of nail art. All the various techniques can be mixed and matched. Foil can be mixed with polish secures, paint mixed with glitter. The possibilities are endless and the only limit is imagination.

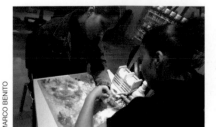

MARCO BENITO

Airbrushing nails in the salon

More Advanced Techniques

Airbrushing

A process that is very popular with some technicians and their clients is airbrushing. Unlike basic nail art, this requires relatively costly equipment and, more importantly, plenty of investment in time for practice. Like artificial nail skills, it tends to look very easy in the hands of an expert, but in reality takes a fair bit of skill.

In the US, airbrushing is rapidly overtaking traditional nail polishing and, believe it or not, some salons no longer offer nail polish as a free service! And of course, the more services your salon offers, the more valuable you are to your clientele! Airbrushing is now one of the fastest-growing nail services. It cannot only create the most amazing designs, but can take the place of traditional nail painting as colour is applied to the nails in such a short space of time.

Airbrushed artwork is a professional skill, which requires specialized techniques and methods of application. There are many products available on the market, and time should be taken to find the right package of equipment. Training courses are essential for this skill as nothing can take the place of practical instruction.

Airbrushed art has been expanding recently into other areas that have become very popular.

- *Body airbrushing*. Designs are painted onto the body using stencils as a decoration, rather like a temporary tattoo.

- *Make-up*. Many professional make-up artists are utilizing the convenience of airbrushing. It is becoming more available in the retail market and is popular for TV work due to High Definition. Used more widely is airbrushing colour onto larger areas of the body. For example, tanning the skin for photographic work and even shading in more impressive acrylonitrile butadiene styrene (ABS)!

- *Tanning*. With so much publicity on the dangers of the sun, artificial tanning is very big business. Self-tanning from any number of products has grown enormously. So has salon tanning and this has now expanded into using airbrushing techniques to apply a thin and even layer of tanning liquid.

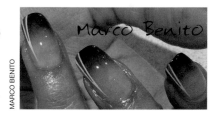

- *Hair*. It is possible to airbrush a design onto hair using a stencil and specialist paint.

An airbrushed design

Equipment
This section is designed to give technicians some idea of what the skill entails and some ideas on airbrushing designs, as well as offering an introduction to how the essential equipment works.

The electrical compressor: Airbrushing requires an electrical compressor to provide the air. These are available in many different shapes, sizes and prices. In essence, there are two main types: the compressor that produces air on demand and that which stores compressed air in a tank that is refilled as the air is used. The air is dispensed under pressure and is therefore potentially dangerous. Care must be taken at all times but note particularly the following two points:

1 Follow all manufacturers' instructions with regard to maintenance. If none are provided, the manufacturer must be asked what the procedures are. The equipment should also be serviced once a year: a faulty compressor can be dangerous.

2 The pressure of the air being dispensed should be around 30 psi (pounds per square inch) and never more than 35 psi. Every compressor should have a psi gauge and regulator to set this level. A pressure of more than 40 psi can push paint (or any other liquid in the airbrush) into the pores of the skin and possibly into the bloodstream.

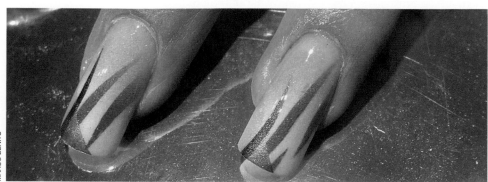

An airbrushed design

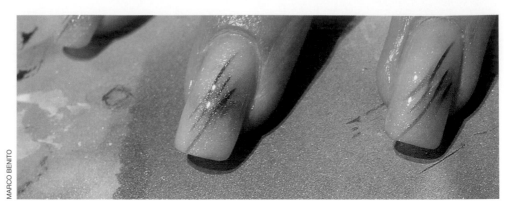

MARCO BENITO

An airbrushed design

Compressors producing air on demand tend to be cheaper, smaller and lighter and are therefore ideal for mobile technicians or salons where airbrushing demands are minimal. The difficulty with this type is that the compressor can only be used for fairly short periods of time before it gets too hot and the amount of air produced is limited.

The storage type of compressor is more suited for use in the salon as it can be used continuously and can often provide air for more than one technician at a time. However, this type is heavier and difficult to move around and is more costly.

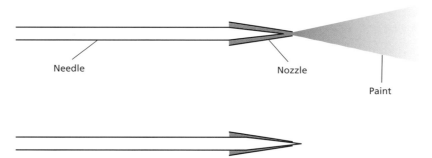

Needle

Nozzle

Paint

Flow of paint in airbrush (a) Needle back in nozzle leaving nozzle open to allow paint through (b) Needle in nozzle sealing nozzle.

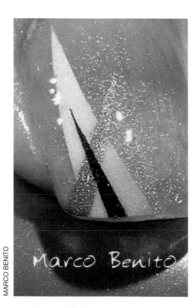

MARCO BENITO

An airbrushed design

There is a certain amount of maintenance required for most compressors, such as draining the tanks and moisture traps and making sure oil levels are right. The least amount of maintenance is obviously better for the user, but always check with your supplier what the maintenance requirements are.

The airbrush: The crucial element is the airbrush itself. This is where the air created by the compressor is mixed with the paint and a fine mist of colour is dispensed onto the nail. There are several different types of airbrush, but the practicalities of dispensing the colour are the same for all.

On the front of the airbrush is a very fine nozzle in a cone shape. A pointed needle fits into this and when the needle is furthest forward the nozzle is blocked but, as the needle is pulled back, more and more air and paint can escape. It is the movement of this needle that regulates the flow of paint from a shut position to a small mist of paint and then to the maximum flow. The trigger that also regulates the flow of air moves the needle. An airbrush suitable for nails is one that has the finest needle and nozzle. Larger versions are better for larger areas such as body painting, tanning and hair colouring.

The air, supplied by a compressor, is fed into the airbrush by a hose that is usually attached under the airbrush. The trigger is sprung and, when depressed, opens a valve to allow the air in and out through the nozzle.

Gravity-fed and bottle-fed paint: The paint is dispensed into the airbrush by one of two methods, depending on the type of equipment:

1   *Gravity-fed*. These airbrushes have a hole in the top or a funnel on the side where small quantities of paint are placed as required. Flushing the old colour through and adding another to the funnel changes the colours.

2   *Bottle-fed*. On some airbrushes there is an attachment on the side where a specific bottle sits, filled with paint colour. Colour changing, after flushing, is done by changing the bottle.

The type used is dependent on the preference of the artist and other factors such as cost, availability, and so on.

Single-action or dual-action operation: The other decision a new artist must make is the type of operation preferred:

1   *Single-action.* The trigger on this type of airbrush can only be pushed down to release the air. The regulation of the amount of paint being dispensed (that is, how far the needle is pulled back from the nozzle to open it up) is set. The needle is set at the beginning of the spraying session to the level that is appropriate for the application. It can be opened up to allow efficient cleaning, but otherwise it remains the same. This type of airbrush is good for beginners as the spraying techniques and designs can be concentrated on. However, most airbrushes of this type need two hands; one to press the trigger, the other to change the regulator and some artists are not keen on this.

2   *Dual-action*. The trigger on these airbrushes can be depressed for air and pulled back to move the needle and therefore regulate the paint. The combination of air to paint regulation is infinitely variable and many artists prefer to have this option. Co-ordination is essential for this operation, and it takes a bit more practice.

3   *Combination*. Some equipment can be used in either of the above ways. The difference in these is that not only do they have a dual-action trigger, but they also have a regulator that can set the position of the needle. This is a good option, especially for beginners. The needle can be set in a position that does not allow too much paint out so no thought has to be given to regulation by the trigger. When the artist is more skilful and confident, the regulator can be left alone and the air to paint ratio can be controlled by the dual-action trigger (and a very delicate finger movement).

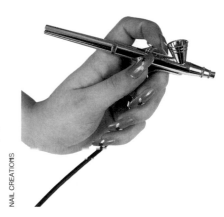

NAIL CREATIONS

A dual-action airbrush

Paint: The paint used in airbrushes for the purpose of nail art is usually water-based acrylic artists' paint that is the consistency of milk. Any thicker and it will keep blocking the equipment; any thinner and coverage will be a problem. Most of the paints available on the market are easily washed off skin with water. Therefore paint that is sprayed over the nail is sealed with a clear topcoat, like nail varnish, and the paint on the skin can be washed off when the sealer is dry. Some paints need to be removed from the skin with a nail varnish remover.

Cleaning the airbrush: Cleaning the airbrush is essential for efficient and correct working. It is something that many artists try to short cut and then they wonder why the airbrush will not work. The paint is air-dried and little flakes of it remain in the airbrush if cleaning is not done thoroughly. These flakes are then dislodged during use and block the nozzle. Flushing through between colours takes a very short time but, more importantly, thorough cleaning after use must be carried out. Manufacturers should supply cleaning instructions and these should be followed to the letter. Most 'broken' airbrushes are caused by:

1 Short-cut cleaning so they are blocked.

2 Short-cut cleaning so needles are removed and poked into nozzles to remove blockages. This results in bent and damaged needles and split nozzles!

For airbrushing beginners, practice and discovery are the keys to good work and enthusiasm. Every beginner should discover their own effects and colour mixes. It is very satisfying!

Techniques of layering colour

Before we look at layering colour, there are a small number of concepts regarding colour that need to be understood. Airbrushing is all about layering colour. Layering one colour on top of another will produce a different colour. This is an effect that will often be required. However, there will also be as many (if not more) occasions when the uppermost colour needs to be a true colour (as with stencil work). In order to achieve this, the lower colour must be covered up to produce a colour-free area. This is achieved by spraying white in the area to mask the lower colour. The top colour can then be added over the white.

EQUIPMENT LIST

- compressor
- air hose
- airbrush
- cleaning brush
- cleaning fluid
- cup of water
- empty paint bottle filled with water
- cleaning unit to spray unused paint and cleaner into (in the absence of a specifically designed unit, a paper cup with disposable towels in it will suffice or, even better, a small cardboard snack tube with disposable towels in it and a hole made in the plastic lid)

- plenty of waterproof protection on desk
- paper towels
- base coat
- topcoat/sealer
- selection of airbrush paints
- plastic tips
- Blu-Tack
- finger rest (optional)
- stencils

Techniques of airbrushing

We shall now look at the basic techniques of airbrushing. This is just the beginning: experimentation and practice (and time) are what produces a skilled artist.

The working area: The first step is to collect all the necessary equipment together and prepare a working area.

Loading and cleaning: Next, base coat plenty of tips ready to practise airbrushing (the paint will not adhere to a plain tip). Practicing loading the airbrush with colour and cleaning it out is very important and manufacturer's instructions should be followed. As a basic guideline the following steps can be taken:

1 Add your chosen colour of paint to a clean airbrush.

2 The paint needs to be 'blasted' through to get it to the nozzle quickly. The method of doing this will depend on the type of airbrush being used. The nozzle needs to be opened to its maximum to let as much paint through as possible and the air also needs to be at maximum strength. This should get the paint to the nozzle quickly. Spray the airbrush onto a disposable towel until the colour appears and then adjust the level of paint spray until there is a fine mist. (Paint should not be seen coming out of the airbrush. If the spray can be seen the level of paint is too high – that is, the nozzle is open too far.)

3 With the colour loaded, practice spraying a fine straight line of dense colour onto the towel by holding the airbrush close to the surface (1). Then practice spraying a thicker, less dense line by holding the airbrush a bit further away. Adjust the amount of paint mixing with the air. Try this several times until you are aware of how the control of air and the control of paint, together with the distance the airbrush is from the surface, affects the results. Far better results are achieved if the colour is built up with several layers rather than trying to create an intense colour immediately.

4 Now practice cleaning in between colours. This should be a very quick process (major cleaning must take place at the end of the session). Spray all the remaining paint into your cup. Add clean water to the airbrush and spray it into your cup. Repeat this a few times until all paint is flushed through. It may be necessary to flush through some of the recommended cleaning fluid. Dip your cleaning brush in water and clean the end of the nozzle to remove any flakes of dried paint that have collected there.

5 Once all the paint has been cleaned away, a new colour can be added.

6 At the end of the session, a thorough clean must be carried out. The manufacturer's instructions for this should be followed, as each airbrush has different removable parts. Never leave your airbrush without this thorough cleaning as it can make the equipment unusable.

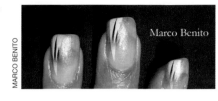

An airbrushed design

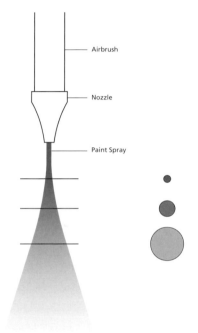

(1) Distance management of airbrush

Gradient blends

- Choose three complementary colours, and have the bottles ready.

- Place at least four base-coated tips on a towel, using Blu-Tack to secure them.

- Get the flow of paint correct by spraying on the towel and then carry the spray across a corner of one of the tips to create a diagonal stripe. Do not spray too close to the tip. Keep spraying across the corner until the colour intensity is dense in the corner but decreasing in density as it goes closer to the centre of the tip. Repeat this on the next tip as a horizontal line, then on the next as a vertical. Finally, try to create small patches of colour on the fourth tip.

- Repeat this on other tips until you achieve lines of colour that are denser on the outer edge than in the centre.

- Clean out the paint and load the next colour.

Diagonal

Horizontal

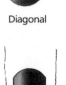
Vertical

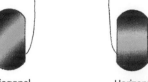
Mixed

Gradient blends

- Spray a line of the new colour close to the first one, but making the dense colour in the centre of the line. Where the thinner colour overlays the first colour there should be another colour created as the two colours mix.

- Repeat for all other tips.

- Repeat the process with the third colour until you have tips with three colours blended on them in various ways.

Overlap

Overlap

Soft Blow

Hard Blow

Double Blow

Double Blow

Triple Blow

Triple Blow

Graduation

Graduation

Overspray

Basing the Background

This technique is often used as a base for many designs in airbrushing, hand painting and other nail art techniques. It is the basis of airbrushing and it is worth spending time mastering it.

Stencils   Stencils are pre-cut shapes in a thin plastic sheet. They can be abstract shapes or specific shapes. The stencil can have shapes cut into the plastic forming holes that the paint is sprayed through, or shapes cut out of the side of the plastic.

There are many ways a stencil can be used. It is not just a case of spraying a blast of paint through a hole. First the stencil must be held properly. A nail curves in two directions and the stencil must be held in such a way that allows for these curves. It must also be held so that you can see what you are doing.

The stencil must be held from the top, away from you so you are not covering your work. Choose the shape of image you want to use; if you are right-handed, you will need to use your left hand (as your right is holding the airbrush); hold your forefinger and middle finger together, then bring your ring finger and thumb together; it is with these fingers that you will need to hold the stencil. Put your ring and middle fingers on one side of the chosen image and your ring finger and thumb on the other side and bring the two sides together. This will make the stencil bend slightly, creating a curve that will sit closely on the nail. Try this a few times until you feel reasonably comfortable holding a stencil.

Have plenty of base-coated tips ready. It is easier if you now use a finger rest and secure the tip onto it. Try holding a stencil on a nail and spraying a colour. See how you get on and keep trying until you can control both the stencil and the airbrush and get reasonable results. Now you are ready to try some stencil techniques:

- *Overlap*. Choose a shape from the centre of the stencil (not the edge) and hold it closely on the nail. Spray. With a different colour, place the same shape on the stencil against the first colour but slightly overlapping and spray. Or choose a shape from the edge of the stencil and repeat the same process.

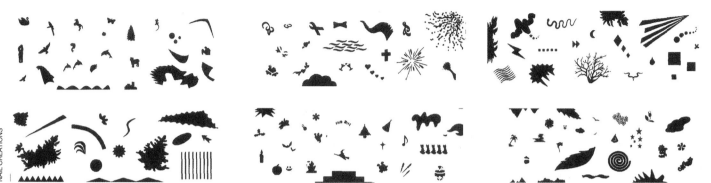

NAIL CREATIONS

Selection of stencils

- *Soft blow*. Hold an image very slightly above the nail and gently spray. The shape produced should have soft edges.

- *Hard blow*. Hold the same image closely on the nail and spray with several layers to build up the intensity of colour. This should produce a strong colour with sharp edges.

- *Double blow*. This is where two colours are used in the one image or shape. The stencil needs to be replaced in exactly the same place to apply the second colour.

- *Triple blow*. The same principle as above, but with three colours.

- *Graduation*. This is similar to the principle of blended colours, but includes the use of a stencil. The image or shape is moved slightly and another colour added.

- *Overspray*. If an image is chosen from the centre of the stencil and the paint is concentrated around the edges, it will produce an image that is pale in the centre and more intense at the edges.

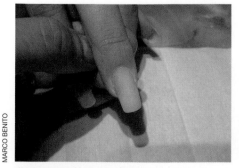

MARCO BENITO

Base the prepared nail with a thin layer of white paint

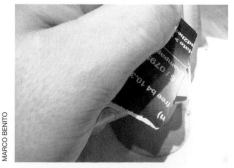

MARCO BENITO

Hold a piece of jagged edge paper at an angle on one side and spray dense white paint

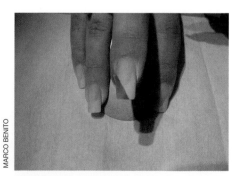

MARCO BENITO

Spray orange in the same way on the other edge

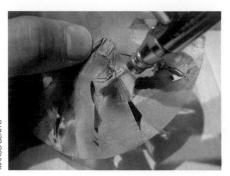

MARCO BENITO

Choose part of a stencil and spray with orange on the white area and white on the orange area

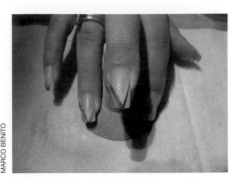

MARCO BENITO

Mist the whole nails with a shimmer white

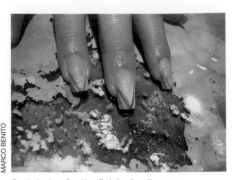

MARCO BENITO

Seal design for the finished nail

- *Basing the background*. This is one of the most important techniques and basic concepts in airbrushing. It is needed if a colour is going to be sprayed over another colour. If this is done without basing the first colour, the two will mix to create a third-colour variation. If the second colour needs to be true this technique must be used. Choose the image for the second colour and place closely on the nail. Spray white until the base colour is covered. Change to the second colour and place the stencil in exactly the same place as before and spray.

Other accessories: Other accessories can be used to create wonderful effects.

As an alternative to ready-made stencils, there is a product called Frisket Film, a sticky-backed plastic that can be used as a mask. This can be cut into any shape with a sharp scalpel and placed onto a nail that has a base colour. Colours can be sprayed over the whole nail and then the film removed. Where the film covered the nail, the base colour will show through. (Striping tape can be used for this. Several strips laid close together and then colours blended over the top look very effective when the tape is removed.)

Another useful accessory is lace. Apply a base colour to the nail. Hold a piece of lace on the nail and base it with white; then spray a second colour and remove the lace. The result is always a surprise.

Thick, fibrous paper can also be very useful if a small piece of it is roughly torn across, a jagged edge will be formed. This edge is ideal for creating effects like clouds (overspray white, move the paper to a different angle and repeat), mountain scenery or sea.

Collection of airbrushed designs using a variety of stencils

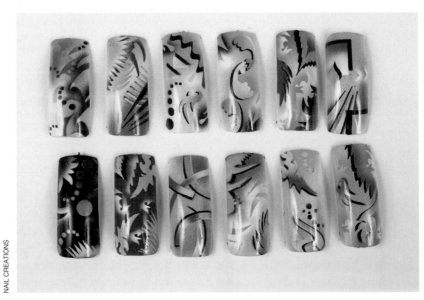

NAIL CREATIONS

French manicure

Airbrushing is a very quick method of applying colour to nails. Some salons have dispensed with traditional nail varnish applications and use their airbrushes entirely.

One excellent application is to provide a 'French manicure' for clients by airbrushing the white tip. Stencils are available that concentrate on these shapes. Various-sized curves, for different finger sizes, and other shapes can create the perfect 'French' smile line without the often bulky white varnish that has a tendency to chip.

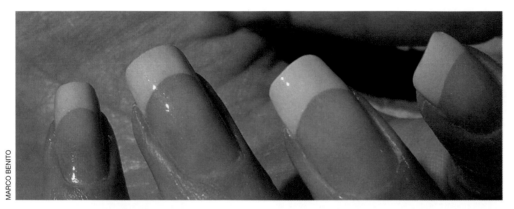

An example of a short nail with airbrushed French

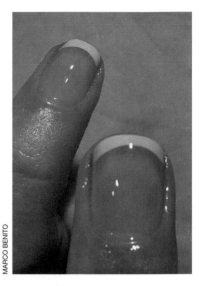

An example of a long nail with airbrushed French

Like all nail art, the limit of airbrushing is the imagination and airbrush artists who practice are capable of creating stunning and original designs that, of course, can help to earn them a good income.

Embedding

Embedding is an interesting technique that does have a place in a commercial salon as it is effective and relatively fast to do. It also has a great advantage for the client: unlike other types of nail art which are as temporary as nail varnish, embedding is much more permanent and, depending on the design, can last many weeks. This will make the additional cost more attractive to the client, particularly if they wear artificial nails anyway.

As the term suggests, things are embedded in the overlay of the nail where they are held and protected by the product. The nature of nails means that any item for embedding must be very small and flat, otherwise the result would be a very ungainly nail. Both liquid and powder and UV gel systems are suitable for this technique (a fibre system would work only if a very thick resin were to be used). UV gel would not be suitable for very delicate items as they are very sticky and it would be difficult not to move a delicate item (such as a feather) once it had been placed.

Ideas for embedding are limited only by imagination (and of course your client's preferences!) together with their size. Craft shops can be a good source of inspiration as can looking around you every day. There are many shapes and sizes everywhere that are small and flat enough to be used. For example, look in a sewing box: threads placed in various shapes, eyelets, pieces of fabric, etc. Look in the kitchen: cooking foil can be cut into shapes. Look on your dressing table: links of broken chains, bits of earrings.

HEALTH & SAFETY

All the relevant health and safety, working practices, client consultation and preparation steps are essential for every application of this kind.

TOP TIP

Make sure any item to be used is perfectly clean before using. Spray with an antiseptic and allow to dry before use.

SOME IDEAS	
polish secures	metal thread
gold or silver leaf	metal chains
Feathers	leaves
Fabrics	lace

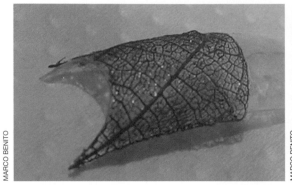

MARCO BENITO

Leaf applied to a clear tip

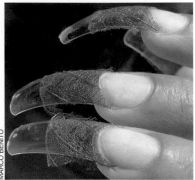

MARCO BENITO

Prepared tips applied to nails

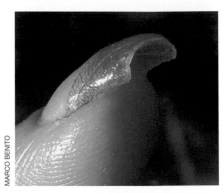

MARCO BENITO

Tips cut, shaped and overlay applied

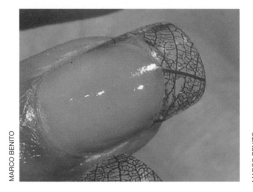

MARCO BENITO

Overlay refined and buffed

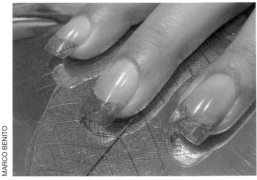

MARCO BENITO

The finished nail

Procedure: Have everything ready to hand before starting.

1 The item to be embedded needs a base before it can be embedded. This can be a plastic tip blended onto a nail, a clear tip so the item can be more visible or a thin base built onto a form of white, clear or coloured product. Prepare the nail in the same way as you would for an artificial nail application and apply the tip or sculpt a thin base.

2 Apply a very small amount of adhesive to the nail (if UV gel is being used, the sticky layer will do the same job) to hold the item in place.

3 Pick up the item using tweezers and place on the nail, using the tweezers to move it into the correct place and flatten it if necessary. Do not use your fingers.

4 Very gently apply a clear overlay, pressing it into the item to make sure all gaps are filled and no air bubbles remain. Ensure that the overlay has the correct curves and is of a sufficient thickness to embed the item after it has been refined and buffed.

5 Finish the nail as usual.

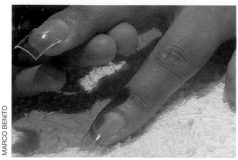

Clear tips applied

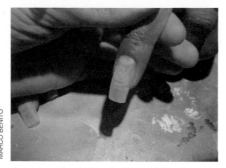

Clear tips blended ready for overlay

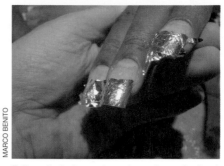

Foil applied after an irregular pattern of adhesive applied to tips

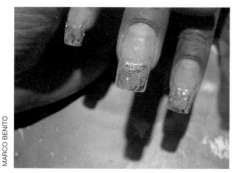

Foil removed to leave pattern on tip

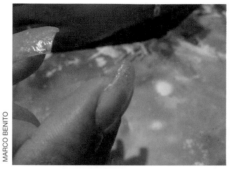

Overlay applied over silver

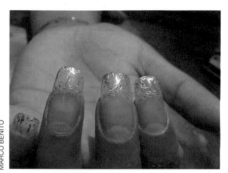

The finished nail

Alternatives   If an item or product to be used is for the free edge only (for example fabric, foil or polish secures) it is possible to apply it to the tip after the contact area has been removed but before applying to the nail.

All the usual aftercare advice and maintenance rules apply to this service. Obviously, the embedded items will grow with the nail and get to a stage where there is no alternative but to remove the artificial nail or buff the overlay off and remove the item.

However much your client wants to keep her design, do not allow the artificial nail to become unbalanced and therefore likely to cause damage to the natural nail for the sake of a piece of nail art.

Coloured overlays

Many of the liquid and powder and UV gel product companies are bringing out their products in many different colours. Like the embedding technique, this has a good advantage for the client in that the designs last much longer.

Warning: A word of warning when using opaque coloured powders or gels on the nail plate: lifting of the overlay or the beginning of any other problem cannot be seen due to the opacity of the overlay. Ideally, the opaque coloured overlay should not be left on for longer than 2 to 3 weeks in case it is hiding a problem that needs immediate attention. This obviously does not apply to transparent coloured overlays.

Every rule that applies to the relevant application of artificial nails also applies to this technique and it is important for every technician to remember that. Just because it is nail art does not mean that any short cuts can be taken.

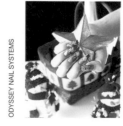

Liquid and powder products with coloured powders

TOP TIP

It is possible, with clever designing, to keep the design through several maintenance visits if the design can be added to the re-growth area without spoiling the effect.

Semi-permanent polish

ALWAYS REMEMBER

Very important: the theory of zones and the stress area must apply to this application too. The finished nail must be balanced and have the correct curves.

The only difference between this technique and that of an overlay or sculpted nail is the sequence of application. Instead of each zone being applied in sequence, in the case of liquid and powder, and the sculpted overlay, in the case of UV gel, the overlay is applied in colours.

There must be a very clear idea of the design, if not a coloured drawing prepared, before starting. The sequence of the coloured application is important. In the case of liquid and powder, the time taken is important as the acrylic will start to cure immediately and UV gels need curing in between applications if sharp definition is needed.

Some wonderful effects can be created by even the least artistic technician using this technique. Blends of colours with or without the use of glitter powders over clear tips can look stunning and are as easy to do as a usual overlay. Or pick up more than one colour acrylic powder on the brush, apply to the nail and see what happens.

Semi-permanent polish

Coloured gels are successfully being used as a semi-permanent polish. All the rules and cautions apply, but the application will last much longer than usual polish and can be infilled if the client still wants to keep the same colour.

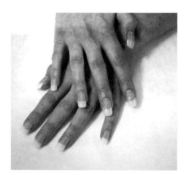

Nails prepared for coloured overlay

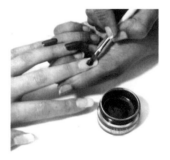

Paint a thin layer of coloured gel, taking care to create neat edges

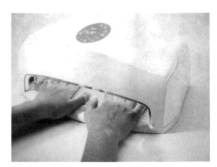

Cure for the recommended time

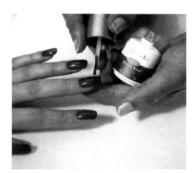

Apply sealer and cure for the recommended time

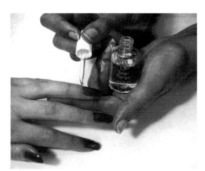

Remove sticky layer and apply cuticle oil

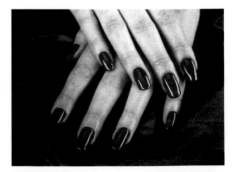

Finished nails

Designs using coloured acrylic powders and UV Gels

Step-by-step autumn nails using coloured L&P

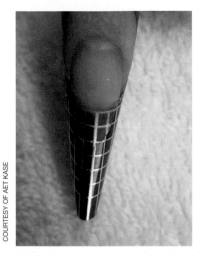

COURTESY OF AET KASE

(1) Start by sculpting a clear free edge with an extended nail plate in opaque powder

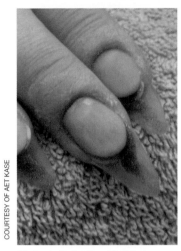

COURTESY OF AET KASE

(2) Apply first coloured glitter

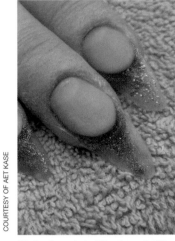

COURTESY OF AET KASE

(3) Continue to build coloured glitters

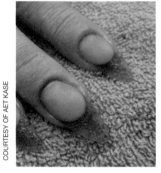

COURTESY OF AET KASE

(4) Cover whole nail with clear layer and refine shape with 240 grit file

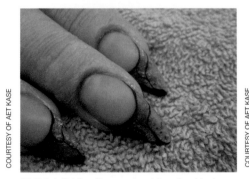

COURTESY OF AET KASE

(5) Paint dividing lines and swirls using black acrylic water-based paint and allow to dry

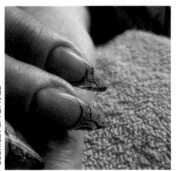

COURTESY OF AET KASE

(6) Seal with gloss polish or a UV topcoat

Step-by-step 'sunny stones'

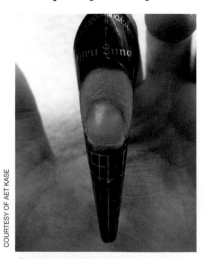

COURTESY OF AET KASE

Start by sculpting a clear free edge

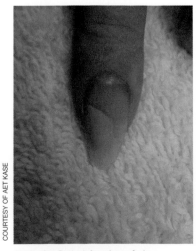

COURTESY OF AET KASE

Apply the first pink colour, fade towards the free edge

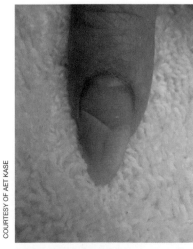

COURTESY OF AET KASE

Apply second pink the same way as first

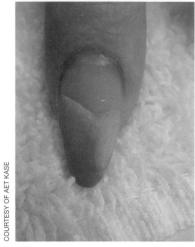

Apply third pink faded from free edge towards the other pinks

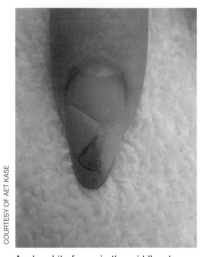

Apply a bit of grey in the middle where pinks meet

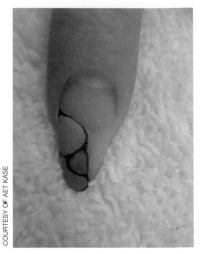

Draw the outlines of the stones with black acrylic/watercolour paint. Only to one side, leave the other empty

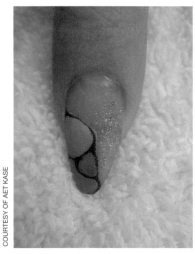

Apply glitter mix and fade

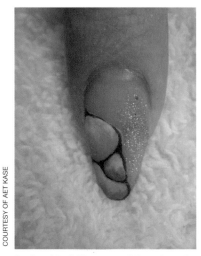

Apply white L&P on top of the colours but only to the 'upper' side. That's where the sun is shining and it leaves a kind of shadow effect

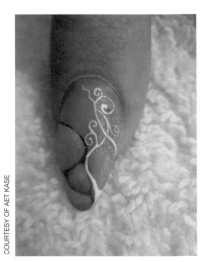

Cover with clear and file to shape

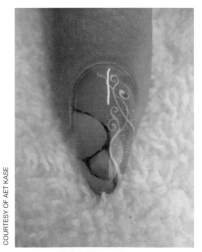

Draw the swirls with white gel/acrylic paint, whatever you like best. Cure if you used gel. For me the white swirls make the stones sunnier

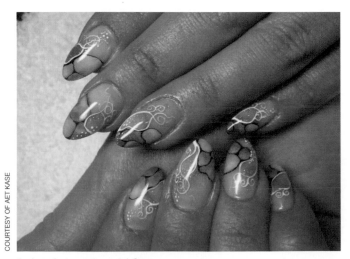

And apply top gel, ready! Cure

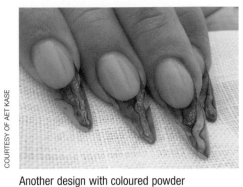

Another design with coloured powder

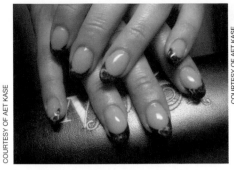

An example of nails using coloured gels

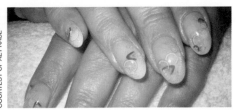

A nail design using Fimo Art Canes (the fruits are thinly sliced from a long 'cane' and applied under UV gel or L&P)

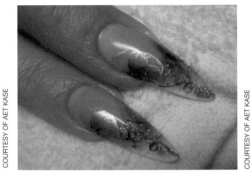

A fabulous gold stiletto using L&P and acrylic paints

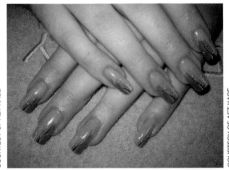

A pink design using similar techniques with some polish secures

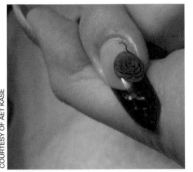

Nail design using a 3D rose sculpted and painted by hand and applied to finished nail design

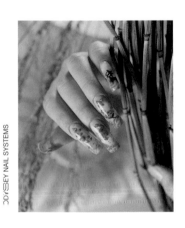
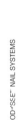
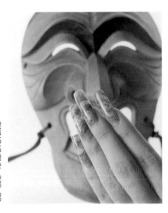
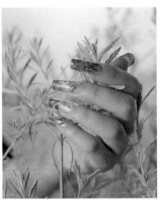

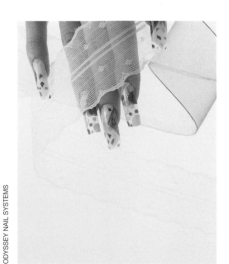
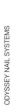
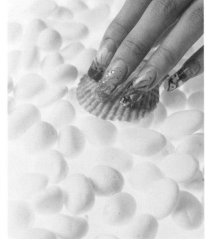

Step-by-step for stiletto nails

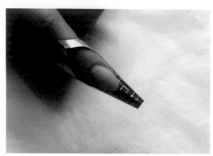

(1) To start this design of stiletto nail, first create a tapered nail with a skin tone opaque overlay (sculpt or tip and overlay for this) and fit a form under it as shown.

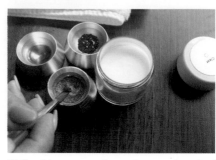

(2) For this we are using a clear powder mixed with pink holographic acrylic powder, large pink holographic sparkles and a clear powder

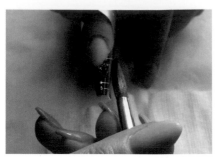

(3) Pick up a medium bead of the pink powder and dip it into the sparkles to pick up a few. Place the bead on the form and start to create one side of the stiletto

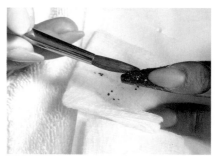

(4) In the same way build the other side of the stiletto

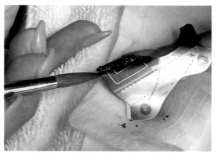

(5) Lengthen the tip and create the point that is in perfect alignment with the finger. Notice that the stiletto at this stage is lower than the free edge of the nail

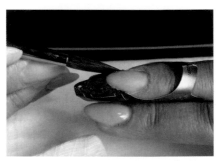

(6) Apply a layer of clear over the stiletto and take a thin layer over the whole nail. Check the structure from all angles

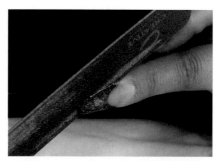

(7) Using a 240 grit file, refine and shape the sides

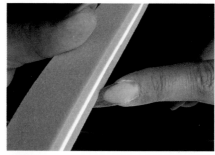

(8) Using a 240 grit buffer (or finer) shape and refine the whole nail

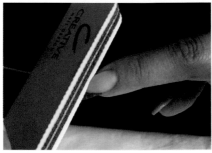

(9) Shine the nail with a three-way buffer or a glosser and apply nail oil

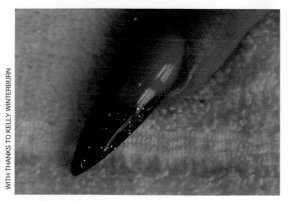

(10) The finished nail!

WITH THANKS TO KELLY WINTERBURN

3D nail art

This is a technique that really is based on ideas rather than professional technique. A creative technician who understands the medium in which they work can create amazing shapes. The base of the nail can be shaped before any overlay is applied to give it a different facet of design.

The simplest way of achieving this is to take a plastic tip, remove the contact area and cut shapes into it with scissors or drill holes and other shapes through it. When you are happy with the shape achieved, buff off the rough edges with a block buffer or file. It is then ready to apply to a natural nail and be overlaid.

Cut-outs on tips are not necessarily practical for clients in a commercial salon but may, rarely, be requested for a special occasion. If this is the case and the client wants to keep them on for a period of time, apply the shaped tip to the nail and apply a strong overlay, taking care to follow the cut-out shape. Where holes have been made, the same drill bit can be used to clean them up.

The shaped tip can be applied to the nail and blended in for a more temporary arrangement, for example, media work or a competition. It can then have a thin overlay applied in any system just to keep it in place. This can be done for speed and ease of removal.

When the shaped tip is in place, any amount of additions can be made: coloured acrylics or gels, polish secures of all kinds, paint, fabrics, etc. This is another design idea limited only by imagination.

This is a technique that utilizes the properties of liquid and powder and UV gel systems and even additional accessories like lace, feathers, etc. As its title suggests, it is creating designs that are in three dimensions and stand proud of the nail. This is a technique that is not so practical in commercial salons, but may be useful for a special occasion and for technicians who want to receive recognition from their peers in nail art competitions.

For a technician who understands the medium in which they work and knows all the necessary health and safety regulations, client care and consultation and correct working practices, this is a subject that only needs the input of ideas rather than teaching. There is no right or wrong way once the basics of nail technology are understood and carried out.

TOP TIP

If using an electrical drill, all the usual regulations for electrical equipment apply. Keep your fingers away from the drill and make sure your hair is tied back if long.

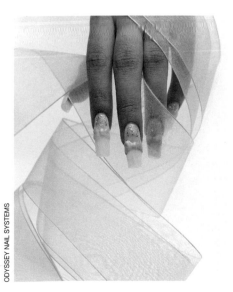

Design of coloured acrylics with cut-outs

3D nails

ODYSSEY NAIL SYSTEMS

There are very few technicians who want to take their craft and skill to the extreme lengths of this type of nail art and even fewer clients who require the service. From an employment point of view, this skill will not make a technician more employable than one without it. A good and intelligent technician who truly understands their products and their application could work out how to create the real fantasy of 3D nail art. For the right technician, it is fun, supremely creative and essential if high level competitions are to be entered.

There is the rare occasion when this type of nail art is required for media work in the commercial world and, as long as safety is observed for all concerned, anything goes!

Competition nail art

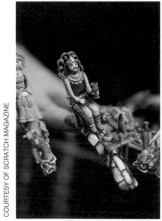

Nails by Claudia Valli (Switzerland) 2nd place Division 3 The Nailympics London 2009

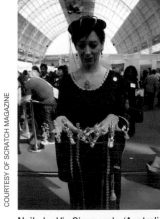

Nails by Claudia Valli (Switzerland) 2nd place Division 3 The Nailympics London 2009

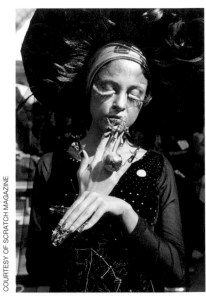

Oksana Bobrova

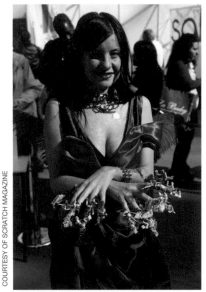

Nails by Viv Simmonds (Australia) 1st Place Division 3, The Nailympics London 2010

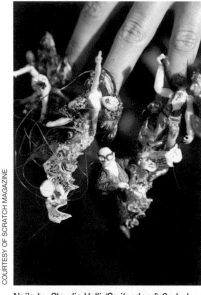

Nails by Viv Simmonds (Australia) 1st Place Division 3, The Nailympics London 2010

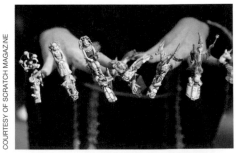

Nails by Viv Simmonds (Australia) 1st Place Division 3, The Nailympics London 2010

Veneers

A relatively new concept in decorating both finger and toenails, veneers, are, with a bit of practice, a very easy and cost-effective service for clients. There are versions that are available for the retail market but these are not as successful and effective as a good professional application.

The professional versions require heat (at approximately 110 °C) to activate the adhesive before application and then a lower level of heat to keep the veneer pliable for a perfect result. This is especially important when sealing them onto the edge of the nail as otherwise they will lift.

Removal also needs heat in order to easily peel them from the nail without causing any damage to the upper layers of the nail plate. When removing them, apply a small amount of heat to the nails, lift a corner of the veneer and peel them away from the nail (DO NOT FORCE) from the sides, not from the cuticle area.

Veneers will last a long time on the toenails but it is not recommended leaving them on for more than 4 to 6 weeks.

COURTESY OF SCRATCH MAGAZINE

Nails by Viv Simmonds (Australia)
1st Place Division 3, The Nailympics
London 2010

Nail 'veneers'

This is a relatively new concept that gives nail professionals an added service to apply a choice of many different designs to the nails. Minx was the first company to launch the concept and it is a film that has an incorporated polymer adhesive. Heat activates the adhesive. The service will last several weeks on the toes and 4 to 8 days on the fingers.

With a bit of practice it is a quick and easy service. It is essential that the nail professional uses an infrared light source and the 'veneers' need to be heated until they are very hot! A lower heat level is then used to mould them onto the nail for a smooth and crease-free finish.

To remove them, heat needs to be applied before they can be peeled off.

Step-by-step nail 'veneers'

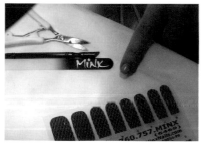

(1) The nails should be prepared by removing any cuticle on the nail plate and then dehydrated to ensure a good bond. Have all the necessary tools ready and give the client a variety of designs to choose from.

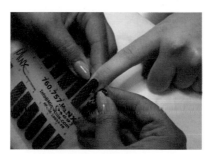

(2) Take the sheet of 'veneers' and place on the nail plate in order to choose the correct size.

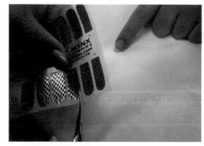

(3) If the nearest size is slightly too wide, pre-tailor it (or wait until it is on the nail and use very fine stork scissors very carefully).

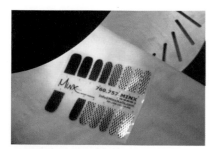

(4) Place the sheet under the lamp for a few seconds.

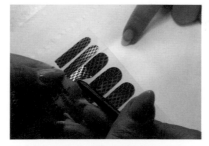

(5) Lift the appropriate 'veneer' from the sheet using the end of a hoof stick (it is better not to touch the adhesive).

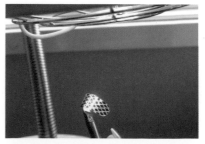

(6) Hold the 'veneer' under the lamp for a few seconds until it becomes soft. This is when the adhesive is activated.

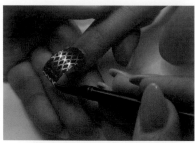

(7) Place the rounded end on the base of the nail as close as possible to the skin.

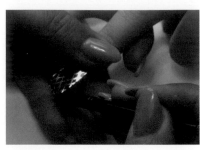

(8) When the 'veneer' is correctly positioned hold in place with your thumb while you remove the hoof stick.

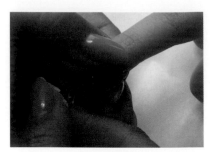

(9) While still holding in place gently pull the 'veneer' over the whole nail.

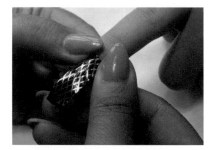

(10) Using your thumbs smooth the 'veneer' so it attaches firmly to the sides of the nail without creases (if there are any creases it can be lifted again and smoothed down).

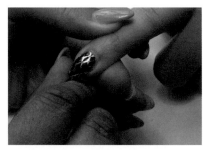

(11) Gently pull the end of the 'veneer' so it fits tightly around and over the free edge. Leave it in place and move on to the next nail.

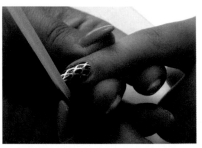

(12) With the file angled under the free edge gently file away the excess. If the free edge is long enough it is better to file down from the edge.

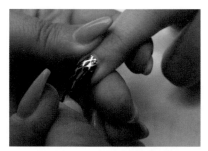

(13) With the finger under the lamp smooth the edges with a hoof stick to make sure they are secure and there are no creases. Mould the free edge with your thumb.

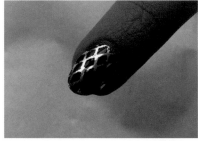

(14) The nail is then finished and needs nothing further. Nail oil can be applied and this will not affect the 'veneer' if it has been applied correctly.

Summary

This chapter has provided information on how to prepare and promote nail art services. It moves from simple steps in nail art to advanced techniques, including airbrushing and embedding.

14

Media work and special occasions

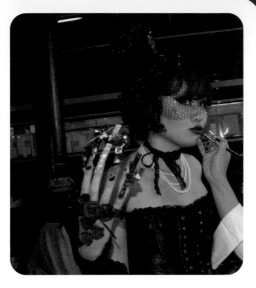

Me gumi Mizuno creates the Fantasy complete look for The Nailympics London 2010

Learning objectives

In this chapter you find out about:

- opportunities for special occasion work as a salon-based technician

- the type of technician suitable for work in the media

- how to start out in the media

- how to create images in preparation for this work

- the roles in media work

- usual technician activities in media work, procedures and tips

- how to plan and provide a nail service for fashion shows

- how images can be created from a brief.

Introduction

As described in the introductory chapter, there are opportunities for technicians to use their skills outside the salon. These could be in connection with the salon, for example, a wedding party might like their nails done at the bride's home, or a local fashion show where the salon can be represented. But there are also opportunities for technicians to use their skills to complement other creative disciplines. Examples of these opportunities could be:

- Fashion shows with designers, hair artists and make-up artists.

- Photographic work for advertising or editorial pictures.

- Visiting technicians (different from a mobile technician).

For straightforward home visits, for example for a wedding party, the usual arrangements for a mobile technician would apply:

- have a full, safe and hygienic kit

- have protection for your client's furniture

- have appropriate insurance for your car (even if you are connected to a salon, the journey and carrying of a kit needs different insurance)

- have an understanding of what is required of you

- leave sufficient time for the journey there and back (especially if you have more clients booked after the visit).

However, this chapter is more concerned with the role of the technician in a commercial media setting, how to create the opportunities, how to maximize them, how to behave, the roles of other people, tips on how to create the various looks, etc. This area of work has definitely developed into a career where very good living can be made by the right person. The main part of the chapter will deal with the higher profile and wider media work as this is such a growing area. However, there are plenty of opportunities for similar work but look for local opportunities, for example:

- local photographers who often use a make-up artist for portrait and commercial work

- freelance make-up artists may need help with nails

- wedding shops who offer a wide range of services to their customers.

A good way to approach this type of work is to have a form of business card made up with a few images of your work. With the latest technology, this need not be expensive. especially with digital cameras. These cards can be taken to various appropriate local businesses and either left for their customers to pick up or used by way of an introduction for you. When creating images for this type of card, try to have a range of examples of your skills, for example, natural nails, artificial nails and nail art.

Media work

A technician doing this type of work should be experienced in all the other areas this book covers, that is:

- healthy and safety issues

- correct handling and storage of products

- **contra-indications** and contra-actions

- a thorough understanding of all relevant products and how to use them correctly and efficiently

- recognition of nail and skin conditions

- providing manicure and pedicure treatments

- application of artificial nails

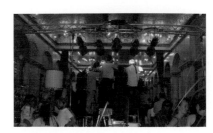

The media at a fashion show

- various nail art techniques

- client care and communication.

In other words, this type of work is not for the complete beginner! It is also important to:

- have the right professional attitude

- be a fast worker

- be able to come up with creative ideas on the spur of the moment

- work as part of a team

- be adaptable to work situations

- be calm

- not be easily upset or hurt

- not be 'precious'!

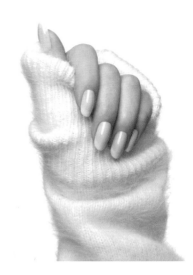

COURTESY: CREATIVE NAIL DESIGN INC

Media work has been around as long as there have been the various media – television, film, newspapers and magazines. Everyone is aware that every actor, presenter, model and celebrity has someone for 'hair and make-up'. Manicurists have often been around, especially in films but not nearly as many as there are hairdressers and make-up artists. This is a situation that is changing and it is much more common for a manicurist to be part of the team now. (It will be a long time before the role is called anything other than a manicurist!)

Hairdressers may be connected to a salon, but most hairdressers in this type of work are specialist 'sessions' hairdressers who only do media work. Many specialize further and only do film or television work or even further specialize in wig making.

Make-up is an essential part of media work and, usually, this is done by a make-up artist who does nothing else. Sometimes they come from stores where they work for specific make-up houses, but usually they specialize in media work only and, like the hairdressers, may only work in film or TV.

It is in this sector that opportunities are opening up more and more for nail technicians. It is quite difficult work to get into and, realistically, it takes some time before earnings are good. But the earning capacity is limitless once a high level of work is reached.

As a general guideline, media work is something like this:

1 *Photographic work* falls into two categories: advertising and editorial.

- *Advertising*: this is work where everyone concerned is paid a daily rate. The rate is agreed at the time of booking and there may or may not be an overtime fee paid at an hourly rate. This is where sessions people (artists) earn the majority of their income. A technician could earn anything between £100 and £1000+ a day. (Good potential pay, but not compared with a top sessions hairdresser who can earn £5000+ per day.) Very few people know who works on specific advertising campaigns as it is not broadcast but neither is it a secret. This work usually follows a relatively strict brief and a sessions team will be booked for their ability and skill to interpret that brief and work well together. Sometimes, individuals are booked because their creativity will bring an extra dimension to the result and their input into the finished images will make a difference.

- *Editorial*: this is work for publications where the names of those creating the image are printed (or credited). Often but not always, individuals are expected to bring their own ideas to make the images more conceptual. This work does not pay! What it does is provide artists with the medium to demonstrate their skills and artistry; all those interested will know who they are and will, hopefully, book them for advertising work. Some of the more glamorous publications pay a small amount of money for this work but it is necessary for all artists to build a reputation and portfolio of work.

2   *TV advertising*. This is very similar to photographic advertising in levels of payment, but it has a different set of rules for working conditions, mostly in terms of hours worked and breaks taken. This is a good form of income and hours can usually be more reliable.

3   *Film work*. Like TV, this has strict working times but can be a guaranteed job for large chunks of time. The big downside, however, is that it involves a lot of hanging around doing nothing.

4   *Fashion shows*. Unfortunately, there is not a great deal of money in fashion (very surprisingly!) and reasonable payment for a fashion show is rare but not unheard of. Payment will depend on how much in demand the artist and their team is. The more usual arrangement is via sponsorship where a company pay the artists to 'do' the show. This may be just the expenses incurred or it may be this plus a little extra for them. Sometimes a company will sponsor a designer to allow their artists to be involved. In return for this, the company can get press coverage for their products. It is an arrangement that suits all but generates little in the way of earnings for the artists. What it does do, however, is get the artists in situations where their skills can be seen. Networking is essential for progress.

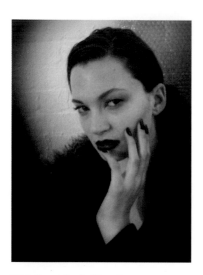

Backstage at a fashion show

> ## ❝ ANECDOTE
>
> As an example of the hours that can sometimes be worked, I have worked on several high profile campaigns and specific numbers of days are booked for the job. The required number of images must be achieved and this is an industry where every individual strives for perfection. My worst ever job in terms of hours worked was a 5-day job with a start time of 9.30am each morning. The finish times for each day went something like this: midnight, 1am, midnight, 2am, 5am. What a 'killer', but the overtime pay was great at double time for every hour after 8 hours!

How to get work in this area

This is rather a chicken and egg situation: a technician needs examples of work to get more work, but cannot get examples without doing the work in the first place!

This is the case for everyone in the industry. Models need to have a portfolio of pictures before they get any work, so 'test' pictures need to be taken at their own expense in order to demonstrate how they look in front of a camera and how versatile they can be.

Those artists who want to work in the image industry need to prove what they can do and need a similar 'book'. A traditional way for hair and make-up artists is to try to assist a working artist in order to gain experience and meet people. This can also work for technicians, as there are now many technicians who work in this field.

Agencies exist that specialize in booking artists for media work. These usually specialize further into areas of media, for example, those that book film work are different from fashion and beauty work. These agencies have a list of artists whom they represent and, depending on the flexibility and popularity of the individual artists, may cover many aspects of media work.

Agencies can be a good starting place for a technician wanting to work in this area. Many agencies now have technicians among their artists or would like to do so. There may be opportunities to assist a working technician and eventually progress to working in their own right. A technician who can produce a good portfolio of images, either genuine or as a series of test pictures, should get a good response from the right agency.

As with any research, a good place to start looking for relevant agencies is on the Internet where a search on hair and make-up agencies should turn up a list. To date there is no agency specializing in nail technicians and the association with other artists is very valuable.

Central to the success of a technician working in any media or special occasion work is their portfolio of images. If a technician is serious in pursuing this area it is worth spending time and money on the creation of a portfolio or 'book'. If these do not occur naturally in the work a technician already does, they must be created and, like the suggestion of a business card earlier in the chapter, they should show a variety of skills.

A good place to start in order to get ideas is the glossy magazines. If you are hoping to earn money from this work then think 'commercial' and see what is used in popular magazines. Also look in the more 'trendy' magazines as these may have images and ideas that are more avant garde. Look at the adverts for fashion and beauty products, in fact any advert that has hands visible. Also look at the fashion and beauty features, as these are important for artists.

Start to plan your portfolio by thinking about the number of pictures and what each image will be. Five or six should be sufficient to start with and these need to show a variety of images and the range of your skills. It is certainly worth getting these pictures taken by a photographer as good pictures of hands and nails are more difficult to achieve than you may think. If you have a digital camera, it is definitely worth experimenting with styling, angles of the hands, lighting, etc. Many high street digital photography printers offer the service of improving digital imaging for a relatively low cost. This would only include things like cropping and colour or lighting improvement, so the image must be good to begin with. Any work that is more involved starts to cost a great deal more money.

Once you have a small collection of images you are ready to approach the many avenues leading to media work.

In addition to the suggestions already given, some others could be:

- Nail magazines. They are always looking for new talent and new pictures. If you already have a stunning picture they may like it for a cover!

- It may be worth contacting the beauty and fashion editors of magazines (their names and the addresses are always inside the magazine). They usually book artists through agencies but sometimes are looking for someone different and would be willing to give a technician a try.

On any media job, whether it is photographic or filming, the technician is part of the team that is there for the model or actor (the person being photographed or filmed is often called the 'talent'). This usually comprises hair, make-up, nails and styling. Depending on the type of shoot, there can be many, many other people. On film work, the numbers can go into

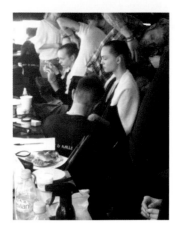

Backstage at a fashion show with nail techs fighting for a bit of space

TOP TIP

You will find that there are many, many more images of nails that are natural or meant to look natural, painted or unpainted, than there are of the more avant garde. Remember that the general media needs to appeal to a very wide audience and that is where the most opportunities for work are found.

 ANECDOTE

A very famous supermodel who now earns millions first started at the age of 16. She had her 'book' of test pictures and went to over 40 castings and 'go-sees' in a strange city on her own. At every place the person she saw flicked quickly through her five pictures, did not even look up at her and dismissed her. She didn't know how to get a bus or train to the next place and no money for a taxi. A very sad but very common story and the majority of young girls do not make it. This one did – and how!

the hundreds, but the technician is not concerned with the vast majority. Occasionally, if a shoot is for hands only, the number involved is drastically reduced, although still may include a stylist and make-up artist.

A guide to the roles that a technician may be involved with:

- *Photographer*. An obvious job, but one of the most important ones. Very often photographers use the same team for most or all of their work. They will certainly have a say in who works on each job. This is not so true in the case of filming as the team is so big.

- *1st, 2nd, 3rd Assistants*. Assistants to the photographer, who can have any number. There are usually between one and three on photographic shoots. Filming involves many different roles assisting the photographer.

- *Art director*. The person concerned with the overall image and how the finished result will look. They work in close conjunction with the photographer.

- *Production*. All filming and most photographic shoots have a production team. These people are responsible for all the logistics of the shoot from booking all the personnel, arranging travel, getting film processed, organizing catering and much, much more. Production people usually know the answer to most things!

- *Make-up artist*. Together with the hairdresser and technician, the make-up artist is part of the small team that creates the 'look' for the model. The nail technician needs to work closely with the make-up artist as the look for the nails must work with the make-up. For example, maybe the nail colour needs to match the lipstick, or the make-up look is very natural so it would usually follow that the nails would need to be also. The make-up artist will often have one or several assistants depending on the job.

The make-up artist is usually responsible for any make-up that needs to go on the hands or feet, but the technician should be prepared with moisturisers and some foundation, especially for a hand or a foot shot.

Almost all make-up artists go on set to keep an eye on the make-up and tidy it up between pictures.

- *Hairdresser*. An obvious role but part of the team central to the model. There will often be an assistant too. The hairdresser will be on set to keep the hair looking perfect and maybe use a wind machine to give the hair some movement.

- *Stylist*. This is the person who arranges all the clothes and accessories for the model. They will decide, in conjunction with the client, the photographer, art director and any other relevant person, what the model will wear. This needs to work with the hair, make-up and nails and it will depend on the subject of the job as to which is decided first. For example, in a commercial for a hair product the hairstyle will be decided first and the styling and overall look will need to fit around that. A fashion shoot will be centred around the fashion so the hair, make-up and nails need to follow that look. The stylist in a shoot for a magazine article will often be the Editor of that section of the magazine, for example Fashion or Beauty Editor or Director. The stylist will dress the model and be on set to make sure the clothes and accessories look right. There is often an assistant.

- *Set designer*. If a set is being created for filming there is always a designer and their team who have built the set and will be on hand to change it.

TOP TIP

It is often the case that the make-up artist is expected to do the nails. Many make-up artists expect this to be the case but times are changing. Not all make-up artists want to do nails and are not very good at it. They certainly are not able to do the more advanced work. Because of this tradition though, 'manicurists' are often considered to be an assistant of the make-up artist. This is not so, but working together as a team is essential.

- *Props stylists*. This is different from a set designer (who will probably provide the props too). Many jobs involve various props, for example, flowers, chairs, curtains, without necessarily involving a full set.

- *The client*. On advertising work there is always a presence from the client who has commissioned the work. This may be the designer of a fashion line, a brand manager of a make-up product or it may be the advertising agency who are creating the campaign or commercial.

When arriving at a job, it is worth introducing yourself to everyone so everyone knows who you are and you can find out who is who. Every job should be preceded by a call sheet. This will give you information about what time to arrive, where to go and who else will be there.

Every job is different and everyone has a different way of working. If possible, try to find out a bit more about the job, such as: what the look is, are the nails likely to be natural or artificial. Most jobs, unless a hand or nail job, could involve anything, so technicians should be prepared! The people most likely to be helpful before the shoot are the stylist, the photographer or the make-up artist. The main focus of the shoot will be discussed primarily, e.g. cosmetics, fashion, a car, fragrance, etc.

For a hand, foot or nail shoot, what is required must be discussed in detail before, preferably with sight of the model's hands or feet. Although a technician must be prepared for most eventualities, a specialist shoot needs preparation as far as possible.

Activities likely on a shoot:

- *Manicure*. This could be for a male or female and requires the technician to tidy the nails and cuticles and make them look as good as possible, however close the camera goes.

- *Pedicure*. Unusual for a man but possible. Very likely for a woman and the technician must always check at the beginning if there is any likelihood of the feet being seen.

- *Painting nails*. If colour is required, a manicure should be given first to provide a good base. Colour may need to be changed during the shoot. Always work with the make-up artist and stylist when deciding what colour to use.

- *Artificial nails*. Artificial nails are often needed, but it is much more likely that they are needed to improve the appearance of the model's nails rather than in their own right. The exceptions to this are shoots for artificial nail products and those requiring an unusual or avant garde image.

- *Nail art or airbrushing*. In the commercial world of media work (as opposed to within the nail industry) nail art and airbrushing are not required very often. Obviously, nail fashions change and unusual designs may be more popular sometimes and may be used to draw attention to or support a theme. From the technician's point of view, it is always good for them and the focus on the subject of nails to do something unusual with the nails but, the most important issue in every job is getting the perfect picture or image on film and that usually involves a lot more than the nails. However, a clever technician will have ideas always available and a kit full of interesting things and be ready to make suggestions that may enhance the image – but will never show disappointment when the idea is not taken up.

TOP TIP

There is usually not enough time for a technician to work with the model alone and it is normally advisable for the nail work to start as early as possible. Artificial nails may need to be applied, which will take time, and polish needs the longest time possible to dry. Also, the feet may need attention. Therefore, it is advisable for a nail technician to work on the model at the same time as the hair or make-up artist. Hair is often prepared first so working with the hairdresser, without getting in the way, is most usual and working with the make-up artist also needs to happen very often. Consideration and teamwork is essential.

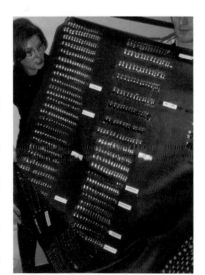

Nails prepared ready for a fashion show

KIT ESSENTIALS

files and buffers	resin and activator
cuticle knives and nippers	tip remover
hand cream and oil	tin foil
varnish remover	nail art products
cotton wool or wipes	wet wipes
selection of colours (as many as you can carry)	orange sticks
tips and adhesive	
tip cutters	

These are the essentials, but there are many things a technician may like to include, especially if travelling by car as this allows many things and equipment to be carried.

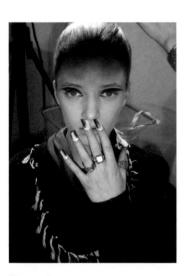

Show nails

General guidelines

- Have a clean, full kit.

- Be prepared for most eventualities.

- Never be late.

- Work as a team where nails are just a part.

- If artificial nails are applied *never* leave without taking them off.

- Work tidily (however much room others take up!).

- For a job of a few days or less, avoid applying full artificial nails.

Working in studios and on locations does not make for ideal working conditions and technicians often have to work out of their kit. The following set of procedures are general guidelines of how good work can be achieved in less that perfect conditions.

> ## " ANECDOTE
>
> The worst situations I have had to deal with (and they are worryingly frequent) are those where the model has had artificial nails put on previously. Very often they have been put on causing damage to the natural nail leaving it thin, sensitive and ridged and very often have not been removed at the end of the shoot, leaving the model to take them off as best she can – which often means biting them off. This makes models very nervous of technicians and what they are going to do to them.

Manicure and pedicure

1 Wipe hands or feet over with a sanitizing wet wipe.

2 Apply oil or cuticle remover to the cuticles of both hands or feet.

3   Shape nails.

4   Remove cuticle and shape nail fold.

5   Buff nails.

6   Clean under free edge.

7   Apply hand cream and leave to be absorbed.

8   With cotton wool on an orange stick or a nail oil pen, wipe around cuticles to provide extra moisture and neaten.

9   During the shoot, occasionally make sure the cuticles are neat and moist and there is nothing under the free edge.

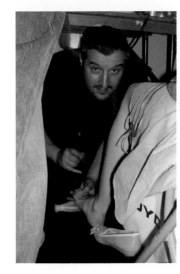

Getting into tight corners to paint nails at a show

Painting

1   After preparing the hands and nails, wipe nails over with a varnish remover that does not have any conditioners.

2   Very carefully, apply the colour making sure the edges are as close to the skin as possible and very neat. If necessary use a different brush from the one in the varnish to make sure of the neatness.

3   Check the varnish in a very good light and if necessary, use a magnifying glass.

4   Clean up the edges if necessary.

5   Apply a quick-dry topcoat.

6   Apply a drop of oil to each nail and leave.

7   Before the model goes on set, check that there is no damage to the varnish (usually there is!).

8   Reapply a topcoat after a few hours to keep maximum shine.

   –   Make sure the model goes to the bathroom before painting!

   –   Undo the top button on jeans for her even after you think the varnish may be dry.

   –   If there is a smudge or dent:

      a.   Wet your finger with remover and gently smooth over the dent.

      b.   Use a quick-dry topcoat and roughly try to smooth the dent (the solvents in the topcoat will soften the varnish a little). Follow this with a good coat.

      c.   Try a smudge repair product.

      d.   If all this fails, take the colour off and re-apply.

TOP TIP

There is often damage to varnish. It takes so long to dry, even with the best quick dryers, that the least-fidgeting models can still have an accident when getting dressed or going to the bathroom. See the tips in this section

Artificial nails   Shoots are temporary situations where the models need to look the best they can for a very short time. If longer nails are needed (or a cover up for bitten or damaged nails) they need to be applied very quickly, with minimum fuss and, most importantly, be removed at the end.

There are many technicians who apply full artificial nails (usually liquid and powder) for a shoot. This takes longer than necessary, takes up more space than necessary, the smell usually offends some people and the results take ages to remove.

It is perfectly acceptable to apply a good set of tips and give them some strength with a layer of resin. This gives a result that is very fast and convenient for everyone, can be left

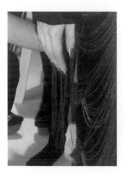

Show nails

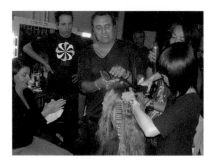

Team backstage

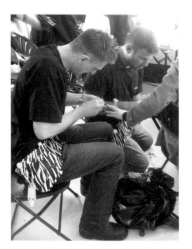

Last minute backstage rush for late arrival

natural or painted, colours can be changed if required and they take 10–15 minutes to remove.

The application is the same as for usual tip application with a layer of resin over them. This is buffed to a shine and colour (if required) and oil applied. This technique can be used whatever the length of the nail, even very long nails for an avant garde image and nail art.

The most convenient method of removal under these circumstances is to soak a cotton wool disc in acetone, place on the nail and wrap in tin foil (foil from a hairdressing suppliers for highlighting is ideal as it is in rolls that are just the right width). Leave this for approximately 10 minutes and remove the foil together with the tip. Apply oil to re-moisturise. If the studio is warm and the model's hands are warm, by the time the last foil is wrapped the first finger is ready to come off.

Nail art and airbrushing

There are no procedures for this other than the safety and hygiene ones. It all depends on what is being done.

Fashion shows

These have a similarity to shoots in that the same people are involved in the central team, that is hair, make-up, styling, designer. They differ in that the time available is usually minimal and the working conditions much worse.

Fashion shows are always carefully planned before the event, but not usually long before. There is always a 'fitting' a day or so before the show. This is where the team get together with a couple of test models and discuss the 'look'. If a technician is involved in a show, it is best to try to get to these fittings even though it takes up more time that is rarely paid for. If the fitting is missed, an opportunity for a suggestion on the nail look is missed and instructions will need to be taken from the make-up artist.

The designer and stylist will discuss what they expect and will have the collection there to see and for the models coming for castings to try on. The hairdresser will try out their suggestions as will the make-up artist. These may change a few times before the final decision is reached.

It is rare for nails to play a big part in fashion shows, but occasionally there is a designer who would like to make a big statement. This is a situation that seems to appear for a short while then go away again. If a *big* statement is required for the nails, then very careful planning needs to be done.

1 Consult with the designer or their stylist exactly what they want. They will usually have a good idea.

2 Create some designs based on their ideas to show them. This can be sketches or drawings, but would be better if it were a selection of ideas on tips. In this way the technician will have the opportunity to try the design out to see if it is practical and the designer/stylist will see the designs for real. It is always best to create a couple of alternatives, especially if a literal interpretation of the original idea is tricky or impractical.

3 Try to find the quickest, easiest and most practical method of creating the design given the time and working condition constraints.

4   Make sure that the producers and the whole team are aware that the application of nails needs the nail team to have time and space to do their work as, in this situation, they are as important as the hair and make-up.

5   Prepare as much as possible before the show so what needs to be done at the show is minimal. For example, prepare tips with the design on ready, if this is possible. They can then just be stuck on to the natural nails. As this is not the close-up work of a photographic shoot, minute perfection is not necessary.

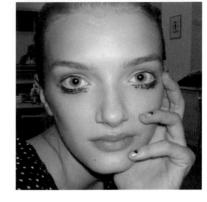

Show nails

TECHNICAL TIP   Do not use nail glue to apply a pre-prepared tip if at all possible. It can take a long time to remove and very often models are rushing off to the next show and do not have time to wait for you. Use sticky pads as these are easily removed with a drop of remover down the back or, sometimes soaking in warm water. These can be obtained from high street chemists or contact the manufacturers of the retail press-on tips.

6   A great deal of airbrushing and application of 3D designs can be done before the show.

7   At the very least, if long nails are required, have them painted or airbrushed and in a variety of sizes. Prepare many more than you think you may need remembering that the middle numbers of tips are used the most. 3D designs can be made before and applied to the tips with adhesive at the show.

8   It is possible to airbrush at a show, but there must be a safe area to do this with an adequate power supply and provision to clean up the fingers after spraying. Space is always at a premium, so this is often not practical and will depend on the venue.

TOP TIP   Some designers feel that by having a definite nail style it looks like they are trying too much. If this is how they feel then a clean shiny nail is fine.

9   Try to check the condition of the nails after the models have dressed as this is when accidents happen. Have replacements ready with pads and adhesive, but remember to take great care of the clothes! Spilling adhesive or varnish on the clothes is not a good idea!

10   Remove all designs after the show. Try to catch the models running out of the door as you will not be thanked for damaged nails and everyone will hear about it.

The more usual situation with shows is that the designer just wants the nails looked after and probably painted a colour. The worst scenario (and it happens frequently) is the requirement for bare nails.

If a colour or colours are appropriate, choose a couple of alternatives for the stylist to decide. Remember to find out if toes will be showing and what is required for them.

Arrive at the venue in plenty of time to get yourself arranged. There may be space to set up a nail area, but this will only work for the early arrivals. Most of the models will arrive without enough time to visit you and you will need to work at the same time as the hair and make-up team.

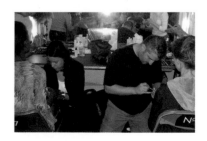

Making the most of opportunities to get nails done

Ask the producer or stylist for a list of models. If there is not one available, go around the clothes rails and make a list of the models that will be on each section. Check you have the right number. This can then be used to tick off each model as they are done so none are missed.

EQUIPMENT LIST

The kit for this type of fashion show can be minimal. There is little time to do much more than paint.

remover

cotton wool

files

nippers

oil topcoat

appropriate colours

TOP TIP

Hands and feet are more moveable and available than heads or faces. A technician at a show is the one who needs to fit into spaces, not hair and make-up.

TOP TIP

Remember NO colour is preferable to the wrong colour.

Make sure you have enough assistants in the nail team to get the job done efficiently and without unnecessary people. As a very general guide, one technician should be able to cope with ten models for simple painting. Anything more elaborate will obviously need more, but never more than one to five.

Make friends with the hair and make-up team and explain that you are there to do the nails, you need to work alongside them but should not get in the way.

Get as many models done as soon as possible and, if necessary, get under the table to do feet!

Don't worry too much about the condition of the cuticles, just apply a little oil at the end but not so much that it could get on the clothes.

Any model who arrives really late will be pounced upon by the hair and make-up teams and there will be little or no room for a technician. Also colour so recently applied will be wet when dressing and just get smudged or on the clothes. When this happens, just remove any existing colour that is wrong and leave it at that. If existing colour is almost right, leave it on. Don't forget the toes.

Keep checking that everyone is done from your list and also all fingers and toes.

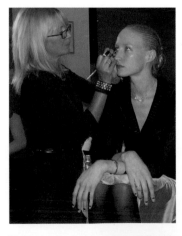

Make-up at a fashion show with nails already done

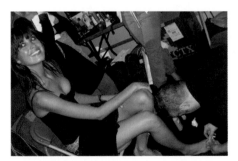

Painting toes at fashion show

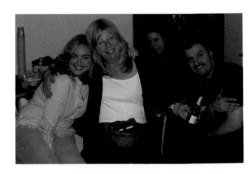

The nail team backstage

Images in the media

It is now a common occurrence for a nail technician to be on a photographic shoot, whether it be beauty, fashion or any other focus. There are also more opportunities for the focus to be on nails. Whatever the focus the brief is important, the team are important and, above all, the finished image is important.

This section of the book takes a small selection of images that have been published in the media that I have worked on. It explains why and how the image was achieved. The images chosen show a range of natural and artificial nails and a range of techniques, including the 'unlikely' in order to demonstrate the versatility of a technician's work.

Media Image 1

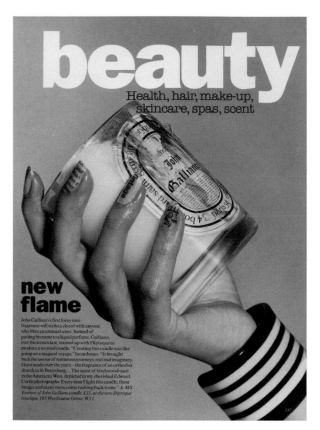

With thanks to British Vogue. Photographers: Barbara Metz, Eve Racine

- *Background*: this page is what is called a 'beauty opener' in a magazine. This means that it is the first page of the beauty section. It can be an introduction to a main feature in the section or a point of interest in its own right. This is editorial work.

- *Brief*: this was a page for *British Vogue* and the editor wanted to show a new and unusual candle that had been developed for the very high class manufacturers, Diptique, by John Galliano, designer for Christian Dior. It needed to be held and a very unusual and bold design for the nails were required.

- *Research*: I happened to be working with John Galliano just before the shoot and had the opportunity of asking him where he got his inspirations for the fragrance. He had the candle sent over for me and explained that the main influences were the Russian orthodox church and native American Indians! The candle was very 'heady' and the base of incense very strong. I also asked the editor what she had in mind for the image and she wanted a very unusual image that maybe involved beads and anything else I wanted. Quite a wide brief then!

- *Ideas*: the Russian church and Indian references created all sorts of ideas in my head of Fabergé eggs and feathers, but I had to remember it was for *Vogue* and I had to be relatively subdued! I decided, having seen the candle, that the base colour needed to be exactly the same as the background of the Galliano packaging, which was a deep creamy colour. This could then be decorated with some chains that loop down the finger, black jets, pearls and some airbrushing. In fact everything. But we would see when we got there what the hand model's fingers and nails were like.

TOP TIP

Any patterned tissue (not waxed) can be used to create a design on nails. Cut a piece of the approximate size and shape of the nail, apply a base coat and, while it is still wet, place the tissue using an orange stick to press it into the wet varnish. Carefully apply a layer of topcoat making sure it soaks into the tissue. When the top-coat is dry, trim the edges with a pair of fabric scissors. The pattern of the tissue will be seen and any areas not patterned will be clear.

● *On the shoot*: this shoot was a good example where all involved should keep an open mind and (hopefully) I have been booked for my ideas and opinions as much as just getting the job done. In the morning I had a bright idea of a completely different look for the nails, but as we had agreed an outline design in principle, that was the one to do first and see if there was time for my alternative.

Having seen the model's hands and nails and discussed the fact that they wanted the candle to look like it had been alight, I decided to use the airbrush to create black half moons over the cream and continue the black up the finger like smoke from a candle. Chains were put down the sides of the nails to drape over the fingers and a few jets and beads applied to the nails. The editor and photographer loved the result and spent ages taking pictures from every possible angle.

I had mentioned my other idea at the beginning and the editor was happy for me to try it if there was time. As the first image took most of the day, there was very little time left, but she felt it was worth a go. My idea was to use the tissue paper that is used in all Galliano packaging that is printed like a newspaper (the Galliano Gazette!) and put it on the nails, using relevant words or pictures where possible. There was a problem as the tissue was waxed and would not soak up the clear varnish but we managed. Once again, everyone loved the nails and many more pictures were taken, but with little time left.

● *The image*: I was hoping the words on the nails would be used because, although the first version was great, the newsprint looked so different and clean. Fortunately that was the one and I love it. There was, however, a bit of tidying up by computer afterwards as the waxed tissue was so difficult.

Media Image 2

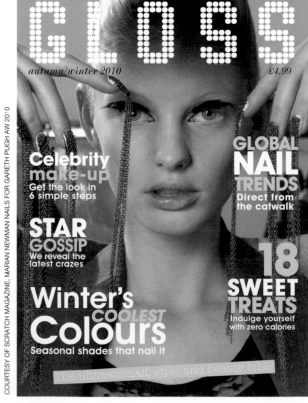

- *Background*: these are nails for a fashion show held in Paris during Paris Fashion Week.

- *Brief*: the nails for all models needed to complement the collection and the hair and make up to create a complete 'look'. The collection was a very strong 'statement' so the look needed to be equally as strong and eye catching.

- *Research*: the designer, Gareth Pugh, provided images of several pieces in the collection.

- *Ideas*: the general silhouette of the collection was strong and angular with diagonal patterns in the fabrics. There were also a few 'main' pieces that had the same silhouette but had draped chains. I created several ideas based on the look of the make up (nude tones with strong accents in black and with faded black on the forehead). All the ideas were versions of black fading into a nude colour which were achieved by airbrushing. There were also different shaped nails to compliment the various designs. In addition, I created several nails using chains that were draped or hanging from the nails.

  All the alternatives were discussed with the designer and his stylist and together we decided on the nails that would be in the show. The choice was long nails but each shaped into a chevron that had its apex between the middle and ring fingers. Diagonal stripes were airbrushed onto the nails to match the shape. For the main pieces with chains, the nails would be the same shape and colour but with the same chains as on the pieces, just smaller. The 'show stopping' pieces would have long chains and the others would have shorter 'day wear' chains!

- *At the show*: all the nails were made before hand. Each model needed a choice of sizes and all had to fit so that the chevron worked on each hand. These prepared nails were carefully organised into boxes so each technician had sufficient nails to fit every model. These were attached immediately before the show with sticky pads so removal would be fast at the end. The chain nails needed adhesive as they were far too heavy for sticky pads.

- *The image*: many pictures were taken backstage before the show and this is one of them. The chain nails certainly caught the imagination of the world's press as they were commented on and featured in many magazines and websites.

Media Image 3

- *Background*: this was an image that was connected with a main feature in the magazine about restaurateurs. As with any cover, it needed to be bold and eye-catching.

- *Brief*: the information I received was that the picture was connected with sushi, had a Japanese feel and the nails were to be used as chopsticks.

- *Research*: sushi is more Japanese than Chinese so I looked at the styles of Japanese chopsticks. They are usually more pointed than the Chinese version and lacquered, often in black.

- *Ideas*: until the shoot, I was not sure if the nails as chopsticks was literal (i.e. looking exactly like chopsticks) or conceptual (used as chopsticks). I favoured the conceptual version as it would be less disturbing for a cover and long nails play a part in Japanese history and tradition. My main idea was very long, tapered nails with a black lacquer on the top and gold leaf on the underside, in keeping with the traditional chopsticks. I considered decoration with Japanese style writing but, as with almost all images, 'less is more'.

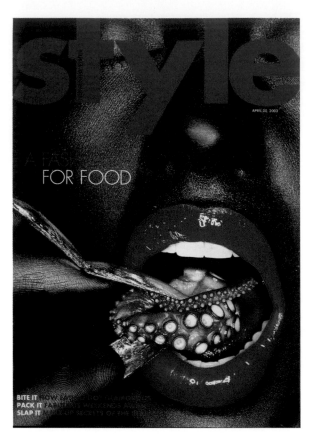

With thanks to photographer Darren Feist and Sunday Times Style

- *On the shoot*: when the team sat around for the brief, I discovered that the image was to have only the colours of black, red and gold, so my black with gold nails fitted very well. Obviously, artificial nails were needed and I spent some time getting the shape right, not too curved and with a smooth and perfect upper arch. With a glossy colour on a nail it is important to spend time on the upper arch as the light reflection on them must be a perfect line (light line). Any irregularities in the surface or shape will show immediately. Painting such long nails with a dense colour like black can be tricky as the varnish becomes tacky and thick very quickly. Keeping the bottle cold and working fast helps. I had applied the gold leaf to the underside of the long free edge first so avoiding the possibility of smudging the varnish.

  The finished nails were amazingly effective and had plenty of time to dry with all the make-up required! They fitted the theme exactly. The photographer spent quite a lot of time taking various angles with hands and mouth (before the sushi was added). Unfortunately for my Japanese chopstick nails, it was really difficult to light the picture in such a way that all detail could be seen and still get the gold underside in and obvious. The only answer was to put gold leaf on the top too so there was sufficient gold in the image to satisfy the brief. That took minutes to do.

- *The image*: well, covers need to be eye-catching! I love the nails and the mouth, but I'm not too sure about the octopus! Another picture inside the magazine was similar but with some sushi covered with yellow caviar!

Media Image 4

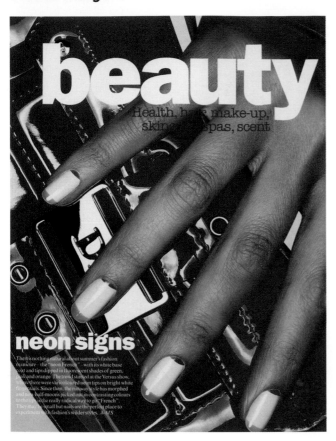

With thanks to British Vogue and photographer Robin Derrick

- *Background*: this was another 'beauty opener' image.

- *Brief*: the brief from the Editor was based on the bold 'acid' and fluorescent colours that were popular and different ways of wearing them.

- *Research*: there had been some fashion and accessory lines that fitted with the brief, so it was just a case of finding some of those for colour combinations. This can be done by looking at the 'look books' of the various fashion shows (the easiest place is style.com).

- *Ideas*: there had been some fabulous jewellery around that was layered Perspex of bright vibrant colours. I liked the idea of lines of colour. Also, from campaigns I had already done, there was some interest in the nail itself with regard to the free edge and half moon. Airbrushing would be the best option as this can give accurate lines and vibrant colours. Although with the airbrush there were many possible variations that could have been more graphic, I was keen on a French variation as this was more recognizable to the readers of the magazine.

- *On the shoot*: I arranged for an assistant to help as I wanted the airbrushing to be as accurate as possible so Marco (see his designs in Chapter 12) came along to help. We had a hand model to work with and a Dior bag as the main prop. After trying out several designs we settled on the version as a variation of a French with lines of colour.

- *The image*: a strong image that is fun too. It is not necessarily a look that readers may try at home, but it does demonstrate that French does not always mean pink with a white tip and the bold, acid colours do not have to be worn all over the nail.

Media Image 5

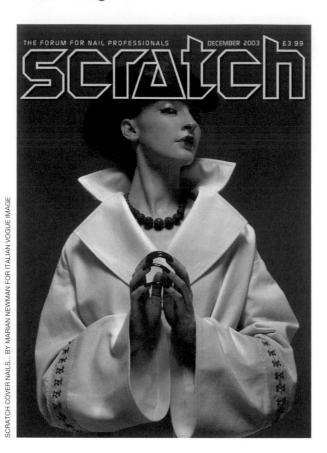

SCRATCH COVER NAILS... BY MARIAN NEWMAN FOR ITALIAN VOGUE IMAGE

- *Background*: this image is from a jewellery shoot for Italian Vogue.

- *Brief*: the editor and photographer wanted very unusual images where the jewellery pieces were in the background to very unusual hair, make up and nails.

- *Research*: there was really no research for this shoot. As often happens on creative shoots such as these, it is a case of developing ideas with the team on the day. There was a very loose 'Kabuki' or oriental theme but there was no real direction.

- *Ideas*: when doing session work it is not always just a good range of polishes that are needed. Sometimes a variety of materials can come in useful. My kit is vast and includes all sorts of unusual things. This particular shoot resulted in about eight images and I used wool, cellophane, beetle wings, diamantes among other more usual nail products.

- *On the shoot*: for this picture, the stylist had decided to use a pale coat and the make up would incorporate red lips. I decided to make the nails red but to create a more visual impact they were joined together! To do this I sized the model's nails with a tip that had a strong curve. Each size then had two more tips added to create the curve and then the joins were blended and the sides tidied up. When all 8 fingers (not the thumbs) were prepared, I joined the two little fingers together, the two ring fingers etc. The join, as before, was blended and the whole structure painted with a very shiny red.

When the model was ready to go on set, I applied the 'structures' with adhesive very quickly. It is rather claustrophobic to have your nails clamped together like this so I was close by with scissors to cut them apart as soon as the photographer had finished.

● *The image*: a very striking image that makes one look twice to see what is happening with the nails! It was one of several very unusual pictures for the 'story' and one that worked particularly well.

Media Image 6

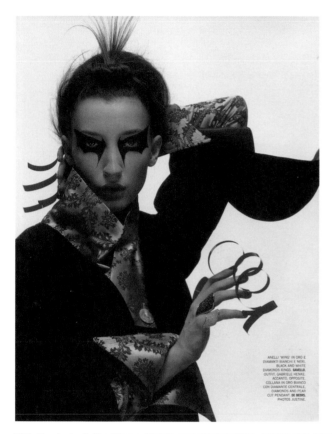

ANELLI 'WING' IN ORO E
DIAMANTI BIANCHI E NERI.
BLACK AND WHITE
DIAMONDS RINGS. **GAVELLO.**
OUTFIT, GABRIELE HENKEL
ACCANTO. OPPOSITE.
COLLANA IN ORO BIANCO
CON DIAMANTE CENTRALE,
DIAMONDS AND PEAR
CUT PENDANT. **DE BEERS.**
PHOTOS JUSTINE.

With thanks to *Italian Vogue Gioiello* and photographer Justine and model Inge Guerts

● *Background*: this is part of a jewellery story in a magazine that likes to present jewellery in an unusual and often surprising way. As it is jewellery, there are often rings and bracelets and therefore hands and nails!

● *Brief*: this story had a '*kabuki*' brief. That is a Japanese feel with strong graphic shapes. There would be lots of images, several models and each look very different from the last.

● *Research*: *kabuki* is a traditional Japanese dramatic art and there are many designs of masks used and graphic shapes. It also involves dance using many strong hand shapes.

● *Ideas*: it was difficult to have many specific ideas without seeing the styling, hair and make-up, but I needed many nails that would be fast to put on and take off. I took my usual vast kit with a few extra bits that may come in useful: beetle wings I found in New York, gold paper doilies, cellophane and glitter pipe cleaners.

- *On the shoot*: myself, the hairdresser and make-up artist managed to come up with about eight totally different looks and I used everything except the pipe cleaners! I had an idea that the cellophane could make long transparent, curly nails somehow. When I tried it the cellophane was too flimsy and the colour not strong enough. Photographers use coloured gels to cover lights for different effects. These gels are like thick cellophane and come on a roll! Strips of this cut to various widths similar to a nail width with one end straight and the other curved could do the job. Because the gel is thick, it was not able to curve onto the nail but it was never meant to look real, so a spot of adhesive did the trick. One hand was left very long and the other cut a bit shorter in order to give the photographer more shapes to work with.

- *The image*: every image in the story was amazing, but this one has made such a feature of the hands and the 'nails' were so quick and simple to do.

Media Image 7

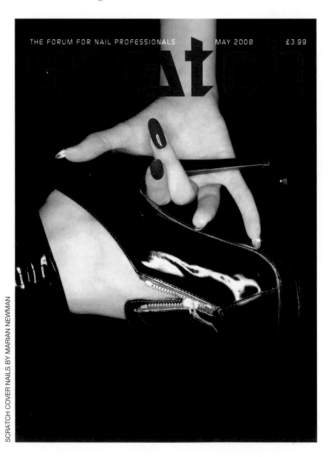

- *Background*: Habia asked me to create a series of images for them that they could use in their printed material and marketing. I asked several technicians to create some images and I worked on a couple too. This is one of them.

- *Brief*: Habia wanted some generic pictures that were not product-based and had some connection with fashion or hair or make up.

- *Research*: I wanted to have a strong image that connected with fashion but still focussed on the nails. The Laboutin shoe is instantly recognisable but I wanted one that is more unusual that the traditional court stiletto. Also, tight PVC trousers have a tough fashion look but are simple in their shape.

- *On the shoot*: I applied tips to give the nail length and shape. Matching the red of the sole was too obvious so a 'clash' was better. Pink is such a popular nail colour so I applied a bold pink on the nails with, as usual, a high shine. To give the nails more interest and demonstrate that colour does not just have to be on the top, I used some real silver leaf under the free edge. This sticks very well to wet polish and gives a flash of metal when the hand moves.

  It was a difficult pose to get right for the photographer. Hands are very difficult to shoot so they look attractive. Add in a foot and part of a leg in such a way that is physically possible for the model makes for a very tricky time!

- *The image*: this is a strong and powerful image that shows the nails off. They are not too extreme, so wearable, but have the quirk of the silver flashes. The expensive shoe and glimpse of the trousers is all it needs to give it a classy fashion feel.

Although most media work is usually very straightforward, these images have been chosen to demonstrate how varied it can be. It is almost that all the rules must be known and understood, but then broken in order to achieve something different. But, while these rules are being broken, the care of the client/model and everyone's safety must be put first.

Summary

This chapter has dealt with an area new to the education of technicians. It has shown where opportunities to work outside the salon exist, how to find them, and how to promote yourself. It has defined various roles in media work and has provided the starting points for many potential areas of work.

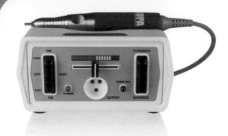

15
Using electric files

Introduction

We have learnt that the early artificial nail products evolved from the dental industry. Drills have also been used by dentists and dental technicians to great effect. It was, therefore, obvious to use similar drills especially with the early products that were very hard once cured.

Drills, electric files or e-files, as they are commonly called in the nail industry, have been in use since the beginning. Their use was almost essential when working with the products available then as buffing the overlays was a difficult, time-consuming and strenuous job.

Other than the salons that use MMA as a monomer that still need the added help of mechanical filing, their popularity has decreased. Modern overlay products are much softer and more flexible and do not necessarily need anything more than light buffing by hand.

However, there are many technicians who prefer to use them and there are a few techniques that can only be done with an e-file. Some technicians have developed RSI (repetitive strain injury) by many hours each day buffing nails. Some have found that using an e-file has helped this condition. RSI is caused by using muscles in the same way for long periods. This can happen with an e-file too!

On balance the use of e-files has a place within the professional nail industry. The decision to use one is purely the choice of the technician. In the hands of a trained and experienced user an e-file is a useful tool. In the inexperienced hands of an uneducated technician an e-file can cause a great deal of damage to the client and pose serious health hazards for the technician.

An important aspect to remember with the use of e-files is this: it is NOT a tool to correct poor application skills! It is a tool, that, in the right hands, can be an optional technique that, with practice, can speed up certain stages of the nail technician's skilful services.

Applying too much product that needs removing or extreme shaping correction is NOT the purpose of an e-file. A technician that uses it for this purpose is an untrained and unskilled technician.

This Chapter is a guideline and reference only. This subject must NEVER be self-taught. A practical training course must be taken and the learner should spend a great deal of time practicing on their own nails before attempting to use an e-file on a client. The technician should also check with their insurers that they are covered for using an e-file.

Uses of the e-file

E-files are usually used on L&P systems as the characteristics of the overlay respond well to an e-file. A UV gel is often too soft but it can be used on gels in exactly the same way, usually with a finer abrasive.

ALWAYS REMEMBER

The NOS do not allow for use of an e-file on the natural nail. The reason for this is the level of damage that can be caused in a split second of lost concentration. Some very experienced users have techniques that are effective but this takes many years of practice and is not recommended for beginners. This chapter does NOT cover any natural nail use of the e-file and includes techniques that help to avoid any contact with the nail plate.

1   *Refining the overlay*. Once an overlay has been applied the shape can be refined ready for the final buffing.

2   *Preparing nails for a maintenance service*. This is one of the most useful uses of an e-file as it can quickly de-baulk a nail, cut a new smile line and reduce length.

3   *Cleaning under the free edge of an artificial nail*. This is very difficult to do by hand and it can be achieved quickly and efficiently by an e-file

4   *Buffing an overlay to a shine*. There are attachments that will shine the nail. However, many users believe that it is quicker to do this by hand.

5   *Nail art*. Some experienced nail artists use special attachments to shape, refine and cut designs.

6   *Pedicures*. Hard skin can be removed with specially designed attachments.

7   *Soak off coloured gels*. These usually require the surface to be etched before removal. An e-file can do this job very quickly.

There are many salons that use e-files inappropriately and are often the salons that use MMA in their L&P system. An e-file is virtually essential as removing this type of overlay by hand is very time-consuming and strenuous.

The following images are of a client's nail that has been damaged at one of these types of salons. The soft nail by the matrix was filed and completely removed in a second. The nail bed was infected and came through the surrounding nail. The first picture was taken

2 weeks after the event when the infection had subsided. The second picture was 2 weeks after that when the nail bed was starting to heal. It is unlikely that the matrix, the nail bed nor the nail will ever recover in this area.

Anatomy of an e-file

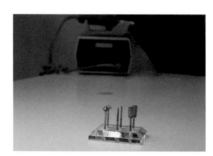

CREATIVE NAIL DESIGN INC

E-filing control unit

A selection of clean bits ready for use. It is usually unnecessary to have more than these three ready for use

There are many e-files on the market. Like any piece of equipment the price will depend on the quality. A serious technician who wants to use an e-file professionally will only buy a good quality product. There are some inexpensive units that would be useful for nail art but for use on clients' nails a good quality unit with several features is essential.

- *Control unit*. This is a box that sits on the desk. The features it should have as a minimum are:

  - power indicator light

  - speed control: an e-file needs a speed adjustment of between 0 up to 30 000 RPM (revs per minute)

  - reverse switch to reverse the direction of the file.

  Most units are mains operated but there are some that are rechargeable and will hold charges for between 2–8 hours of use. Like any electrical equipment, this should be regularly checked by a qualified electrician.

- *Handpiece*. Connected to the control unit by a lead, this holds the 'bits' in the 'chuck' and drives the spinning action of the abrasives. It is full of moving parts and it is impossible to prevent dust from entering it. It needs regular maintenance to clean it and replace worn parts. This should be done by a qualified person and not attempted by a nail technician.

  There are a few different methods of releasing the chuck (the mechanism that holds the bit in place) and this is down to personal choice.

  When buying an e-file it is important to choose carefully. The handpiece should sit comfortably in your hand, feel balanced and, most importantly, have little or no vibration. A handpiece that vibrates will cause RSI eventually!

- *Holder*. There should be a holder for the handpiece either as a separate stand or attached to the control unit. The handpiece should not be placed on a desk top while the bit is in place.

- *Foot pedal (optional)*. For those technicians who use an e-file a great deal there is an option to have a foot pedal to turn the e-file on and adjust the speed.

- *Bits*. These are the parts that actually do the job of filing. There are many to choose from both in shapes and surface.

  - Surface materials:

    - *Carbide*: these bits have cutting flutes that 'scoop' the surface rather than grind it. There are various grades of abrasive from fine to course. This is generally considered to be preferable for several reasons:

      - The dust created is larger, heavier particles that will fall to the desk surface rather that float in the air which is a health hazard.

      - They need little or no pressure to be effective so are efficient and quick.

      - The lack of pressure means that there is little heat generated on the nail.

- *Swiss carbide*: a higher quality version of carbide that is made from a finer material that will stay sharp for longer.

- *Diamond*: made from diamond particles of various sizes depending on the grade of abrasion. These grind the surface and create a great deal of fine dust. There are various grades available from course through to very fine for buffing. However, due to the level of fine dust created, carbide bits should be considered and buffing carried out by hand.

- *Sanding bands*: these are similar material to normal files and are fitted to a mandrel (a bit with a smooth barrel that holds the sanding band). They are available in different abrasive qualities and are disposable. A new band should be used for every client. Like the diamond bits, they create a lot of dust.

- *Shapes*. There are many, many shapes of bits all performing a slightly different job. The choice of bit is mostly personal opinion and dependent on the type of work a technician wants to use their e-file for. There are delicate shapes that are used for artwork that will make fine and precise lines. There are larger bits that are designed to use during pedicures.

  Realistically, a technician using an e-file for general nail work only needs three types of bits:

  - A medium carbide barrel for shortening and shaping.

  - A French fill diamond carbide (or similar) for cutting new smile lines (the diamond refers to the shape not the material).

  - A cone or UNC (under the nail cleaner) carbide that is long and thin.

Cleaning

All the equipment must be kept clean and free from dust and a wipe with a damp cloth after every use should suffice.

The handpiece should be regularly and professionally cleaned to remove any dust that has found its way inside the seals. If this is not done the moving parts will seize up or it will overheat when least expected.

The bits need careful cleaning. A clean bit should be used for every client. If you are able to buy several of each of the bits you are using, keep a closed box for used bits and one for clean bits. (A desk stand is useful to have each of the bits you will be using with a client available for a quick change.)

A used bit should be washed in soap and water using a nail brush to remove all debris. Then it should be immersed in a disinfectant solution. Follow the manufacturer's instructions about the minimum immersion (usually 10–15 minutes) and do NOT leave the bits in longer than this as they will rust. Take them out, dry on a disposable towel and place in a covered container ready for use. Carbide or titanium bits are best cleaned in acetone as it dissolves acrylic particles that block up the cutting flutes. They can then be immersed or sprayed with disinfectant solution.

Disposable sanding bands should be discarded after every client.

If bits are made of any other type of material, such as a fabric, follow manufacturer's instructions for disinfecting.

HEALTH & SAFETY

1. *Electrical equipment*. All electrical equipment must be checked annually by a qualified electrician.
2. *Decontamination*. Follow the cleaning guidelines above.
3. *Injuries*.
   a Make sure the handpiece has little or no vibration.
   b Some bits can be hot after use so care must be taken when removing them straight after use.
   c Do not use on the natural nail or even close to the nail plate.
   d Keep the e-file away from soft tissue.
   e Always have hair tied back as there is a high risk of it being caught up in the handpiece.
4. *Dust*. This is the single most important issue when using an e-file. Carbides are the safest bit to use as they generate less dust and particles are heavier. However, all e-files create dust. Dust is one of the most hazardous problems of a nail salon (see Chapter 3).

   It is essential to use a dust extractor when using an e-file. Ideally this should be set in the desk top where the dust will be pulled downwards as it is being generated and not upwards through your breathing space.
5. PPE (see Chapter 3):
   a *Dust mask*. A technician is working in a dusty environment all day. It is essential to wear a dust mask when using an e-file especially as the technicians face is so close to where the dust is being generated. A correctly fitted mask with a nose clip should be used.

(Continued)

Dust masks should also be available for clients especially those who suffer from asthma.

b *Eye protection.* Suitable eye protection should be worn as large particles can fly straight up into the eye and cause damage that can be long-term. Spectacles will provide some protection but even these should be covered by suitable eye pieces.

c *Gloves.* Newly applied overlays will have some unreacted monomer in the dust. Continual contact with this will eventually result in an allergic reaction. Nitrile gloves should be worn.

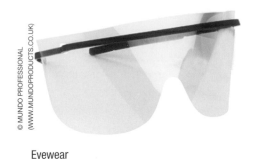

Eyewear

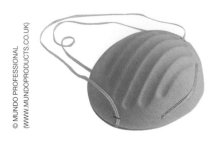

Cone mask

TOP TIP

Pressure = heat
There is no need to put any pressure on the nail while filing. The correct bit used at an appropriate speed will not require pressure.

TOP TIP

Never leave the e-file running when you are not using it! Always turn it off before you put it down in its holder.

TOP TIP

Do not leave a bit in the chuck when the e-file is not in use. If it falls the bit could snap off in the chuck.

Safe techniques for using an e-file

When you are first practicing with an e-file, start at slower speeds and take longer. Raise the speeds and complete the stages faster only when you are confident that you are holding the file at the right angle and there is no possibility of touching the nail plate or surrounding skin.

When you are confident and can safely raise the speeds the job will be done efficiently in seconds. This comes with practice so take it slowly.

Reversing the e-file

The nail should always be filed in the opposite direction to the spin of the bit in order to remove the surface efficiently and avoid you losing control of it around the underside of the nail.

Imagine looking down the handpiece at the spin of the bit. If the bit is spinning in the 'forward' position it will spin clockwise. In this position you should move the e-file over the nail from the right side wall (as you look at it) to the left side wall. NOT backwards and forwards.

If you file in the direction of the spin, you will lose control of the file as it will spin around the finger and could damage the skin. (It is also frightening for the client!)

While you only file in this one direction it is not necessary to reverse the e-file and this saves a great deal of time.

If you are left handed it may be more comfortable to work from the left side wall over to the right (as you look at it). If this is the case, keep the e-file in the 'reverse' position.

The only technique that requires you to reverse the e-file is cleaning under the nail (see step-by-step).

Holding the client's finger

When using an e-file, the client's arm should be comfortably resting on a support. The technician should have both arms resting on the desk.

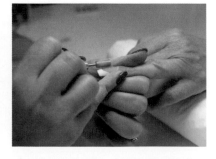

How to hold the client's finger when using an e-file. Notice the finger is held between the technician's finger and thumb and the little finger of the hand holding the e-file is used to steady the hand.

If right handed, the technician's left hand should *firmly* hold the client's finger that will be worked on between their forefinger and thumb while keeping the skin out of the way.

The e-file should be held comfortable in the right hand like a pen. The little finger should be used as an anchor to steady and control the use of the e-file.

ALWAYS REMEMBER

Do not prepare the natural nail with the e-file and do not blend tips with an e-file.

Finishing a new overlay

Aim to work at speeds of around 20 000–30 000 RPM for this but start at around 10 000 and take longer while practicing.

1 When the overlay has been applied to all nails you are ready to use your e-file to shape and refine the nails.

2 Place a medium grit carbide barrel bit in the handpiece.

3 Hold the e-file at the correct angle for Zone 1, start slightly in from the side of the free edge (if you start on the edge you will lose control of the e-file and it will go under the nail) and refine and thin the overlay by making 2–3 strokes from right to left. No pressure should be needed!

4 Adjusting the angle, move back to Zones 2 and 3, again from right to left only and, with just a few strokes, refine the overlay but leaving the side walls untouched.

5 Take extra care in Zone 3 not to touch the skin or margin of nail plate!

6 Each zone should need only 2–3 strokes.

7 Twist the finger to expose the right side wall. Starting just behind the extreme edge, file down the side wall towards the cuticle area. One stroke should be enough.

8 Twist the finger to expose the left side wall. File up from the cuticle area to the free edge.

9 Refine the corners of the free edge that have been deliberately missed. (By working in this pattern it is not necessary to reverse the e-file.)

10 Unless you are intending to change the bit two or three times and buffing every nail with each bit, the nails should now be a perfect shape and ready for buffing with a three-way buffer to a high shine.

TOP TIP

Remember most of the shaping should be done with your brush not your file or buffer.

TOP TIP

The e-file should be kept parallel to the surface of the nail! Keep the structure of the upper arch in mind while doing this. Do not stay in one place, keep the e-file moving or a flat area will be created. Do not exaggerate the angle of the file, just follow the gentle upper arch.

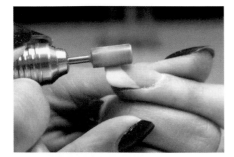

The correct angle for the e-file to refine Zone 1.

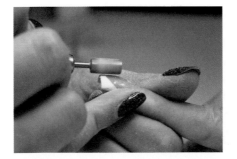

Notice the e-file has started just in from the side wall.

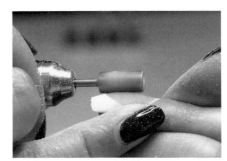

Moving back over Zones 2 and 3.

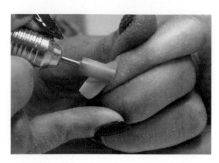

Refining the right side wall. Start just back from the free edge working back to Zone 3.

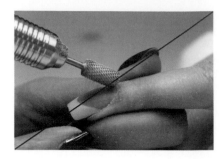

The WRONG angle in Zone 3. Never angle the e-file into the cuticle area as this will cause massive damage to the nail plate.

Maintenance using an e-file

This essential service for all artificial nail clients can benefit from the use of an e-file. As maintenance preparation mostly requires 'removal' the process can be very quick using e-file techniques.

If a client has a pink and white overlay, a maintenance service requires the smile line to be replaced in the correct position. Using an e-file can make this service very quick as the whole overlay does not need filing down (de-baulking).

However, fast preparation with an e-file only works successfully if the original set of artificial nails were applied correctly! It is not so useful in correcting mistakes and poor application.

Any lifting can be removed by an e-file. The lifted areas can be 'cut out' but blending the remaining overlay to the nail plate must be done manually.

The following techniques are concerned with use of the e-file only. All other preparation steps such as cuticle removal, nail plate dehydration, primer/bonder use should be followed according to manufacturer's and system instructions.

Remove length

On a maintenance service, length of the nail should be shortened back to the original application length. This can be easily and quickly done by an e-file.

Aim to work at speeds of 20 000–30 000 RPM

1   Use a medium carbide barrel bit.

2   In one stroke, remove the length of the free edge (the shape can be refined later) by using the e-file pointing downwards towards the floor and holding it against the free edge from the left towards the right. If left handed, use the e-file from right towards the left in reverse motion.

Infill/rebalance preparation

Aim to work at speeds of 10 000–20 000 RPM

1   Using a medium barrel carbide bit and keeping the e-file parallel to the surface of the nail (the upper arch) de-baulk the overlay by a half of its original thickness.

2   Leave a thin line of untouched overlay in Zone 3. this will ensure that the nail plate is not touched by the e-file. File this manually.

3   if there is no new smile line to apply and no lifting to deal with, the nail is ready for a new, thin overlay to be applied.

Cleaning the underside

Sculptured nails often have a slight ridge where they have grown out after 2 weeks as do tips with overlays. Also, artificial nails with a growth of natural nail under the free edge sometimes needs cleaning up.

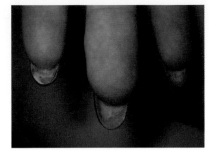

Artificial nails with a growth of natural nail under the free edge

Aim to work at speeds of around 10 000 RPM

NB Do not let the e-file touch the skin or get close to the hyponychium!

1   Using a cone or UNC bit turn the client's finger over to expose under the free edge. Hold the client's finger firmly and ensure you hold the underside of the skin with your thumb pulling it away in order to be able to get as close as possible without touching the skin or hyponychium.

2   With the e-file in the 'forward' position, start at the centre of the nail and work out to the left side (as you look at it).

3   Reverse the e-file.

4   From the centre, work out to the right side.

5   Under the free edge should now be smooth and clean.

Cutting out lifting

An e-file will cut out lifting (with practice). Minor lifting can be dealt with quickly and easily. Major lifting can be cut out but will need further blending with hand filing.

Aim to work at 8000–15 000 RPM. This is the only time the edge of the barrel bit is angled into the nail! Extreme care must be taken. If done correctly, it takes a second of filing!

1   Use a medium carbide barrel bit.

2   Place the edge of the file on the join line of the lifting area on the overlay NOT over it, i.e. the edge of the white area. Cutting on product that is still adhered to the nail will not allow it to fall or break away easily. Cutting on the lifted area will leave a small white line and you will then need to hand file with natural nail exposed which may cause damage.

3   A second of filing should cause the lifted area to fall away DO NOT PRISE! But it can be lifted away gently if it does not break away itself.

4   If this is unsuccessful then use a hand file BEHIND the line of lifting otherwise you will be 'chasing the line' (this is a term used when buffing the lifted area keeps going further and further up the nail).

5   With practice this can be done in a second!

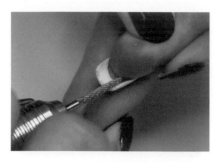

Preparing to clean and tidy under the free edge during a maintenance service.

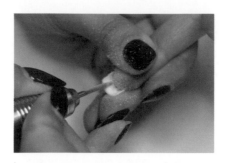

Smoothing any step created by a sculptured nail and cleaning under the free edge of the natural nail. Start in the centre and work to the left. Reverse the e-file and work from centre to right.

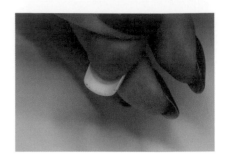

A clean and tidy nail before a maintenance.

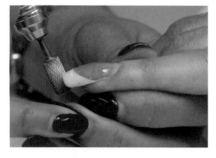

The correct angle of the e-file for removing length.

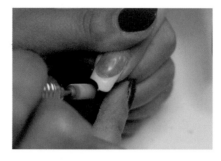

Removing length in preparation for a maintenance service.

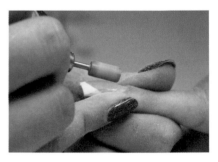

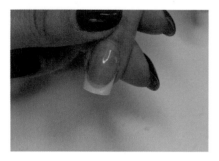

Length removed in a few seconds.

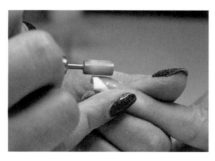

De-baulking Zone 1.

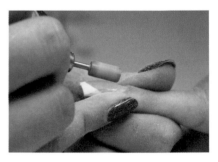

De-baulking Zones 2 and 3 but avoiding the edge and therefore any possibility of filing the nail plate. Make sure a thin line of shiny overlay remains in this area.

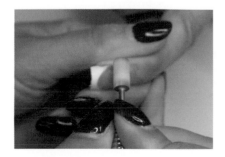

Turn nail and refine left side wall. Work from the base up to the free edge. Avoid the corner of the free edge.

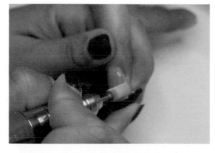

Refine the other side wall avoiding the corner of the free edge. Start from just below free edge down to Zone 3.

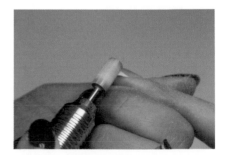

Thin the corners of the free edge.

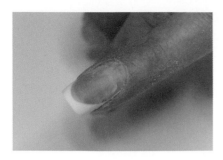

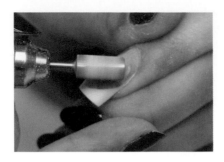

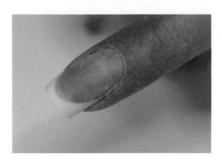

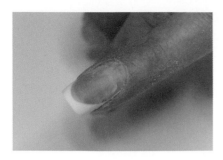 A small area of lifting that needs removing (lifting that is bigger than this needs attention to the initial preparation!).

File 'behind' the area of lifting not over it! About 1 second of filing will result in the lifted area falling away.

Lifted area removed.

Cutting a new smile line

Pink and white overlays after 2 to 4 weeks need the smile line to be replaced as it will have grown up onto the free edge. This needs to be replaced (depending on the type of overlay) to its natural position, i.e. at the end of the finger.

Some technicians are only capable of a straighter smile line; some clients prefer a straighter smile line. A smile line that elongates the nail bed without having a long nail has a more exaggerated curve. The same technique works for both but the pictures accompanying this step-by-step is of a more graceful smile line.

Aim to work at speeds of 8000–15 000 RPM

1 De-baulk the overlay as described above.

2 Using a 'diamond French' carbide bit, mark the placement of the new smile in the centre of the nail. This will provide a depth guide when cutting the line.

3 Twist the finger to expose the right side wall (as you look at it).

4 Cut the new smile line from this edge to the middle.

5 Notice you have created a 'trench' that has three lines:

   a. The new edge of the smile line.

   b. The base of the 'trench'. When you see the specs of white at the base of this trench you know you have reached the correct depth. No specs and it is too shallow, a solid white and it is cutting into the natural nail.

   c. An edge in the white that will be removed.

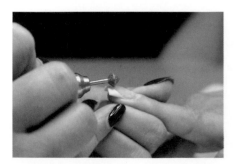

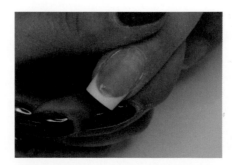

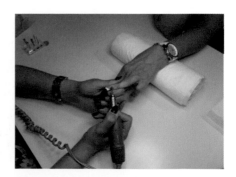

The correct angle of a diamond French bit for cutting the smile line.

Mark the centre of the placement for the new smile line.

How the finger should be held for accurate smile line cutting.

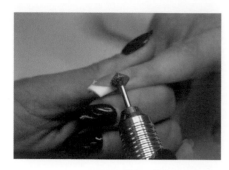

Turn the finger and cut a new smile line from one side wall to the centre mark.

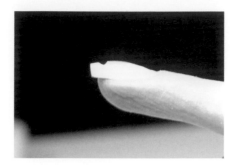

Side view of a correctly cut 'new smile'. This is the apex of the nail and where the overlay is at it's thickest.

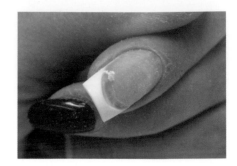

Continue the new smile line around to the other side wall paying particular attention to the 'new smile' sharp edge and correct depth.

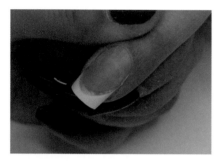

A new smile cut in and ready for overlay

6 Twist the finger to expose the left side wall.

7 Continue the new smile line from the centre marker to the side wall that mirrors the opposite side.

8 It is important to try and create the new smile line in long sweeps from side to centre rather than stopping and starting otherwise you will create untidy edges which will be obvious when the new white is applied.

9 Change bits to the barrel carbide (speeds for this can be up to 20 000 RPM).

10 Remove most of the remaining white tip to prevent any possibility of shadowing using 'forward' and starting at the right side of the free edge.

Apply new overlay

After following all of the above techniques, the nail is ready for a new pink and white overlay.

1 Apply white to the prepared Zone 1.

2 As the white is being smoothed and shaped to the 'C' curve it will automatically fall into the prepared new smile line and will not need any shaping.

3 Apply a thin layer of overlay to Zones 2 and 3 and blend over Zone 1.

4 Refine the shape as described in 'Applying a new overlay' above.

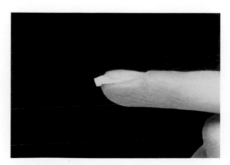

Side view of the nail with Zone 1 ready for application.

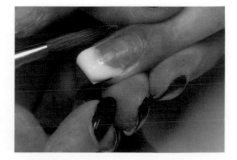

Apply white L&P to the prepared Zone 1.

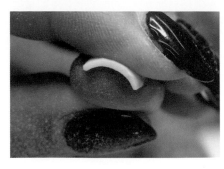

The thickness of the shortened nail's free edge which must be thinned.

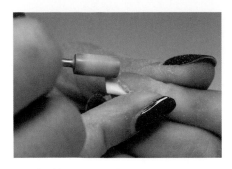

Thinning Zone 1 ready for a new application. Notice the sharp edge of the overlay ready for the 'new smile'.

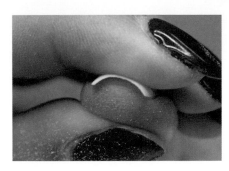

The thinned free edge ready for the new application.

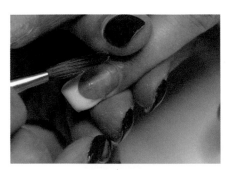

Shape Zone 1. Notice how the white L&P sits against the 'new smile' without any effort.

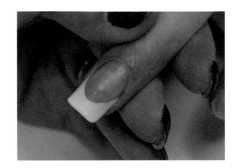

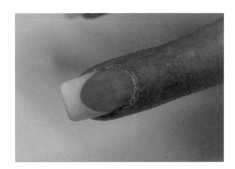

A thin layer of L&P over Zones 2 and 3, ready for finishing.

Summary

This final chapter has dealt with how to use e-files safely, how to finish artificial nail overlays and how to use an e-file effectively for maintenance services. As explained earlier in this chapter, the e-file can be used for other tasks. Those described here are those that should be the most useful to a professional nail technician.

Glossary of terms

This glossary of terms relates to the words shown in bold in the book on their first use and the context in which they have been used. Many of the words have several meanings. Other definitions can be found in a dictionary or encyclopaedia.

Abductor   to move away from the centre of the body

Abrasive   material used to shape, polish and remove the surface of natural and artificial nails

ABS   acrylonitrile butadiene styrene; a polymer from which most plastic tips are made

Absorption   in this context, one of the nail 'routes of entry' into the body; that is, through the skin

Acetone   a solvent commonly used as a tip remover and nail varnish remover

Acids   substances that have pH values of less than 7.0; the opposite of alkaline

Acid mantle   a mixture of sweat and sebum on the skin that has a pH value of 5.5 and acts as a protection against bacteria

Acrylates   a 'family' of organic chemicals

Acrylics   in this context, a 'system' that uses two components, liquid monomer and powder polymer, to create an artificial overlay

Activator   one of the components in the 'fibre system'; this is a liquid that speeds up the polymerisation of a cyanoacrylate resin

Adductor   to move towards the centre of the body

Adhesion   a force that makes two surfaces stick together

Adhesives   chemicals that cause two surfaces to stick together; the most common adhesive in the nail industry is cyanoacrylate

Aftercare   the advice given to clients following a treatment

Age related ridges   longitudinal lines on some or all nails

AHA   Alpha hydroxy acid. Relatively mild fruit acid used as an ingredient in some skincare products. It can assist exfoliation and encourage healthy cell renewal

Albinism   a skin condition where the skin cells do not produce any melanin

Alkaline   the opposite of acid. 8–14 in the pH scale

Allergen   a substance that causes an allergy

Allergic reaction   the reaction of the body to an invasion of a chemical substance or foreign body that could be harmful or that the body has developed a sensitivity to. Can be topical (restricted to an area) or systemic (affects the whole body)

Amine   a type of chemical compound

Amino acids   small molecules that the body uses as building blocks for proteins

Anaemia   blood disorder affecting its ability to transport oxygen

Anterior   relating to the front

Antiseptic   a sanitiser, the lowest level of decontamination, usually suitable for skin use

Aorta   large artery leading from the heart

Apocrine gland   one of the two types of gland found in the skin. This one is only found in the armpit and groin area and is controlled by hormones

Arteries   blood vessels that carry the blood from the heart to other parts of the body

Arthritis   a disease affecting the joints

Assessor   person qualified to assess the performance of an NVQ candidate

Atom   smallest unit of matter that is recognisable as a chemical

Atrium, right and left   the two upper chambers of the heart that receive blood from the lungs and venous system of the body

Autonomic nerves   nerves that are not consciously controlled

Autonomic nervous system   the part of the nervous system that is not under conscious control

Bacteria   single-cell, vegetable-like organisms; some are capable of causing disease

Bacterial infection ('Greenies')   bacteria forming between an overlay and the nail plate

Beaded ridges   longitudinal lines with little bumps usually associated with circulatory problems

Beau's lines   horizontal lines on nail plate

Bed epithelium   the epidermis that makes up the nail bed

Benzoyl peroxide   a heat-sensitive catalyst often found in powder polymers

Blue nails   a condition usually associated with circulation problems where the nail bed appears blue rather than pink

Brachial artery   artery of the arm

Brittleness   the condition of a substance that determines how likely it is to break

Bruised nails   an area of skin beneath the nail that has suffered some form of trauma causing blood from local vessels to leak into surrounding tissues

Bunion   misaligned toe joint

'C' curve   the curve of the nail from side wall to side wall

Calcaneus   one of the tarsal bones in the ankle

Callus   area of hard skin, usually caused by pressure or rubbing

Capillaries   the smallest blood vessels that carry blood to all parts of the body

Carbon dioxide   a waste product of the body, collected by the blood and expelled by the lungs

Cardiac muscle   a type of muscle found only in the heart

Cardiovascular   the system of the body that relates to the circulation of the blood

Carpals   bones in the wrist

Cartilage   a strong fibrous tissue in joints

Cartilaginous joints   a type of joint

Catalyst   a chemical added to a substance to promote, speed or control the chemical reaction or polymerisation; a catalyst does not take part in the chemical reaction

Cell   the smallest unit capable of life

Central nervous system (CNS)   part of the nervous system that includes the brain and spinal cord

Checklist   a comprehensive list for verification purposes

Chemicals   matter; everything except light and electricity is a chemical

Chemical bond   the bonds between the atoms and molecules of a chemical

Chemical reaction   a process of two or more chemicals combining to create a different substance

Chiropodist   practitioner qualified to give treatment to the feet that has a more medical rather than a cosmetic focus (also known as a podiatrist)

Cleaning   removal of dirt, stains or anything else that could contaminate you and/or your client or the work area

CNS   central nervous system

Collagen   fibre proteins found in the skin that help provide support to the structure of the skin and surrounding tissues

Constriction   a narrowing

Contact area or well   refers to the area of a plastic tip that is adhered to the nail plate

Contamination   unwanted or foreign substances on an implement, surface or in a product

Contra-actions   action to be taken to correct an adverse reaction

Contra-indication   an indication against performing a treatment

Copolymer   a polymer made from two or more different monomers

Corns   patch of hard skin on toes, usually caused by pressure

Corrosive   substances capable of causing rapid and sometimes irreversible damage to human tissue or other surfaces

COSHH   Control of Substances Hazardous to Health

Cure   polymerisation

Curing   the process of polymerisation

Cuticle   a very thin layer of skin growing from under the lateral nail fold that adheres to the nail plate

Cut-outs   a technique used in unusual nail art that involves cutting away shapes in the plastic tip

Cyanoacrylates   the family of acrylates used in adhesives and resins

Cytoplasm   the gel-like contents of a living cell that contain the cellular structures

Decontamination   the process of reducing the risk of harm from pathogenic microorganisms

Dehydrate   to remove water from the surface of the natural nail plate

Deoxygenated blood   blood returning to the lungs that is depleted of oxygen

Dermatitis   non-specific skin inflammation

Dermis   lower layer of skin, below the epidermis

Desquamation   the shedding of non-living cells

Digestive system   one of the systems of the body, deals with the breaking down and assimilation of food

Digital arteries and veins   blood vessels in the fingers

Dilation   opening, widening

Disease   an unhealthy condition of the body

Disinfectant   substance capable of killing some micro-organisms and inhibiting the growth of others; second level of decontamination

Disinfection   a level of decontamination that kills some living organisms and inhibits the growth of others. Suitable for hard surfaces and implements.

Distal   refers to the part of a structure that is furthest from the centre of the body

Dorsal   relating or belonging to the back. In this context it refers to the back of the hand

Eccrine glands   one of the two types of gland found in the skin. Found all over the body except in the armpit and groin. Help eliminate waste products and control body temperature

Eczema   a skin condition, usually with a genetic basis

Effleurage   a movement in massage. A stroking movement

Eggshell nails   thin delicate nails, usually curving under at the free edge

Elastin   fibre of protein found in the skin that helps the skin maintain its elastic properties and return to shape

Elements   the smallest part of a chemical that can recognisably exist

Embedding   a technique used in nail art that uses small items within the overlay

Epidermis   upper layer of skin, above the dermis

Eponychium   the skin fold and seal that is at the base of the nail plate

Ethyl cyanoacrylate   one of the acrylate-based family of adhesives, usually used as a nail adhesive

Ethyl methacrylate (EMA)   a monomer most commonly used in acrylic nail systems

Evaporation   the conversion of a liquid into a vapour

Exfoliation   the mechanical removal of dead skin cells from the surface of the skin

Exothermic   heat-producing chemical reaction

Extensions   artificially extending the length of a fingernail

Extensor   extends or straightens

Fabric mesh   usually a silk or fibreglass fabric used in a fabric 'system' to provide extra strength

Fan-shaped nail   a nail plate that is wider at the free edge than at the cuticle

Femoral artery   main artery in the upper leg

Femur   bone of the upper leg

Fibre   in this context, the 'system' that uses a fibre (e.g. silk, fibreglass) with a cyanoacrylate resin to create an artificial overlay

Fibreglass   a fine mesh of fibreglass used to strengthen a cyanoacrylate resin system

Fibrous joints   a type of joint

Fibula   a bone of the lower leg

Filaments   a structure in striated muscle

Flexibility   the property of a substance that determines how much it will bend

Flexor   flexes or bends

Foiling   a technique in nail art that uses a foil to decorate the nails

Follicles   found in the skin; the hair follicle is where the hair is formed

Free edge   the part of the nail plate that extends past the end of the finger

French manicure   a method of painting nails using a white colour on the free edge and a transparent natural colour over the nail bed

French white tips   plastic tips that are an opaque white to provide the French manicure effect in artificial nails

Frictions   a movement in massage, for active, deeper effect

Fumes   particles suspended in smoke

Fungus (fungi)   microscopic plant; can colonise or grow on or under the nail plate and skin, and can lead to medical problems

Furrows   longitudinal ridges on the nail plate

Gel   thickened liquids; can refer to a thick adhesive or a UV-cured material

Gel stage   refers to the start of the polymerisation process of an 'acrylic' system when the liquid and powder react forming a 'gel-like' substance before hardening or curing

Glues   often used to describe adhesives; its true meaning is an adhesive that is protein-based, usually animal-derived (e.g. bones, hides, etc.)

Grit   used to describe the abrasiveness of files and buffers; the higher the number, the finer the abrasive – a level of not less than 240 grit should be used on the natural nail

Habia   Hairdressing and Beauty Industry Authority

Habit tic   an habitual action that damages the matrix of a nail. Usually seen on the thumb where the forefinger picks at the nail fold

Hair follicle   structure in the skin that produces a hair

Hairless skin   version of skin found on the palms of the hands and soles of the foot. Has no hair follicles.

Hairy skin   a version of skin with hair follicles

Hangnail   sharp piece of nail in the side walls that is separated from the nail plate

Hardness   a measure of how easily a substance can be scratched

HASAWA   Health & Safety at Work Act

Hazardous   substances that may be capable of causing physical or health-related injury

Heart   part of the cardiovascular system that pumps the blood around the body

Histamine   a chemical released by the body as a defence mechanism to protect against harm from an unwanted substance that causes an irritation or other type of reaction

Hooked (or claw) nail   a nail plate that has an extreme upper arch and curves under at the free edge

Hormones   a substance secreted by glands that stimulates organs into action

Humerus   bone of the upper arm

Hyperidrosis   overactivity of the sweat glands of the feet

Hyponychium   the distal edge of the nail bed; a seal between the nail plate and nail bed

Infections/inflammation   the detrimental colonization of the host organization by a foreign parasite species. If condition is present, do not treat the client

Infill   a treatment than compensates for the natural nail growth after the application of artificial nails. Usually required 2–3 weeks after application

Ingestion   one of the main 'routes of entry' into the body; that is, via the mouth

Inhalation   one of the main 'routes of entry' into the body; that is, via the lungs

Initiator   a chemical that starts the chemical process of polymerization

Intercellular fluid   a clear fluid that bathes all cells of the body and supports cell function

Iron   mineral necessary for efficient oxygen transportation by the blood

Irritants   substances capable of causing inflammation of the skin, eyes, nose, throat or lungs

Irritation   general description of a mildly inflammatory condition

Isometric contraction   a muscle put under tension but not altering its length

Isotonic contraction   a muscle put under tension and shortening

Keratin   protein created by the body and one that is formed when skin cells have become keratinised to form the nail plate

Keratinized   the description of a skin or nail cell that has lost its contents and transformed into the protein keratin

Koilonychia   flat, spoon-shaped nails usually with a systemic cause

Lamellar dystrophy   peeling, splitting layers of the nail plate

Lateral   to the side

Lateral nail fold   skin on either side of the nail plate

Lateral and medial plantar artery and vein   blood vessels in the foot

Leucoderma   patches of skin that do not have any pigmentation

Leukonychia   white spots on the nail plate; usually caused by trauma to the nail plate but may have other medical causes

Lifting   term used to describe the separation of an artificial nail overlay from the nail plate

Ligaments   fibrous tissue supporting joints

Lipid   a natural fat produced by the skin; this helps to form part of the intercellular cement that holds keratinised skin cells together

Liquid   the most common definition is a physical state, e.g. solid, gas, liquid; in the context of nail products, it refers to the monomer in a two-component acrylic system

Low odour sometimes used in the context of acrylic monomers; means that they have a lower evaporation rate or are not so easily detected by the human sense of smell; does not refer to degree of safety

Lower arch the curve of the lower part of the free edge when viewed from the side

Lunula whitish area at the base of the nail plate where keratinisation is incomplete; often referred to as the 'half moon'

Lymph a clear fluid circulating the body via the lymphatic system whose main functions are to fight infection and remove waste

Lymph node structure in the lymphatic system that filters lymph

Lymphatic system one of the systems of the body; involved in protection

Lymphocytes one of the white blood cells

Lymphoedema a constriction in a lymph vessel causing localised excess of lymph fluid

Macrophage type of blood cell that destroys harmful microorganisms

Manicure a treatment involving the skin and nails of the hands and lower arm

Mantle the area of skin that covers the matrix; proximal nail fold

Marbelling a technique used in nail art that mixes two or more colours together

Massage the rubbing, kneading and stimulating of muscles and joints of the body

Matrix area below the proximal nail fold where the process of keratinisation of skin cells takes place to form the nail plate

Medial relating to the middle

Medial plantar artery and vein blood vessels in the foot

Melanin a pigment created by specialist skin cells to protect the lower layers of skin from sun damage

Melanocytes adapted skin cells that produce the pigment melanin

Metacarpal arteries and veins blood vessels in the wrist

Metacarpals bones in the hand

Metatarsals bones in the foot

Methacrylic acid an acid commonly used as a primer in many nail systems

Methyl methacrylate (MMA) monomer no longer used as a component of an acrylic system except as a 'co-polymer' with ethyl methacrylate (EMA)

Mist fine liquid particles produced by spraying

Mitosis the process of cell division and reproduction

Molecule a specific arrangement of atoms to create a specific chemical

Monomer one unit or molecule; individual chemical units that can react to form a polymer

Motor nerves nerves connected to muscles that cause them to move

Mould a term often and incorrectly used to describe nail infections, usually pseudomonas (green infection between the nail plate and overlay)

MSDS Material Safety Data Sheet; forms that provide various information relating to safety issues

Mucocutaneous a variation of skin that secretes mucous for either protection or lubrication

Mucous membrane the internal version of skin that secretes mucous, e.g. lining of the gut

Multiple sclerosis a disease associated with the nervous system

Myofibrils structures in muscle

Nail bed area of skin that lies directly under the nail plate

Nail enamel a term sometimes used to describe a product used to apply colour to the nails

Nail lacquer see Nail enamel

Nail plate the hard layers of keratinised skin cells that form a 'plate' on the end of each finger and toe

Nail polish see Nail enamel

Nail unit the area at the end of the finger that includes all parts of the fingernail

Nail varnish see Nail enamel

Nail wraps most commonly, a fibre system used to overlay the natural nail; can refer to any system

National Occupational Standards (NOS) the level and detail of the various competencies required by specific industry sectors that make a person capable of carrying out specific work, laid down by the industry sector

Natural nail the finger nail that is formed in the matrix to make a nail plate

Natural nail overlays artificial nail products used to coat a natural nail plate

Neurones a nerve cell

No-light gel a cyanoacrylate-based gel

Nutrients a substance providing nourishment

NVQ National Vocational Qualification; a qualification based on the National Occupational Standards and strongly promoted by the Department for Education and Employment (SVQ in Scotland)

Odour presence of a chemical that can be detected by the sense of smell. Is not an indication of degree of danger or quantity of chemical

Oedema condition involving the inefficient function of the lymphatic system

Oligomers chains of monomers that are considerably shorter than a polymer

Onychocryptosis ingrowing nail

Onychodermal band seal between the nail plate and the hyponychium

Onycholysis separation of the natural nail from the nail bed

Onychomadesis loosening of the nail plate at the proximal nail fold; usually due to trauma

Onychomycosis lifting, discoloration or rotting of the nail plate

Onychophagy the habit of nail biting

Onychorrhexis longitudinal splitting of the nail plate; often associated with furrows

Optical brightener an additive that makes colours look brighter and white look whiter

Oval a shape of the free edge of the nail that is rounded

Overlay   a coating applied to the natural nail or blended plastic tip and natural nail

Oxygenated blood   blood from the lungs rich in oxygen

Palmar arches   arteries in the hand

Parkinson's disease   a disease associated with the nervous system

Paronychia   inflammation caused by damage of foreign body around the edges of the nail plate

Patella   bone protecting knee joint, also known as kneecap

Pathogen   a microorganism capable of causing disease

Pedicure   a treatment involving the skin and nails of the feet and lower leg

Peripheral nervous system (PNS)   the nervous system of the body excluding the brain and spinal cord

Petrissage   a movement in massage; an active, stimulating movement

Peyer's patches   structures in the lymphatic system

pH value   a measure used to determine the level of acidity or alkalinity of a substance; 7 is neutral, 1 is the most acidic and 14 is the most alkaline

Phalanges   bones in the fingers

Photoinitiator   a chemical that responds to specific types of light to start a chemical reaction

Pitting   a description of the surface of the nail plate that has small dips in it. Often a sign of a skin condition such as psoriasis

Plantar arch   blood vessels in the sole of the foot

Plasma   the clear liquid part of blood

PNS   peripheral nervous system

Podiatrist   an alternative name for a chiropodist

Polish secures   accessories in nail art that stick to the nail using nail varnish

Polymers   literally 'many units'; very long chains of chemically bonded monomers or units. It can refer to the acrylics used in artificial nails; it also refers to any other polymer, e.g. hair, that is made up of chains of amino acids

Polymerization   a chemical reaction that creates polymer chains from monomers or oligomers

Popliteal artery   artery in the leg

Posterior   relating to the back

Powder   materials that have been finely ground; in this context, powder generally refers to powder polymers which are tiny beads of polymer

Ppm   parts per million; a general measure of ratio; in this context, it can be the number of molecules of vapour in 1 million molecules of air

Pre-tailor   to shape a plastic tip before application to create a better fit and shape

Primer   a substance used to improve the adhesion between the nail plate and artificial products

Prioritize   make a list of tasks that need to be carried out and then rearrange them with the most important or urgent at the top

Pronator   muscle movement that turns hand down

Protein   chemical substances created by the body from long chains of amino acids

Proximal   nearest to the centre of the body

Proximal nail fold   the fold of epidermis covering the matrix and extending onto the nail plate

Psoriasis   a non-contagious skin condition

Pterygium   an abnormal condition where the skin adheres to the nail plate and is stretched by the nail growth

Pulmonary   relating to the lungs

Radial artery and vein   an artery and vein in the lower arm

Radius   a bone in the lower arm

Rebalance   corrects position of apex when it has moved because natural nail has grown

Receptors   type of nerve cell that receives a stimulus

Resin   refers to a version of cyanoacrylate used in the fibre system

Resin activator   a product that speeds up the cure time of a cyanoacrylate resin

RIDDOR   Reporting of Injuries, Diseases and Dangerous Occurrences Regulations

Risk assessment   a requirement of COSHH that assesses potential hazards

Routes of entry   the three ways a chemical can enter the body: ingestion (mouth), inhalation (nose), absorption (skin)

Sanitization   to kill or reduce the numbers of pathogens to a level considered safe by public health standards

Saphenous vein   vein in the leg

Sculptured nails   artificial nails created by building the nail onto the natural nail and extending it over a form rather than a plastic tip

Sebaceous gland   gland associated with the hair follicle that produces sebum

Sebum   a natural oil produced by the sebaceous glands attached to hair follicles that moisturises and lubricates the skin and plays a protective role

Sensitivity   a condition that causes the body's immune system to react

Sensitization   the biological process of becoming sensitive to a chemical that usually results in an allergic reaction

Sensory nerves   a type of nerve that receives stimuli

Side wall   the soft tissue along the sides of the nail plate

Skeletal muscle   the type of muscle connected to the skeleton

Ski-jump nail   a nail plate that curves upwards from the cuticle area to the free edge

Smile line   the curve that is created naturally by the hyponychium or by a coloured artificial overlay or nail varnish

Smooth muscle   a type of muscle. Found in arteries, digestive tract, etc

Solehorn   epidermis attached to the underside of some natural nails; more often seen on nails that are almond shaped: it has a blood and nerve supply, so should not be removed

Solvents   substances capable of dissolving other substances; water is the 'universal solvent'

Spleen   organ in the lymphatic system

Splinter haemorrhage   small black streaks under the nail plate

Square   a shape of the free edge of a nail that has a straight edge with corners and parallel sides

Squoval   a shape of the free edge of a nail that has corners and parallel sides but a rounded edge

Sterilization   the process that achieves the complete destruction of all living organisms

Stop point   the part of a plastic tip that fits around the free edge of the natural nail

Stratum corneum   uppermost layer of the epidermis consisting of keratinised skin cells

Stratum germinativum   base layer of the epidermis where new skin cells are formed

Stratum granulosum   one of the mid layers of the epidermis where the process of keratinisation starts

Stratum lucidum   one of the mid layers of the epidermis apparent in the palms of the hands and soles of the feet

Stratum spinosum   one of the mid layers of the epidermis where some cells are connected together

Strength   the ability of a substance to withstand breakage if force is applied

Striated muscle   skeletal muscle

Subcutaneous layer   below the dermis of the skin where fat is stored

Sun damage   damage to the skin where the skin has created permanent melanin discoloration, e.g. freckles

Supinator   a muscle movement that turns the hand up

Sweat   a liquid produced by the sweat glands in the skin; one of the main functions of sweat is to help regulate body temperature

Sweat gland   structure in the skin that produces sweat

Synovial joints   a type of joint; moveable joint

System   in this context, this refers to the 'system' used to overlay the natural nail or plastic tip, e.g. acrylic, UV gel, fibre

Systemic disorder   caused by one of the systems of the body and affecting many areas

Talus   bone in the ankle

Tapered   a shape of the free edge of a nail that becomes thinner towards the distal edge

Tapotement   a movement in massage; stimulating movement involving tapping

Tarsals   bones in the ankle

Tendons   tissue that connects muscles to bones

Thixotropic   the ability of a liquid to become thinner in viscosity when agitated, returning to its original viscosity when agitation stops

Tibia   a bone of the lower leg

Tonsils   structure in the lymphatic system at the back of the throat

Toxic   the description of a substance that can adversely harm humans at measured levels

Trauma   excessive force

Turnover   the money value of total sales over a set period

Ulna   a bone of the lower arm

Ulnar artery and vein   an artery and vein in the lower arm

Ultraviolet (UV) light   an invisible part of the spectrum above the colour violet in the visible light bands

Upper arch   the curve of the nail from the cuticle area to the free edge

UV absorbers   additives that act like sunscreens

UV block   a chemical ingredient that prevents UV rays from affecting the product or underlying skin tissues

UV gel   one of the 'systems' of artificial nails; it uses a pre-mixed 'gel' and UV light to create the overlay

UV Light cured   the process of polymerization using a photo-initiator to start the chemical reaction, usually UV light

Vapours   molecules of a chemical in air created by evaporation of the substance

Varicose veins   a condition affecting the blood vessels. Usually seen in the legs

Vein   blood vessels that return the blood to the heart

Vena cava   large vein leading to the heart

Ventilation   the process of changing the air in an area and therefore removing dust and vapours

Ventricle, right and left   the two lower chambers of the heart that pump the blood to the lungs and arteries of the body

Verruca   similar to warts, but ingrowing, usually found on the feet

Viruses   a wide group of microorganisms that can only reproduce in living cells and can cause a vast range of diseases

Viscosity   the measure of a liquid's ability to flow, that is, its thinness or thickness

Vitamin D   a vitamin formed in the body and essential for the efficient absorption and use of calcium

Vitiligo   a condition of the skin where it is not able to produce the pigment melanin

Volatile   describes a substance that easily evaporates in air

Voluntary nervous system   the part of the nervous system that is under conscious control

Warts   lumps of usually hard tissue on the skin caused by a viral infection

Wetting   the ability of a liquid to spread out to cover a surface

White-tip powder   a colour of acrylic powder used to create a white free edge on an artificial nail

Whitlow   localised and painful swelling at the edge of the nail plate

Yeast   a type of fungus; some yeasts can cause fungal infections

Zones   the three areas of the artificial nail referred to when creating the correct artificial structure

Index